Nutrition Curriculum Activities Kit Level 1

Paul E. Bell, D.Ed.
Carol Byrd-Bredbenner, Ph.D.
Lily Hsu, M.S.
Idamarie Laquatra, Ph.D.
James Rye, M.S.
Karin Rosander Sargrad, M.S.

Illustrated by Eileen Gerne Ciavarella

THE CENTER FOR APPLIED RESEARCH IN EDUCATION, INC.
West Nyack, New York 10995

Acknowledgments

This curriculum has been a collaborative effort of the College of Human Development and the College of Education at The Pennsylvania State University; it was sponsored by the Nutrition Foundation and supported by the Heinz Endowment. The School Nutrition Education Curriculum Study was conducted under the direction of Helen Guthrie and Barbara Shannon.

Many individuals, too numerous to mention by name, have contributed to the development of the nutrition education materials in this kit. We would like to acknowledge their contributions and hope that they are as excited as we are to see the fruits of their labor in print. A special thanks goes to JoAnn Daehler and to Lisa Oesterling for technical assistance. A very special thank-you goes to Norma Woika for the preparation of the manuscript and for her never-failing optimism about this project.

10   9   8   7   6   5

Library of Congress Cataloging-in-Publication Data

Nutrition curriculum activities kit.

  1. Nutrition—Study and teaching (Elementary)
2. Diet—Study and teaching (Elementary)   I. Bell,
Paul E.   [DNLM: 1. Child Nutrition—education.
2. Curriculum.   WS 18 N9767]
TX364.N87   1986   372,3'7   86-4203
(level 1)

IBSN 0-87628-617-1

Printed in the United States of America

About the Authors

The *Nutrition Curriculum Activities Kits, Level 1* and *Level 2,* are based on the nationwide "Pennsylvania State University Nutrition Education Project" conducted from 1974 to the present. The Project consisted of several studies, done at each grade level, that examined nutrition knowledge and attitudes, and also the dietary behavior changes that occurred because of nutrition education. The content material was field-tested in Pennsylvania public schools. Authors of the materials are:

Paul E. Bell, D.Ed., Curriculum and Superivision, is an Associate Professor of Science Education at The Pennsylvania State University. Dr. Bell has many years of experience in elementary and secondary science education, curriculum development, and supervision. An active lecturer and consultant, he has made presentations to the Association for Supervision and Curriculum Development, the School Science and Math Association, the National Science Teachers Association, and the California Dairy Council. He has also contributed nutrition education articles to *Today's Education* and the *Journal of Nutrition Education.*

Carol Byrd-Bredbenner, Ph.D., Home Economics Education, is an Assistant Professor of Nutrition at Montclair State College, Montclair, New Jersey. She is an ADA Registered Dietitian and a member of the American Home Economics Association and the Society for Nutrition Education. Dr. Byrd-Bredbenner has presented research papers to the Society for Nutrition Education, the American Home Economics Association, the International Congress of Nutrition, and the American Dietetic Association. Her nutrition education articles have been published in the *Journal of Nutrition Education, Thresholds in Education,* and the *Home Economics Research Journal.*

Lily Hsu, M.S., Nutrition, is an Instructor in Nutrition at The Pennsylvania State University. She is an ADA Registered Dietitian and a member of both the Society for Nutrition Education and the International Reading Association. Ms. Hsu has made nutrition education presentations to the Society for Nutrition Education and the International Reading Association and has published nutrition articles in the *Journal of Nutrition Education, Thresholds in Education,* and *Highlights for Children.*

Idamarie Laquatra, Ph.D., Applied Nutrition, is a Corporate Nutritionist with the Heinz Corporation. She is a frequent nutrition counseling workshop leader and speaker. She is an ADA Registered Dietitian and a member of the Society for Nutrition Education. Dr. Laquatra has published articles in the *Journal of the American Dietetic Association* and the *Journal of the Medical Society of New Jersey.* She has presented papers at the American Dietetic Association and for the New Jersey and the New York affiliates of the American Heart Association.

James Rye, M.S., Nutrition, is Chairperson of the Dietetics Department at Viterbo College in LaCrosse, Wisconsin. He is an ADA Registered Dietitian and a member of the Society for Nutrition Education. Mr. Rye was a team member responsible for delivering the Special Supplemental Feeding Program for Women, Infants, and Children throughout Arizona and has helped to implement a cardiovascular risk factor intervention program. His nutrition articles have been published in the *Journal of Nutrition Education* and the *Journal of the American Dietetic Association.*

Karin Rosander Sargrad, M.S. Nutrition, is a Nutritionist at The Pennsylvania State University. She has extensive experience counseling pregnant and breast-feeding women, mothers of infants and children, and children. She is involved in a variety of nutrition education projects, including nutrition courses by correspondence. Ms. Sargrad is a member of the Society for Nutrition Education and is an ADA Registered Dietitian. She has published nutrition research articles in the *Journal of Nutrition Education* and has made presentations to the Society for Nutrition Education.

About the
Nutrition Curriculum Activities Kits

The *Nutrition Curriculum Activities Kits, Level 1* and *Level 2*, are unique aids designed to provide a complete nutrition education activities program for grades 5 through 12 in two self-contained kits. The kit for Level 1 includes twenty carefully planned nutrition-teaching lesson/units for grades 5 through 8 with over 140 pages of reproducible lesson materials composed of nutrition information, student worksheet activities, tables, tests, and other evaluation devices.

The scope and sequence of the kits were developed to provide students with the knowledge and skills necessary to make personal dietary decisions. The basic premise of the kits is that nutrition education should encompass three aspects of learning: cognitive, affective, and psychomotor. In order to improve their eating habits, students must understand certain nutrition information (cognitive), must choose and apply these ideas within their personal value systems (affective), and must develop the skills to carry out these tasks (psychomotor). In this spirit, the first units in Level 1 of the kits introduce basic nutrition concepts as a firm foundation on which to teach subsequent units in diet planning, special diets, meal planning and preparation, and nutrition issues. In Level 1, the emphasis is on nutrition knowledge, while Level 2 emphasizes the application of nutrition knowledge and skills in higher-level lessons.

In the beginning, students accumulate firsthand experiences through the lesson/units in order to broaden their perspective on food and nutrition. Attention is also given to the development of sensory skills, to familiarity with food variety, to the nutrient content of food, and to the relationship of food to various social settings. Students also learn the food sources of several nutrients as well as how their bodies use nutrients. Here the focus is on the individual and on his or her food choices. Finally, the units deal with nutrition issues and controversies and with the application of nutrition knowledge. Topics of interest to teenagers are presented in order to spark their interest and to encourage them to explore nutrition. In Level 1, topics such as fad diets, the athlete's diet, and food advertising are among those included.

The *Nutrition Curriculum Activities Kits* offer several unique features. The kits were developed to encompass the nutrition concepts that were identified in a nationwide survey conducted by recognized nutrition educators and that should be studied in grades 5 through 12. Going beyond an introduction to the Basic Food Groups, the kits include teaching units devoted to nutrients and to their food sources and also to the application of nutrition knowledge and skills in personal diet decision making.

Each lesson/unit in the kits provides:

- A detailed teacher's guide that includes all of the background information and step-by-step directions needed for teaching the unit. Discussed also are "Concepts" the unit will develop, the specific learning "Objectives" of the unit, and a "Teacher's Unit Introduction" that can be used, as is, to present the unit in class. The guide also provides reproducible student nutrition information sheets that open the unit topic for class discussion and includes tips on classroom implementation to help maximize learning.

- A "Basic Activity," in easy-to-follow lesson plan format, that spells out the "Time Needed," the "Materials Needed," and step-by-step procedures for carrying out the activity in class. All materials for teaching the unit are provided within the pages of the spiral-bound kit, including student worksheet, table, information, and evaluation pages designed to be copied directly, for immediate distribution, with no additional teacher preparation.

- Full-page, reproducible student worksheet activities pages, which students use to apply the nutrition knowledge and skills learned in the "Basic Activity." These activities give students practice in interpreting the various nutrition tables and charts included in the kit.

- "Advanced" and "Follow-Up" activities for students who want to learn more about the unit topic. These activities give students the opportunity to become involved in activities like interviewing, library research, and out-of-class preparation for presentations such as demonstrations and food fairs.

- An "Evaluation" device for each unit with a complete "Answer Key" (printed at the end of the kit). The devices include a wide range of formats such as multiple-choice and short-answer tests, attitude scales, writing exercises, word searches, and crossword puzzles. The "Evaluation" devices may be used for a pre- or postassessment of student understanding of the unit material.

In short, each teaching unit provides all of the elements required for a well-organized, easy-to-use nutrition lesson. All you need to do to get started is either to reproduce the student materials for classroom distribution or to make acetate copies for projection on an overhead projector.

The following chart defines the scope and sequence of the *Nutrition Curriculum Activities Kits, Level 1* and *Level 2*.

Nutrition Curriculum Activities Kit Level 1

Section I   Basic Nutrition Concepts

Unit 1	Nutrition Overview: Proteins, Carbohydrates, and Fats
Unit 2	Nutrition Overview: Vitamins, Minerals, and Water
Unit 3	RDA Doorway to Good Health
Unit 4	RDA Meterstick to Good Nutrition
Unit 5	The Three Bs: Meeting Your RDAs
Unit 6	Your RDA for Energy
Unit 7	RDA in the U.S.A.
Unit 8	Identifying Nutrient-Rich Foods
Unit 9	Determining Nutrient Density in Food

Section II   Diet Planning

Unit 10	Eating Right, Feeling Well
Unit 11	How Do You Stack Up Nutritionally?
Unit 12	Start the Day Better with Breakfast
Unit 13	Your School Lunch
Unit 14	The Good Goodies
Unit 15	Designing a Personal Diet Plan
Unit 16	Discovering Foods with Your Senses

Section III Special Diets

Unit 17	Energy Balance and Fad Diets
Unit 18	The Athlete's Diet

Section IV Meal Planning and Preparation

Unit 19	Interpreting Ingredient Labels

Section V   Nutrition Issues

Unit 20	A Close Look at Food Advertising

Nutrition Curriculum Activities
Kit Level 2

How to Use This Resource

Using the *Nutrition Curriculum Activities Kits* in Your Program

The *Nutrition Curriculum Activities Kits, Level 1* and *Level 2,* are designed to facilitate and promote nutrition in grades 5 through 12. These kits will save lesson preparation time and energy by providing imaginative, new nutrition units ready for immediate use in the classroom. The kit for Level 1 contains twenty ready-to-use, self-contained nutrition lesson/units complete with student worksheets, charts, information sheets, and evaluation devices to be reproduced by copier for distribution to students.

The two kits comprise a full sequential nutrition education curriculum for grades 5 through 12. Ideally, students would begin their exposure to nutrition education at the preschool level and continue through the twelfth grade. Since this continuity is not always possible within a school district, a review of the basic nutrition content usually presented in the earlier grades is provided in the first two units of *Level 1:* "Nutrition Overview: Proteins, Carbohydrates, and Fats" and "Nutrition Overview: Vitamins, Minerals, and Water." These two units serve as an introduction to nutrition for students who have had little or no exposure to nutrition education. These units also serve as a review for students who have been taught nutrition in earlier grades, thus providing a common starting point for all students in the class.

Classroom Implementation of the Nutrition Units

The nutrition units can be used in sequence to provide a complete nutrition education program, or they can be used to supplement the existing curriculum. The units are equally appropriate for individuals, small groups, or the entire class.

Each unit follows the same easy-to-use format:

- The "Unit Title" introduces the unit.

- Specific "Concepts" to be developed in the unit are listed. Generally, a unit addresses several related concepts, encompassing both nutrition content and practical applications.

- Specific behavioral "Objectives" that students should be able to achieve throughout the unit are listed. There are also several objectives and concepts for each unit that include affective and cognitive goals.

- The "Teacher's Unit Introduction" provides background information on the nutrition topic of the unit and may be used, as is, to introduce students to the unit. Although the information presented is not comprehensive, enough material has been provided to spark students' interest in the topic and to facilitate the teaching of the unit. Further investigation of the topic is encouraged. The thorough References/Resources section at the end of this kit offers sources of additional materials (books, booklets, audiovisuals, software, and other printed matter) pertinent to each unit. Following each "Teacher's Unit Introduction" are specific implementation tips and suggestions for the unit, along with references to material in other units in *Level 1* that may be useful in instruction.

- The core of each unit is found in the sections entitled "Basic Activity," "Advanced Activity," and "Follow-Up Activities." The "Basic Activity" and "Advanced Activity" appear in the same easy-to-follow format that indicates the "Time Needed," the "Materials Needed," and numbered step-by-step procedures for carrying out the activity in class. The "Basic Activity" is designed for students who have little or no background in the nutrition topic, and the "Advanced Activity" and "Follow-Up Activities" are for students who want further study or challenges in the topic area. Generally the "Advanced Activity" requires additional reading, writing, or intellectual skills and may require out-of-class assignments. The "Follow-Up Activities" consist of short descriptions of teaching ideas that may be used in addition to either the "Basic Activity" or the "Advanced Activity." Due to their supplemental nature, the "Follow-Up Activities" do not contain as much detail and are not as fully developed as either of the other two activity types.

The following activities are presented in a wide variety of formats to stimulate student interest and expression:

taste-testing parties	interviews
field trips	panel discussions
puzzles and games	guest speakers
library research	debates
learning centers	diet and activity diaries
bulletin board preparation	roleplaying
lab experiments	case studies
contests	demonstrations
unique meal planning and preparation	ad writing
attitude surveys	practice shopping
	menu planning

- Following the step-by-step activity directions is a section of reproducible student materials, including information sheets, charts, worksheets, and evaluation devices. Each of these appears on a full page and may be photocopied for distribution to the class. "Answer Keys" for worksheets and evaluation devices are located at the end of this kit.

- "Reproducible Student Charts and Tables" are also located at the end of this kit. Within the nutrition units, you will find references to these charts and tables. As the need arises, provide students with individual copies of them and instruct students to keep them on hand for reference.

The student reference charts and tables include:

Chart A	Recommended Dietary Allowances
Chart B	Daily Food Guide
Chart C	Key Nutrients in Food
Chart D	Food Composition Table for Selected Nutrients
Chart E	Dietary Calculation Chart
Chart F	Height/Weight and Recommended Energy Intake
Chart G	Calorie Expenditure by Activity

The *Nutrition Curriculum Activities Kits* promote a well-rounded study of nutrition, in new and interesting ways, in order to stimulate student involvement. The nutrition skills taught in these units will serve your students for a lifetime!

Contents

> This section lays the groundwork for all other nutrition instruction by focusing on these basic nutrition concepts: the six classes of nutrients, the Recommended Dietary Allowances, and nutrient density. The information presented in this section will facilitate the students' application of nutrition knowledge in personal diet decision-making.

> This section gives students experience in applying basic nutrition concepts when making snacking and meal decisions. These units help students explore how an individual's food selection is influenced and observe associations between eating habits and good health. Students are also given the opportunity to design a personalized diet plan and to conduct a sensory evaluation food lab.

> This section expands the concepts introduced in Section II by examining the special dietary needs of athletes and of individuals on weight-control diets. These lessons give students the opportunity to rate various types of diets and to evaluate their nutritional safety.

SECTION IV   MEAL PLANNING AND PREPARATION   201

> This section focuses on nutrition consumerism and the food supply. The increasing number of new food products marketed each year causes consumers to be faced with more and more food decisions. In order to make wise food choices, students must begin by developing nutrition label reading skills.

SECTION V   NUTRITION ISSUES   215

> This section promotes critical thinking and the application of nutrition knowledge and skills. The skills developed in this section will help students discriminate between nutrition information and misinformation and prepare them to deal with other nutrition-related controversies outside the classroom.

APPENDICES   233

Reproducible Student Charts and Tables

References/Resources

Section I

BASIC NUTRITION CONCEPTS

Unit 1: Nutrition Overview: Proteins, Carbohydrates, and Fats

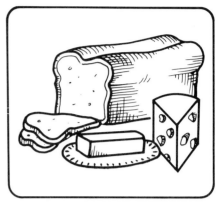

CONCEPTS

–Nutrients are nourishing substances found in food having specific functions in maintaining the body. Nutrients are materials that your body usually cannot supply in sufficient amounts to meet its need.

–There are six classes of nutrients: proteins, carbohydrates, fats, vitamins, minerals, and water.

–Proteins are nutrients that provide building blocks for making and for repairing tissue and blood cells; proteins can also provide energy for all body functions, such as breathing, digestion, and physical activity.

–Proteins are found primarily in foods from the Meat-Poultry-Fish-Beans group (meat, poultry, fish, eggs, legumes, nuts, seeds) and from the Milk-Cheese group (milk, yogurt, cheese).

–Carbohydrates are nutrients that provide energy for all body functions, such as breathing, digestion, and physical activity.

–Carbohydrates are found primarily in foods from the Bread-Cereal group (breads, biscuits, muffins, waffles, pancakes, cereals, macaroni, spaghetti, noodles, rice, oats, barley) and from the Fruit-Vegetable group (fruits and vegetables). Sugar, honey, and other sweets from the Fats-Sweets-Alcohol group are also rich sources of carbohydrates.

–Fats are nutrients that provide energy for all body functions and carry the fat-soluble vitamins A, D, E, and K.

–Fats are found primarily in oil, butter, margarine, and other fats from the Fats-Sweets-Alcohol group, in most foods from the Meat-Poultry-Fish-Beans group, and in many foods from the Milk-Cheese group.

–Iron CaPAC is a term used to summarize the most important nutrients in Units 1 and 2. It represents the nutrients iron, calcium, protein, Vitamin A, and Vitamin C.

OBJECTIVES

–Students will be able to determine the effects of calories and exercise on body weight.

–Students will learn that carbohydrates, fats, and proteins provide energy.

–Students will be able to identify sources of these nutrients.

–Students will be able to to state the roles and functions of carbohydrates, fats, and proteins.

–Students will be able to describe the relationship of a nutritious diet to health.

3

TEACHER'S UNIT INTRODUCTION

Nutrition has recently claimed the nation's attention. Consumers are clamoring for nutrition information and entrepreneurs are seizing the opportunity to provide the public with massive amounts of literature pertaining to food and nutrition. Since many authors and publishers do not have a solid foundation in the basics of nutrition, they often give inaccurate theories and so-called "facts." If consumers and educators are to sort through the stacks of nutrition-related material, they must learn the nutrition basics.

Nutrition is the relationship between foods, nutrients, and health. We all know what foods are: fruits, vegetables, breads, cereals, meats, eggs, nuts, milk, cheese and anything else you can think of that is edible. Since we all have an idea of what health is, let us just say that optimum health is not merely the absence of disease but also the realization of an individual's full potential. When it comes to defining nutrients, though, many of us have to stop and think a minute. Let us look at a definition of nutrients. *Nutrients* are defined as nourishing substances that are found in foods and that have specific functions in maintaining the body. *Essential nutrients* are materials that the human body cannot supply in sufficient amounts to meet its needs, and so they must be provided by the diet. Carbohydrates, proteins, fats, vitamins, minerals, and water are all nutrients. For many essential nutrients, a Recommended Dietary Allowance (RDA) has been established. For others, as well as for calories, an estimated range has been given for the amount considered to be adequate (see Chart A, "Recommended Dietary Allowances," and Chart F, "Height/Weight and Recommended Energy Intake").

Simply stated, nutrients are the basis of life. Without nutrients, our bodies cannot perform their thousands of separate yet vital functions. Breathing, muscle contraction, heartbeat, nerve transmission, and regulation of body temperature. All of these events are controlled by nutrients. And from where do we get these nutrients? From food! The "Daily Food Guide" (Chart B) gives recommendations for planning daily diets that provide for our nutrient needs.

This unit will develop students' understanding of the energy-yielding classes of nutrients, including their functions and their sources. A complete understanding of the concepts taught in this unit will pave the way for an in-depth understanding of the concepts taught in the other units in this kit. If students have a good background in nutrition, this unit and Unit 2 are ideal as a review. This unit is designed to be completed as a class activity, or as an individual self-instructional activity. Unit 1 presents the macronutrients, that is, the energy-yielding nutrients: proteins, carbohydrates, and fats. Unit 2 presents the micronutrients: vitamins, minerals, and water.

BASIC ACTIVITY

Time Needed: Two class periods

Materials Needed: Sheets 1-1 through 1-4: "All About Energy-Yielding Nutrients"
Sheets 1-5 through 1-11: "Laying a Good Foundation"
Sheet 1-12: "Laying a Good Foundation Summary Chart"
Quiz Sheets 1-1 through 1-2

Class Period 1

1. Distribute Sheets 1-1 through 1-4, "All About Energy-Yielding Nutrients," and provide an introduction, if necessary, that includes the reason why we study nutrition, the relationship between foods, nutrients, and health, and the overall role of nutrients.

2. Have the students read Sheets 1-1 through 1-4; "All About Energy-Yielding Nutrients." You may wish to either read the sheets aloud or else to ask students to take turns reading aloud.

Class Period 2

1. Distribute Sheets 1-5 through 1-11, "Laying a Good Foundation," and have students complete the worksheets. This activity is designed as a self-instructional package. Students should be permitted to work at their own rate. However, you may also wish to have students work in either small groups or in a large discussion group. Students should be encouraged to keep these sheets for future reference. As a package, Sheets 1-1 through 1-11 provide a useful reference booklet.

2. After the students have completed Sheets 1-5 through 1-11, conduct a class discussion to complete the first three sections of Sheet 1-12, "Laying a Good Foundation Summary Chart." Students should keep Sheet 1-12 to complete in Unit 2. You may wish to draw Sheet 1-12 on the board or on an overhead transparency and to complete the sheet as students provide answers. This large-group activity will provide an opportunity both to informally assess students' understanding of the concepts in this unit and to help identify students' strengths and weaknesses.

3. **Evaluation:** Distribute Quiz Sheets 1-1 through 1-2 and have students complete them independently. Discuss the answers together in class.

ALL ABOUT ENERGY-YIELDING NUTRIENTS

PROTEINS

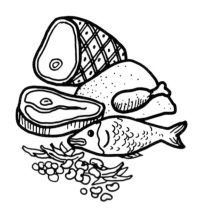

Proteins are a part of all living things. Proteins are needed for the growth and repair of body tissues such as muscles, blood, bones, hair, skin, and nails. Enzymes, hormones, and antibodies (things needed for your body's operation) are also proteins.

Amino acids are the so-called "building blocks" of proteins. In your food and in your body, twenty amino acids form, break down, and re-form into a lot of different proteins. Nine of these amino acids cannot be made in your body and so must be eaten in food; these amino acids are called *essential amino acids*. Your body will not be able to make new proteins if any one of these nine essential amino acids is lacking in your diet. The other amino acids can be made from the carbon, oxygen, nitrogen, and other things in your diet.

A protein in food _____ is broken down into amino acids during digestion

and forms a different protein in your body.

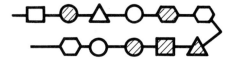

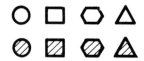

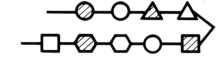

Example: whey, a protein in milk

_____ hemoglobin in blood

Foods that have what we call *complete proteins* are ones that contain just the right amounts of all nine essential amino acids. Animal sources of protein (meat, poultry, fish, eggs, milk, and milk products) contain complete proteins. Plant sources of protein (dried beans and peas, nuts, breads, and cereals) contain *incomplete proteins*. These protein foods are low in one or more of the essential amino acids. However, it is possible to add together two or more plant sources of incomplete protein to form a complete protein. Eaten together, beans and grains, for example, become a complete protein (see the diagram on the next page). An amino acid that is low in one food may be found in adequate amounts in another, and vice versa.

Both the amount and type of protein in the typical American diet is more than we need to live and grow. The amount of protein we need each day can be found in two small servings of protein-rich foods. A tuna salad and a cup of cooked beans, or two eggs plus one half of a chicken breast would provide more than half of your body's protein needs for a single day. The rest of your protein needs could be provided by foods that are not generally thought of as high-protein foods. These include foods from the Bread-Cereal group and the Fruit-Vegetable group.

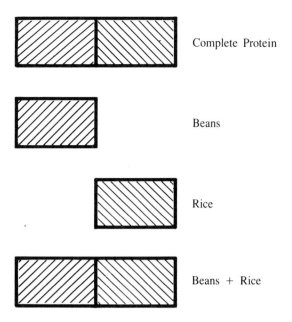

Complete Protein

Beans

Rice

Beans + Rice

Many Americans, especially athletes, believe that the more protein they eat, the healthier and stronger they will be. Not so! If you eat more protein than you need, the extra protein is changed to glucose (blood sugar) and is either used for energy or stored as fat. Extra protein will not help build bigger muscles or give special extra energy. In fact, diets really high in protein may do some harm if foods high in other important nutrients, such as Vitamin A and Vitamin C, are neglected.

Knowing how much protein you need is important. A good rule of thumb is to consume 10 to 22 percent of your daily calories from protein.

SAMPLE CALCULATION OF PROTEIN INTAKE:

2200 calories/day $\times$ 10% = 220 calories from protein

220 calories $\div$ 4 calories/gm protein = 55 gm protein

Eating more than fifty-five grams of protein is wasteful. The extra protein will either be used for energy or else will be made into fat. Remember: Protein is an expensive and wasteful source of energy. Carbohydrates, on the other hand, are a more direct and less expensive source of energy.

CARBOHYDRATES

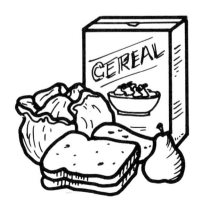

The popular idea that carbohydrates are fattening or otherwise "bad" causes people to avoid foods rich in carbohydrates. The fact is, carbohydrate-rich foods, especially those rich in complex carbohydrates, are excellent sources of energy, are low in calories, and have plenty of vitamins and minerals as well.

There are two types of carbohydrates: simple and complex. *Simple carbohydrates* are made of one or two sugars. Examples of foods containing primarily simple carbohydrates include table sugar, brown sugar, honey, jams, jellies, milk, and many fruits. *Complex carbohydrates,* on the other hand, are composed of many sugars hooked together to form a long chain. Two examples of complex carbohydrates are starch and fiber. Foods high in starch include vegetables, breads, and cereals. Food sources of fiber are bran, whole-grain breads and cereals, and the skins of fruits and vegetables. In addition to providing complex carbohydrates, these foods also supply essential vitamins and minerals.

It is important to choose your carbohydrates carefully. Choosing foods high in refined sugars (such as table sugar, candies, jams, jellies, soft drinks) may give you carbohydrates, but they give you few, if any, other nutrients. These foods provide "empty" calories. *Empty-calorie* foods are ones that have a lot of calories in proportion to the nutrients they offer. They are usually high-calorie foods with very few vitamins, minerals, or proteins. Better choices of carbohydrate-rich foods would be whole-grain breads and cereals, milk, fresh fruits, and fresh vegetables. These foods would give you vitamins, minerals, protein, and, in most cases, fiber as well as calories.

About 46 percent of the calories in the typical American diet come from carbohydrates, with 18 percent of the total calories coming from refined and processed sugars. It is suggested that Americans increase their total carbohydrate intake to 58 percent of their total calorie intake, but reduce the intake of refined and processed sugars to 10 percent of the total calories they consume. In terms of foods, this means eating more whole-grain breads and cereals, fresh fruits and vegetables (complex carbohydrates), and eating less sugar, candy, jams, jellies, soft drinks, and other sugary foods.

FATS

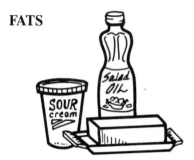

Some fat is needed in the diet, but most Americans eat enough or too much fat. Fats supply a concentrated source of energy, with more than twice as many calories, ounce for ounce, as proteins or carbohydrates. The fat-soluble vitamins A, D, E, and K need fat to transport them in your food and in your body. Fats supply an essential fatty acid (linoleic acid), which is needed for the growth, maintenance, and functioning of many tissues, including the skin and nerves. A minimum amount of fat needed in the diet has not yet been set, but even one tablespoon of vegetable oil per day is probably enough to supply the essential fatty acids needed for health.

The American diet typically contains more fat than is needed, with about 42 percent of its calories coming from fat. It is recommended that the amount of fat be reduced to 30 percent of the total calories.

Besides being found in oils, fats are found in butter, margarine, and lard. Fats are also "hidden" in fatty meats such as bacon, in the marbling of meat, in the butterfat of milk and cream, in salad dressings, in nuts and seeds, and in cakes and pastries.

There are several different types of fats worth talking about because of the controversies that surround them. The terms *saturated* and *unsaturated* refer to the chemical structure of two different types of fat (see the diagrams on the next page). All fats are composed of a carbon chain. The carbon chain of saturated fats is full of (or saturated with) hydrogen atoms. These fats are generally solid at room temperature. Examples are coconut oil, stick margarine, lard, butter, and most animal fats. Unsaturated fats, on the other hand, do not have all of the chemical bonds in the carbon chain full of hydrogen atoms. These fats are generally liquid at room temperature and are of vegetable origin. Examples include corn oil, soybean oil, cottonseed oil, sesame oil, safflower oil, and sunflower oil.

Cholesterol is another kind of fat. Its chemical structure is very different from the saturated or unsaturated variety. It is needed by the body for several reasons. Making bile acids and nerve tissues are two functions of cholesterol. Your body makes enough cholesterol to meet your needs. There is some evidence, however, that infants and young children may need a small amount in their diets. Cholesterol is found in many foods of animal origin; the richest sources are eggs and organ meats (liver, for example), red meats, butter, and milk products. No plant foods contain cholesterol. Typical American diets include plenty of cholesterol.

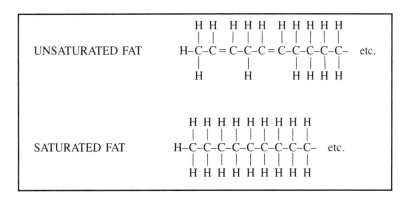

For most Americans, diets that are high in saturated fat and cholesterol raise blood cholesterol levels. Americans tend to have higher blood cholesterol levels than do people in countries where the diet is low in saturated fat and cholesterol. The amount of heart disease is also high in America. Research has shown that a high blood cholesterol is a strong risk factor in heart disease. Thus, it is wise for the American population, as a whole, to cut back on saturated fat and cholesterol consumption. Even in early childhood, smaller intakes of these substances are recommended for the following reasons:

1. Childhood eating patterns are often carried over into adulthood.

2. The deposition of cholesterol in artery walls, which can eventually lead to heart disease, starts early in life.

LAYING A GOOD FOUNDATION

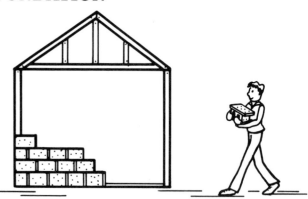

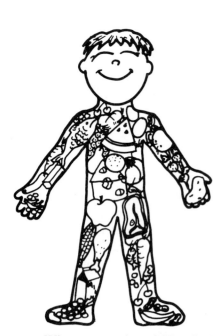

Did you ever hear the saying, "You are what you eat"? Do you think it is true or just a tall tale? If it is true, what does it mean?

Sheets 1-5 through 1-12 will help you find out that the food you eat really does affect your health and how you feel. You will discover that food has something to do with your weight, your height, your skin, your smile, your eyes, and many other parts of you. The way you feel is related to food and nutrition.

What is nutrition all about? *Nutrition* is the way your body uses food to make you grow, to give you energy, and to keep you healthy. Nutrition is also the relationship between foods, nutrients, and health.

What are nutrients? You find *nutrients* in foods, but you cannot really see them or taste them. A nutrient usually cannot be made by your body. Examples of nutrients are proteins, carbohydrates, fats, vitamins, minerals, and water.

YOUR GENERAL HEALTH

Your health and how you feel determine, in a big way, how much you get out of life. Nutrition helps keep you healthy and feeling well. The six nutrients just mentioned—proteins, carbohydrates, fats, vitamins, minerals, and water—each has a job to do in helping to keep you healthy. It is pretty amazing to think that something in your food, something that you cannot see or taste, can be so important.

Maybe you still do not believe it. Nutrition cannot be all that important, you may say. Well, read on . . . you may just change your mind!

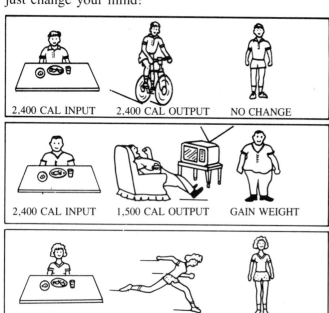

2,400 CAL INPUT   2,400 CAL OUTPUT   NO CHANGE

2,400 CAL INPUT   1,500 CAL OUTPUT   GAIN WEIGHT

2,400 CAL INPUT   3,000 CAL OUTPUT   LOSE WEIGHT

If you are like most people, you are probably interested in calories and in watching your weight. Calories measure food energy; your weight is a measure of your body size. Basically, there are two things you need to know when watching your weight. One thing is how many calories you eat or take in from your food. The other thing is how many calories you use up by exercising. Keep the number of calories coming in the same as the number of calories going out if you want to stay the same weight. If you want to lose weight, eat fewer calories than you use up. If you want to gain weight, eat more calories than you use up. This chart illustrates how food intake and exercise levels affect weight. In the chart, the word *calorie* is abbreviated as *cal*.

THE BALANCING ACT

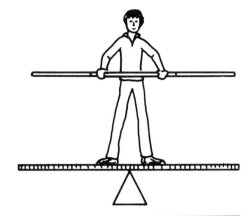

Your weight is a simple matter of balance. Balance is the difference between the calories that come in and the calories that go out.

WHAT IS THE ANSWER?

Directions: Fill in the blanks below with *more, less,* or *the same* (number of):

If I want to lose weight, I need to eat _____ calories

and/or exercise _____ .

If I want to gain weight, I need to eat _____ calories

and/or exercise _____ .

If I want to stay the same weight, I need to eat _____ calories

and/or exercise _____ .

Directions: Now see if you can figure out the "balance" of each of these people. If you think the person will stay the same weight, write *NC* (no change) in the blank. If you think the person will gain weight, write ▲ (increase) in the blank. If you think the person will lose weight, write ▼ (decrease) in the blank.

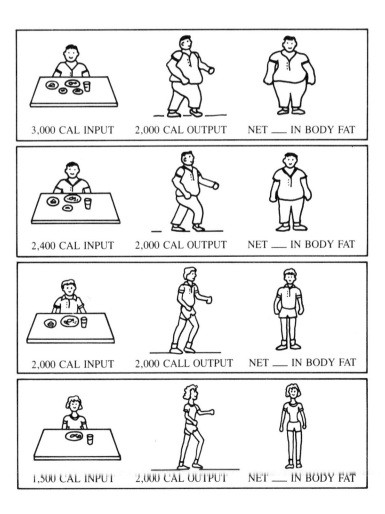

3,000 CAL INPUT   2,000 CAL OUTPUT   NET ___ IN BODY FAT

2,400 CAL INPUT   2,000 CAL OUTPUT   NET ___ IN BODY FAT

2,000 CAL INPUT   2,000 CALL OUTPUT   NET ___ IN BODY FAT

1,500 CAL INPUT   2,000 CAL OUTPUT   NET ___ IN BODY FAT

NUTRIENTS AND CALORIES

Let us stop and think for a minute. Where do all these calories come from? What do you need them for anyway? Calories come from the many foods you eat. To be more specific, calories come from three different nutrients. These nutrients are called carbohydrates, proteins, and fats. Remember, nutrients are the many substances in food that are needed by your body. Carbohydrates, proteins, and fats are needed by your body to give you energy.

WHICH THREE NUTRIENTS GIVE YOU ENERGY? 1. _____

2. _____ 3. _____

Energy is the ability to do work. Energy gives your body the ability to breathe, to digest your food, to move your muscles, and to do all kinds of other activities.

List some activities that require energy: _____

_____

_____

Carbohydrates, proteins, and fats all provide calories. So why do you need all three? Can you get all the calories you need just from proteins? Or just from carbohydrates? Or just from fats? The answer is *no*. These three nutrients have other jobs, too. You see, they work double-time or triple-time!

Carbohydrates' exact second job is unknown, but it is known that you will become sick if you remove carbohydrates totally from your diet. Carbohydrates are the *best* way to get your calories, though. They are the most efficient form for your body to use, plus they are the least expensive form to buy. So, all around, carbohydrates are a bargain!

Another job of proteins, which is really their main one, is to help make and repair tissues all over your body. Proteins are important in blood cells, in bones, in muscles, and in every other part of your body.

Fats' second job is to carry certain vitamins in your body. These vitamins are called fat-soluble because they dissolve in fat. These are vitamins A, D, E, and K. Certain fats also provide you with linoleic acid, which your body needs for healthy skin.

Now, back to calories. Calories and nutrients work together to give your body energy. The calories in your food are provided by the three nutrients, carbohydrates, proteins, and fats. Any food that contains these nutrients has calories. There are other nutrients important to your body's need for energy. The B vitamins are needed to help your body *use* its energy, that is, to burn its calories. Other nutrients help "break up" calories so they can be used by your body for energy.

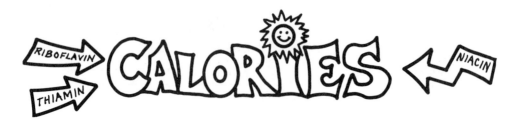

The Food Chart, on Sheets 1-8 and 1-9, tells you which foods have the three energy-containing nutrients—carbohydrates, proteins, and fats. It also tells you how many calories there are in a serving of each food.

FOOD CHART

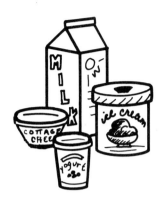

Food	Serving Size	Calories	Carbohydrate	Protein	Fat
cheese, hard	1 ounce	95		X	X
cottage cheese, creamed,					
small curd	½ cup	130	X	X	X
ice cream	⅔ cup	180	X	X	X
milk:					
whole	1 cup	160	X	X	X
2%	1 cup	125	X	X	X
skim/nonfat	1 cup	85		X	
buttermilk	1 cup	85	X	X	
evaporated	1 cup	330		X	X
yogurt, plain, made with skim					
milk	1 cup	125	X	X	

Meat-Poultry-Fish-Beans Group

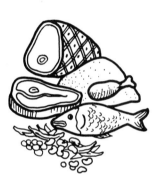

Food	Serving Size	Calories	Carbohydrate	Protein	Fat
egg, raw	1 medium	80		X	X
fish/seafood:					
clams	2 ounces	55		X	X
crabmeat	2 ounces	60		X	X
fish	2 ounces	110		X	X
oysters	2 ounces	50		X	X
tuna, drained	2 ounces	110		X	X
lean meat:					
beef	2 ounces	110		X	X
veal	2 ounces	120		X	X
lamb	2 ounces	110		X	X
pork	2 ounces	130		X	X
liver, beef	2 ounces	130		X	X
kidney, beef	2 ounces	135		X	X
legumes:					
dry beans, cooked	1 cup	210	X	X	
dry peas, cooked	1 cup	290	X	X	
lentils, cooked	1 cup	210	X	X	
peanut butter	2 tablespoons	180		X	X
peanuts, roasted	¼ cup	210		X	X
poultry:					
chicken	2 ounces	110		X	X
turkey	2 ounces	110		X	X

Fruit-Vegetable Group

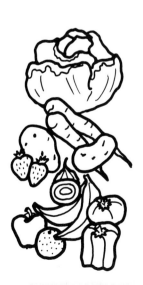

Food	Serving Size	Calories	Carbohydrate	Protein	Fat
apple	1 medium	80	X		
apricot, raw	8–10 halves	80	X		
artichoke, cooked	1 medium	45	X		
banana	1 medium	100	X		
beets, cooked	½ cup	30	X		
berries	1 cup	90	X		
broccoli, cooked	½ cup	20	X		
cantaloupe	½ medium	80	X		
carrot, raw	1 whole	35	X		
cauliflower, cooked	½ cup	20	X		
celery, raw	1 stalk	5	X		
chard, cooked	⅗ cup	20	X		
cherries	1 cup	105	X		
collards, cooked	½ cup	30	X		
corn, cooked	½ cup	70	X		
cucumber, fresh	½ medium	15	X		
dates, dried	8–10	220	X		
eggplant, cooked	½ cup	20	X		
grapefruit	½ medium	40	X		
green beans, cooked	½ cup	15	X		
lemon	1 medium	20	X		

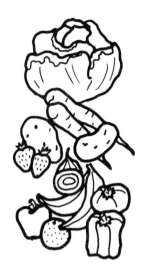

Food	Serving Size	Calories	Carbohydrate	Protein	Fat
Fruit-Vegetable Group *(continued)*					
mustard greens, cooked	½ cup	20	X		
okra, cooked	½ cup	25	X		
onions, cooked	½ cup	30	X		
orange	1 medium	65	X		
parsnips, cooked	½ cup	50	X		
peach, fresh	1 medium	40	X		
pear, fresh	1 medium	100	X		
pepper, green, raw	1 medium	35	X		
plum, fresh	1 medium	20	X		
potato, baked	1 medium	145	X		
prunes, dried	8–10	240	X		
raisins	½ ounce (1 pk.)	40	X		
rhubarb, cooked, sugar added	½ cup	190	X		
rutabaga, cooked	½ cup	35	X		
spinach, cooked	½ cup	20	X		
strawberries	½ cup	30	X		
summer squash, cooked	½ cup	15	X		
sweet potato, baked	1 medium	205	X		
tomato, raw	1 medium	30	X		
turnip greens, cooked	½ cup	15	X		
winter squash, cooked	½ cup	15	X		
Bread-Cereal Group					
bread	1 slice	65	X	X	
cereal, cooked	1 cup	110	X	X	
cereal, ready-to-eat	1 cup	110	X	X	
crackers (saltines)	4–5	60	X	X	
hamburger roll	1 roll	120	X	X	
macaroni	1 cup	160	X	X	
muffin, roll, biscuit	1 medium	120	X	X	
pancake	1 cake	60	X	X	
rice	1 cup	220	X	X	
Fats-Sweets-Alcohol Group					
beverages, alcoholic*					
beer	12 fl. ounces	360	X		
whiskey	1½ fl. ounces	100	X		
wine	3½ fl. ounces	85	X		
beverages, carbonated, sweetened (soft drinks)	12 fl. ounces	145	X		
butter	1 Tablespoon	100			X
honey	1 Tablespoon	65	X		
jelly/jam	1 Tablespoon	55	X		
lard	1 Tablespoon	115			X
margarine	1 Tablespoon	100			X
oils	1 Tablespoon	120			X
salad dressings:					
French	1 Tablespoon	65			X
Italian	1 Tablespoon	80			X
thousand island	1 Tablespoon	80			X
mayonnaise	1 Tablespoon	100			X
sugar	1 Tablespoon	40	X		
syrup	1 Tablespoon	50	X		

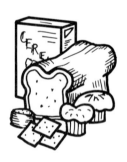

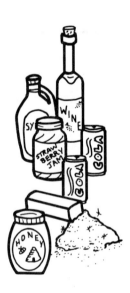

*Although the calories in alcoholic beverages come primarily from the alcohol and *not* from the carbohydrates, the body uses the alcohol in a manner similar to the way it uses carbohydrates. Therefore, for purposes of simplicity, alcoholic beverages will be considered rich sources of carbohydrates.

CAN YOU FIND THE FOODS RICH IN THESE NUTRIENTS?

**WHICH FOOD GROUPS PROVIDE
A LOT OF CARBOHYDRATES?**
_____
_____
_____

**WHICH FOOD GROUPS PROVIDE A
LOT OF PROTEINS?**
_____
_____

**WHICH FOOD GROUPS PROVIDE A
LOT OF FATS:**
_____
_____
_____

Directions: The names of the foods in this list are found somewhere in the accompanying puzzle. They may be printed going up, down, across, or diagonally. Circle each word you find.

CARBOHYDRATE CORNER

BANANA

BREAD

CABBAGE

CARROT

CEREAL

CORN

CRACKER

HONEY

NOODLE

ORANGE

RAISIN

RICE

ROLL

SUGAR

TOMATO

A	M	L	O	S	T	R	B	A	T	C	L	O
Y	R	H	O	R	H	N	B	M	O	A	L	N
O	R	O	L	L	A	L	N	A	R	T	S	O
G	L	N	A	P	Q	N	S	G	N	B	C	E
T	E	E	L	C	U	U	G	L	S	A	D	N
T	O	Y	Y	R	I	C	E	E	A	C	N	C
M	T	O	M	A	T	O	E	S	R	I	L	A
B	R	O	B	C	R	R	L	C	S	D	E	B
N	P	Q	R	K	A	N	L	I	G	A	B	B
A	K	R	E	E	N	R	A	R	F	H	L	A
S	U	G	A	R	L	R	R	O	D	O	I	G
I	M	I	D	T	S	N	O	O	D	L	E	E
E	D	C	E	R	E	A	L	S	T	P	E	P

Directions: The names of the foods in each list below are found somewhere in the accompanying puzzle. They may be printed going up, down, across, or diagonally. Circle each word you find.

PROTEIN PAD

CHEESE

EGGS

FISH

LEGUMES

MEAT

MILK

NUTS

POULTRY

SEEDS

YOGURT

```
Y O C O T N S
O S H A L U M
G E E N O T U
P M E L P S Y
L M S B C E D
L O E F I S H
N E E D O G L
O I S G L S T
P D P D G E M
D A L C B S O
L E G U M E S
O E T H G E A
B U T L H D M
Y R E E D S N
P O U L T R Y
S U G O N P Q
T L A U N I U
M I L K R O S
M S S L O T S
```

FOODS WITH FAT

```
M A R M A R G A R I N E L
C H L E O X Y M N A P S M
H A N O I L R B I K U E E
E T M E A T R N U I D E S
E G G S L Z N U M T O D L
S O A U T U R T Y M T S O
E L O L T F I S S W R E N
T Q W H O L E M I L K T R
```

BUTTER

CHEESE

EGGS

MARGARINE

MEAT

NUTS

OIL

SEEDS

WHOLE MILK

LAYING A GOOD FOUNDATION SUMMARY CHART

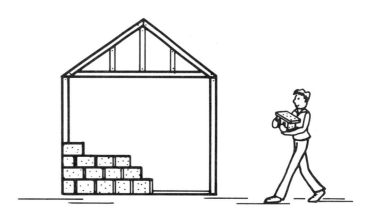

Directions: Fill in the columns in the chart below using nutrition information you learned in Units 1 and 2.

Nutrients	Functions	Food Sources
Proteins		
Carbohydrates		
Fats		
Vitamin A		
Vitamin C		

B Vitamins
  Thiamin
  Riboflavin
  Niacin		

Calcium		
Iron		
Water		

QUIZ
NUTRITION OVERVIEW: PROTEINS, CARBOHYDRATES, AND FATS

1. Figure out the "balance" of each of these people. If you think the person will stay the same weight, write NC (no change) in the blank. If you think the person will lose weight, write ☛ in the blank. If you think the person will gain weight, write ☝ in the blank.

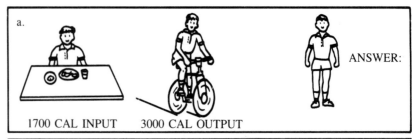

a.

1700 CAL INPUT   3000 CAL OUTPUT   ANSWER:

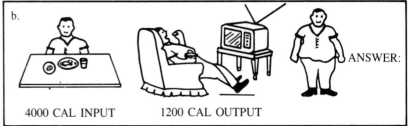

b.

4000 CAL INPUT   1200 CAL OUTPUT   ANSWER:

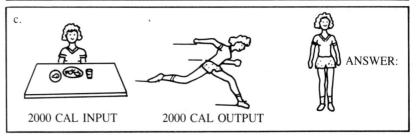

c.

2000 CAL INPUT   2000 CAL OUTPUT   ANSWER:

_____ 2. Sally eats 1,800 calories a day. She wants to lose weight. How many calories should she eat?

    a. 2,500   c. 1,800
    b. 2,000   d. 1,500

_____ 3. If you always eat 2,400 calories and use 3,000 calories, what will happen?

    a. You will lose weight   c. Your weight will stay the same
    b. You will gain weight   d. Nothing

_____ 4. To keep your weight the same you should

    a. Eat fewer calories than you expend
    b. Eat the same number of calories as you expend
    c. Eat more calories than you expend
    d. None of the above

_____ 5. To gain weight, you should
    a. Eat fewer calories than you use
    b. Eat the same number of calories as you use
    c. Eat more calories than you use
    d. None of the above

_____ 6. Which nutrient(s) provide calories?
    a. Proteins, vitamins, and minerals
    b. Vitamins, carbohydrates, and fats
    c. Carbohydrates, fats, and proteins
    d. Carbohydrates, fats, and minerals

FOR QUESTIONS 7, 8, AND 9 YOU MAY CHOOSE MORE THAN ONE RIGHT ANSWER.

_____ 7. Which food group(s) are rich sources of carbohydrates?
    a. Bread-Cereal group
    b. Fruit-Vegetable group
    c. Fats-Sweets-Alcohol group
    d. Meat-Poultry-Fish-Beans group

_____ 8. Which food group(s) are rich sources of protein?
    a. Bread-Cereal group
    b. Fruit-Vegetable group
    c. Meat-Poultry-Fish-Beans group
    d. Milk-Cheese group

_____ 9. Which food group(s) are rich sources of fats?
    a. Fruit-Vegetable group
    b. Milk-Cheese group
    c. Meat-Poultry-Fish-Beans group
    d. Fats-Sweets-Alcohol group

_____ 10. Joshua has been told he needs more protein. Which foods will help him get more protein?
    a. Squash
    b. Carrots
    c. Hamburger
    d. Sherbet

_____ 11. A rich protein source is
    a. Milk and cheese
    b. Meat and fish
    c. Fruits and vegetables
    d. Answers a and b

_____ 12. Salad dressing is found in which food group?
    a. Fruit-Vegetable group
    b. Milk-Cheese group
    c. Fats-Sweets-Alcohol group
    d. None of the above

13. Name the functions of each of the following nutrients:

    a. Proteins: 1. _____

                       2. _____

    b. Fats: 1. _____

                       2. _____

    c. Carbohydrates: 1. _____

                       2. _____

Unit 2: Nutrition Overview: Vitamins, Minerals, and Water

CONCEPTS

–*Iron CaPAC* is a term used to summarize the most important nutrients in Units 1 and 2. It represents the nutrients iron, calcium, protein, Vitamin A, and Vitamin C.

–Vitamins are nutrients that help regulate body functions.

–Vitamins are found in nearly all foods from the Daily Food Guide.

–Vitamin A helps us to see, especially in dim light, and promotes healthy skin and bone growth.

–Vitamin A is found primarily in dark-yellow fruits and vegetables and in dark-green vegetables.

–Vitamin D helps build bones and teeth; it allows calcium to be used by the body.

–Vitamin D is provided primarily by sunlight and is found in many fortified foods.

–Vitamin C strengthens blood vessels, helps in wound healing, and contributes to bone and tooth formation.

–Vitamin C is found primarily in citrus fruits and juices, and in many other fruits and vegetables.

–The B Vitamins are needed for healthy nerves. They also help the body utilize the energy contained in fats, carbohydrates, and proteins.

–The B Vitamins are found primarily in foods from the Meat-Poultry-Fish-Beans group. Foods from the Bread-Cereal group also provide B Vitamins. In addition, foods from the Milk-Cheese group provide riboflavin.

–Minerals are nutrients that also help regulate body functions. Iron helps the blood carry oxygen. Calcium is a part of bones and teeth and helps muscles and nerves work together. Fluorine helps strengthen bones and teeth.

–Minerals are found in nearly all foods from the Daily Food Guide. Iron is found primarily in foods from the Meat-Poultry-Fish-Beans group and from the Bread-Cereal group. Calcium is found primarily in foods from the Milk-Cheese group and in dark-green leafy vegetables, sardines, and some seafoods. Fluorine is usually provided in drinking water, and may also be found in some fish products and in some vegetables.

–Water is a nutrient needed for the life of all cells. Water makes up between 60 percent and 70 percent of the body's total weight. Water is the main vehicle for transporting materials through the body. Water also helps the body eliminate wastes.

–Water is found in many foods and beverages.

OBJECTIVES

–Students will be able to identify sources of vitamins, minerals, and water.

–Students will be able to describe the roles and functions of vitamins, minerals, and water.

–Students will be able to describe the relationship of a nutritious diet to health.

TEACHER'S UNIT INTRODUCTION

Vitamins, minerals, and water contain no calories. This does not make them second-class nutrients, however, since their roles are vital to the normal functioning of the body. Let us look at some of the specific vitamins and minerals, their functions, and their food sources. We will also consider the important role of something we often take for granted, water.

This unit is devoted to a further examination of nutrients—specifically vitamins, minerals, and water—and to a study of their functions and food sources. For information on carbohydrates, fats, and proteins, refer to Unit 1. Chart C, "Key Nutrients in Food," provides you with additional information on food sources and nutrient functions. Chart D, "Food Composition Table for Selected Nutrients," provides detailed nutrient analysis for an array of foods. You may choose to use these charts as student handouts or for your own reference.

BASIC ACTIVITY

Time Needed: Two class periods

Materials Needed: Sheets 2-1 through 2-6: "All About Vitamins, Minerals, and Water"
Sheets 2-7 through 2-14: "Laying a Good Foundation"
Sheet 1-12: "Laying a Good Foundation Summary Chart"
Optional: Sheets 2-15 through 2-17: "Word Search One," "Word Search Two," and "IronCaPAC Anagrams"
Quiz Sheets 2-1 through 2-2

Class Period 1

1. Distribute Sheets 2-1 through 2-6, "All About Vitamins, Minerals, and Water," and provide an introduction. The introduction could focus on a brief summary of the concepts presented in Unit 1 and on a discussion of why vitamins, minerals, and water are equally important.

2. Have students read Sheets 2-1 through 2-6; "All About Vitamins, Minerals, and Water." You may wish to have students take turns reading aloud or else to have them read the sheets silently.

Class Period 2

1. Distribute Sheets 2-7 through 2-14, "Laying a Good Foundation," and have students complete them. This activity is designed to be self-instructional and can be completed individually or in small groups. Students should be encouraged to keep these sheets and to add them to the ones kept from Unit 1. The worksheets from Units 1 and 2 provide a useful reference.

2. After the students have completed Sheets 2-7 through 2-14, "Laying a Good Foundation," conduct a discussion to complete Sheet 1-12, which was begun in Unit 1. You may wish to draw Sheet 1-12 on the board or on an overhead transparency and to complete the sheet as students provide answers.

3. **Evaluation:** Distribute Quiz Sheets 2-1 through 2-2. The quiz can either be used as a test or can be completed as a small-group activity. The crossword puzzle includes information from both Units 1 and 2 and helps to conclude the information given on nutrients.

FOLLOW-UP ACTIVITIES

1. If students need additional practice or more review of the nutrients, Sheet 2-15, "Word Search One", Sheet 2-16, "Word Search Two", and Sheet 2-17, "IronCaPAC Anagrams" may be helpful.

    a. Students should complete Sheet 2-15, "Word Search One" (concerned with food sources of Vitamin A, Vitamin C, and calcium) and Sheet 2-16, "Word Search Two" (concerned with food sources of iron and protein).

    b. Optional aids for students who may find the puzzles too difficult are:

        1. Show students where the names of the hidden nutrients occur so that they need to find only the names of the foods.

        2. List the names of the foods for which the students are searching.

    c. Students should complete Sheet 2-17, "IronCaPAC Anagrams." This worksheet presents vocabulary words associated with nutrition and reviews the functions of the nutrients.

2. Set up a role-play situation in which each student takes on the part of a nutrient and makes up a personal name. For example, one student might be Theodore Thiamin, another might be Cal Calcium. A group of students should also become members of the Board of Directors of The Human Body Machinery Company. It is the task of the nutrients to apply for jobs at the HBM Company. Each nutrient will describe why he or she is vital to the company. The Board of Directors will decide if the applicant is qualified.

3. Bring in labels from vitamin/mineral supplements (pills or powder). Ask students to make up sample labels that describe the kinds and amounts of food needed to supply these same nutrients. Is it more expensive or less expensive to eat the food? Are there other things in the food that are not in the supplements? Are supplements a good idea?

4. Design a bulletin board on how nutrition affects appearance. Choose pictures of healthy boys and girls with special emphasis on topics discussed in the lesson (general health, weight, height, skin, smile, eyes, nerves, and blood).

ALL ABOUT VITAMINS, MINERALS, AND WATER

Vitamins

Vitamins are a class name for a group of nutrients that share some similar properties but that perform a variety of functions and have a variety of chemical structures. In general, vitamins are organic substances (meaning they are composed of carbon, hydrogen, oxygen, and other elements) that perform specific essential functions in the body, yet cannot be produced by the body. Vitamins must be ingested, either in the diet or as supplements (pills or tonics).

The functions of vitamins are as diverse as their names. Vitamins are generally used to assist the body in using food. Vitamins are part of enzymes and coenzymes (large protein molecules) that bring other substances together in biochemical reactions. Vitamins help speed up these reactions so that life can be maintained.

Vitamins have traditionally been grouped as being fat-soluble or water-soluble. The charts below list the major vitamins in each category.

Fat-Soluble Vitamins
Vitamin A (retinol)
Vitamin D (calciferol)
Vitamin E (tocopherol)
Vitamin K

Water-Soluble Vitamins
Vitamin C (ascorbic acid)
Vitamin B_1 (thiamin)
Vitamin B_2 (riboflavin)
niacin
Vitamin B_6 (pyridoxine)
Vitamin B_{12} (cobalamin)
folacin

FAT-SOLUBLE VITAMINS

Fat-soluble vitamins are absorbed with fats. They are transported throughout the body in small "fat packages" called chylomicrons.

Fat-soluble vitamins can be stored by the body, and sometimes fatal reactions occur when excessive quantities of vitamins A and D are consumed. The excessive intake is usually the result of taking large amounts of vitamin supplements. Toxic symptoms due to high intakes of vitamins E and K are less well-known, but excess dosages of these vitamins may lead to health problems. Let us now consider the known functions of the fat-soluble vitamins A, D, E, and K.

Vitamin A. Vitamin A plays a vital role in vision. It is needed for the adjustment that occurs when you go from bright to dim light. For example, think of the last time you were driving in a car at night. You could probably see very well until an approaching car flooded you with light. After the car passed, you eyes had to adjust to the dimness of the road. The process of adjustment involves Vitamin A. In a dietary deficiency of Vitamin A, the adjustment to the change in intensity of light is delayed, resulting in a condition called *night blindness*. If the deficiency is severe, eye changes occur and blindness results. Severe Vitamin A deficiency is not common in the United States, but it is a common cause of blindness in Indonesia and in other tropical countries where Vitamin A is lacking in the diet.

Vitamin A also plays a role in maintaining the health of the skin and in the growth of bones. The vitamin also helps mucous membranes stay healthy. Mucous membranes line the nose, mouth, lungs, intestines, and other parts of the body. A lack of the vitamin will cause the skin to become dry, rough, and cracked, and little mucous will be secreted from the mucous membranes.

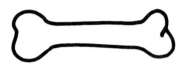

Vitamin D. Vitamin D has been called the "sunshine" vitamin because not only can it be found in foods, but it may also be obtained from the sun! Actually, a substance that can be converted to Vitamin D is present in the skin, and when the ultraviolet rays of the sun reach the skin, Vitamin D is formed.

The major function of Vitamin D is to help bones use calcium to become hard. Vitamin D and calcium work together to build strong bones.

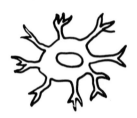

Vitamin E. Although numerous functions of Vitamin E have been promoted by health hucksters, none have been substantiated through scientific investigation. The only role of Vitamin E currently known is that it prevents the breakdown of polyunsaturated fatty acids (PUFAs) in the body. It is believed that Vitamin E helps to maintain the strength of cell walls since cell walls contain many PUFAs. A Vitamin E deficiency results in fragile cell walls that break easily. This condition is most common in newborns. The role of Vitamin E in aging, cancer, heart disease, and sexual performance has not been supported in controlled experiments, and a deficiency in humans is rare.

Vitamin K. Vitamin K is essential for the clotting of blood. After an injury, Vitamin K works to produce a number of factors that are needed to form blood clots. If Vitamin K were not available, any simple cut would bleed continuously and become a serious matter. In fact, a bleeding injury in the presence of a severe Vitamin K deficiency could be fatal. An RDA (see Chart A) for Vitamin K has not been established. This is partially due to the ability of bacteria living in the intestine to produce Vitamin K. Food sources of Vitamin K are listed in the following table.

Food Sources of the Fat-Soluble Vitamins				
Vitamin A	acorn squash beet greens broccoli cantaloupe carrots collards kale	liver mustard greens pumpkin spinach sweet potatoes turnip greens	**Vitamin E**	corn oil cottonseed oil safflower oil soybean oil wheat germ oil

Vitamin D	eggs
	fish liver oils
	fortified milk
	liver
			Vitamin K	cabbage
				egg yolk
				milk
				spinach and
				    other leafy
				    greens
				whole wheat

WATER-SOLUBLE VITAMINS

The water-soluble vitamins are not stored by the body to any significant extent. Intakes in excess of bodily needs are excreted in the urine, making excessive supplementation a waste of consumer dollars. Further, extremely high doses may have harmful side effects and endanger health.

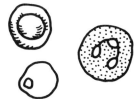

Vitamin C. Probably no other vitamin has received as much publicity as Vitamin C, also known as *ascorbic acid.* Vitamin C's involvement in the prevention of colds and heart disease is an intense area of scientific investigation.

The best-known function of Vitamin C is its role in the formation of *collagen,* a kind of "body cement." Collagen binds body cells together and is important in the growth and repair of body tissues and blood vessels. A Vitamin C deficiency known as *scurvy* results in poor collagen formation, and the physical symptoms are especially noticeable in the gums and on the skin.

Although a Vitamin C deficiency serious enough to cause scurvy is not common in the United States, it has been discovered that blood levels of Vitamin C are decreased by cigarette smoking, the use of oral contraceptives, and physical stress (such as an injury). Still, large doses are not recommended, because excess Vitamin C may cause kidney stones and the breakdown of red blood cells.

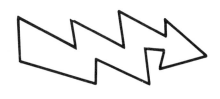

Thiamin, Riboflavin, and Niacin. The B Vitamins—thiamin, riboflavin, and niacin—are involved in the body's use of proteins, carbohydrates, and fats. Food sources of these vitamins are listed in the table on Sheet 2-4. Enrichment of grains and cereals has increased the amount of these vitamins in the food supply of the United States.

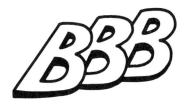

Other B Complex Vitamins. Vitamin B_6, Vitamin B_{12}, and folacin are included under the umbrella term *B complex* vitamins. Vitamin B_6 has many functions, including the building of and the breaking down of proteins, the production of antibodies, and the normal functioning of the nervous system. Vitamin B_{12} is essential for red blood cell formation.

Folacin is also required for the formation of red blood cells. Since a folacin deficiency is often seen in pregnant women, it is recommended that a folacin supplement be taken during pregnancy. Sources of the B complex vitamins are shown in the table on Sheet 2-4.

A widely held belief about vitamins is that if a little is good, then more is better. Your body, however, has fixed reactions that take place in fixed amounts of time. If you have too few vitamins, your body will not operate at full capacity. However, if you have more than you need, your body will discard the water-soluble vitamins and store the fat-soluble ones. Neither of these situations is beneficial. Think of a car's gas tank being filled to capacity and having the trunk filled with more fuel. The excess fuel will either leak out onto the pavement or will get into the trunk and might cause eventual damage. That excess fuel was a waste of money! Vitamin supplementation generally works in a similar way. At best, it is a waste of money; at worst, it may be damaging to your health.

Food Sources of the Water-Soluble Vitamins

Vitamin C	asparagus broccoli brussels sprouts cabbage cantaloupe	cauliflower collards grapefruit grapefruit juice green pepper	lemon mustard greens orange orange juice pineapple	potato strawberries tomato turnip greens watermelon

Thiamin	brazil nuts
	Canadian bacon
	ham
		liver
		peas
		pecans
			pork
			whole-grain or enriched
			   bread
				whole-grain or enriched
				   cereal

Riboflavin	almonds
	avocado
	broccoli
	chicken
		lamb
		liver
		milk
			pork
			whole-grain or enriched
			   bread
				whole-grain or enriched
				   cereal
				yogurt

Niacin	beef
	chicken
	halibut
	ham
	lamb
		liver
		peanuts
		peanut butter
		pork
		potato
			salmon
			sardine
			tuna
			turkey
				whole-grain or enriched
				   bread
				whole-grain or enriched
				   cereal
				veal

Vitamin B_6	banana beef cabbage cheddar cheese egg yolk	ham lamb lima beans liver	pork potato salmon spinach	strawberries veal whole-grain bread whole-grain cereal
Vitamin B_{12}	beef liver cheddar cheese chicken	egg frankfurter	lamb oyster	pork shrimp
Folacin	asparagus banana cabbage carrot	cottage cheese cucumber egg liver	onion orange juice peas potato	rice whole-grain bread whole-grain cereal

MINERALS

Mineral elements are found in trace amounts in your body. Of the more than 100 elements found in nature, approximately 96 percent of your body is composed of only four of these elements: oxygen, carbon, hydrogen, and nitrogen. The remaining 4 percent of your body is made up of at least sixty different mineral elements. Many of these minerals have a known function in the human body. Others may perform an essential function that we are unaware of. Still others are toxic to the body in large quantities.

Minerals play an important role in the body by being constituents of vitamins, enzymes, hormones, and structural tissues. They are classified according to the amount which is present in the body. *Macronutrient minerals* are those minerals that are present in body tissues in relatively high amounts. *Trace minerals,* as the name implies, are present in very small quantities; nonetheless, they are essential.

MACRONUTRIENT MINERALS

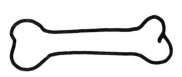

Calcium. The importance of calcium in bone formation was mentioned in the discussion of Vitamin D. Calcium is needed throughout life—not just in childhood when the bones are growing. Bones are active; calcium is constantly being deposited and withdrawn from them. Some researchers believe that the decline in calcium intake in the adult years may be a contributing factor in the development of *osteoporosis*, a bone disease that affects one-third of all females over sixty years of age.

Calcium's role extends beyond the maintenance of healthy bones. It is also needed for the formation of teeth, the transmission of nerve impulses, and the contraction of muscles.

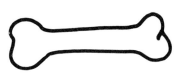

Phosphorus. Like calcium, phosphorus plays an important role in bones and teeth. Approximately 85 percent of the phosphorus in the body is located in these two areas. Calcium and phosphorus in the body exist in a delicate ratio. The optimal ratio is maintained through internal regulation and dietary intake. The RDAs for calcium and phosphorus are identical, since it is believed that optimal calcium and phosphorus utilization is possible with this ratio. Recently, concern has grown regarding the excessive consumption of phosphorus.

The high phosphorus content of soft drinks and processed foods has contributed to increasing the amount of phosphorus in this country's diet. Disproportionate phosphorus intakes may upset the calcium : phosphorus ratio and they may have detrimental effects on the body's ability to use calcium. Some studies with humans suggest that high phosphorus/low calcium diets may result in bone loss; however, more research is needed in this area.

TRACE MINERALS

Iron. Just about everyone has heard of iron-poor blood. The taking of tonics to relieve this condition has long been promoted. Iron is needed in order for red blood cells to be able to carry oxygen. Specifically, iron permits oxygen to reach body tissues. Oxygen is necessary for tissues to live; without oxygen, body cells die.

Failure to consume adequate iron leads to the condition called *iron deficiency anemia*. This problem affects women and children more often than men since these two groups have a greater need for iron. Everyone has a small loss of iron each day, and this loss must be replaced. In addition to this small daily loss, women lose iron during menstruation. Because of this loss during menstruation, women need to consume nearly twice the amount of iron as men. Iron needs are also increased during periods of growth, since an increase in blood volume accompanies growth periods. Body iron increases ten times from infancy to adulthood, and the RDA for iron reflects this need.

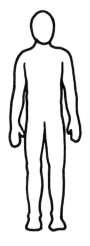

Zinc. Zinc is present throughout the entire body. This wide distribution is indicative of the many functions zinc performs. Zinc is a vital part of numerous enzymes. These enzymes are involved in digestion, bone maintenance, liver function, and maintenance of the acid-base balance in the body.

Zinc deficiency has been associated with reproduction problems, delayed wound healing, loss of the sense of taste, and growth failure. The better food sources of zinc are animal (flesh) foods. The zinc contained in whole-grain breads and cereals is not well absorbed.

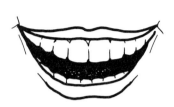

Fluorine. Fluorine is widely distributed throughout nature. Its role in the prevention of tooth decay was established in 1942. Fluorine produces tooth structures more resistant to attack by the acids that cause cavities. In order to decrease the number of cavities, a major public health problem in the United States, many communities have fluoridated their public water supplies. Reductions in decayed, missing, and filled permanent teeth range from 35 percent to over 90 percent in communities with fluorine added to the water. Fluoridated water provides the greatest protection to those who consume it from infancy. Still, benefits do extend into middle and later life. Unfortunately, not all areas fluoridate their public water supply. Presently, thirty-two of the fifty states, or approximately 50 percent of the population, uses public water supplies with natural or added fluorine. Food sources of fluorine and the other minerals are provided in the following table.

Food Sources of Minerals				
Calcium	cheese collards milk	salmon sardine yogurt	Zinc	beef cheddar cheese chicken clams egg lima beans oysters shrimp turkey wheat germ
Phosphorus	beef cheddar cheese chicken egg	milk navy beans pork tuna		

Iron	beef
	broccoli
	dried apricots
	fortified cereal
	lima beans
	molasses, blackstrap
	mustard greens
		oysters
		pork
		raisins
		spinach
		whole-grain and
		   enriched
		   bread
			Fluorine	egg
				fish
				milk
				soybean
				water (fluoridated)

WATER

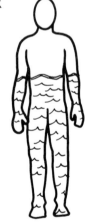

Water may be the most vital, yet most ignored, nutrient of all. Many people do not consider water a nutrient because of its abundant presence in this country. *Water* fits the definition of a nutrient because it serves an essential role in health and life, and because it comes from outside the body. Water composes approximately 60 percent of total body weight. Infants are born with about 75 percent of their body weight as water; by age sixty only 50 percent of total body weight is water.

Water is a constituent of every cell in the body. Water also performs a variety of functions: it transports nutrients and wastes within the body; it participates in many biochemical reactions; it helps lubricate body parts; and it helps regulate body temperature.

Water is everywhere. It is found in beverages such as milk, tea, juice, and coffee, and also in soups, in fruits, and in vegetables. Even "drier" foods, such as bread and beef, contain a relatively large percentage of water (36 percent and 47 percent, respectively). Thus, it is difficult to become dehydrated. However, severe loss of water through strenuous exercise, certain weight-loss diets, use of diuretics, high environmental temperatures, fever, or diarrhea may cause dehydration in a relatively short period of time. In the total absence of water, an individual can survive only two or three days.

LAYING A GOOD FOUNDATION

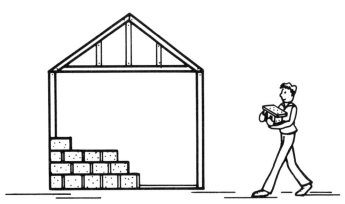

YOUR HEIGHT

Your height is determined by many things. It depends on the heights of your mother and father and your grandmothers and grandfathers. It also depends on what you eat. Some nutrients can make a difference in how fast your bones grow.

Five nutrients that are very important for bone growth are protein, Vitamin A, calcium, Vitamin C, and Vitamin D. These same nutrients also affect the strength of your bones even after you have finished growing.

TRUE OR FALSE

_____ Nutrients are the only things that make me grow taller.

_____ How tall I grow depends partly on the foods I eat.

_____ Calcium, protein, and vitamins A, C, and D help bones grow.

List three foods rich in protein:

_____

_____

_____

List three foods rich in Vitamin D:

_____

_____

_____

List three foods rich in Vitamin C:

_____

_____

_____

Where can you find calcium, protein, and vitamins A, C, and D? These nutrients are found in a variety of foods.

Calcium is found in foods such as milk, cheese, yogurt, ice cream, pudding, and in any other foods made with milk. Besides calcium, protein is also found in these same foods and it is additionally contained in meat, fish, poultry, and beans.

Vitamin A is found in dark-yellow and orange fruits and vegetables and in dark-green vegetables. Examples of dark-yellow and of orange fruits are cantaloupe, apricots, and peaches. Examples of dark-yellow and of orange vegetables are carrots, winter squash, and sweet potatoes. Examples of dark-green vegetables are spinach, turnip greens, and broccoli.

LIST THREE FOODS RICH IN CALCIUM:

_____

_____

_____

LIST THREE FOODS RICH IN VITAMIN A:

_____

_____

_____

Vitamin C is found in citrus fruits, citrus juices, and in many other fruits and vegetables. Examples of *citrus fruits* are oranges, grapefruits, lemons, and limes. *Citrus juices* are the liquids squeezed from these fruits. Examples of other fruits and vegetables that have Vitamin C are strawberries, cantaloupe, tomatoes, spinach, turnip greens, and broccoli.

Vitamin D is found in fortified milk, and it can also be made in the skin when the skin is exposed to sunlight. Other rich sources of Vitamin D include eggs and butter.

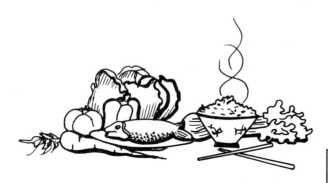

Ku Sung's Story

Ku Sung is a young girl who lives in California. Her grandparents grew up in Korea and moved to the United States soon after they were married. They said goodbye to their families and friends and left behind many customs and habits in Korea.

In Korea, Ku Sung's family ate a diet mainly of rice, soybeans, fish, and many vegetables. In the United States, her grandparents adopted many American ways, including the American diet. The American diet included meat, poultry, and fish; milk and milk products; many fresh fruits and vegetables; and whole-grain breads and cereals. They enjoyed their new diet.

When Ku Sung's parents were born, they were healthy and strong. They ate the American diet, too. When Ku Sung was born, she was longer and bigger than most babies born in Korea. When she grew older, she was taller than most of the young girls in Korea. Ku Sung's other Korean-American playmates were also taller than most girls and boys in Korea.

Many people think that the American diet made the girls and boys grow taller. What do you think? Write your answers in these boxes.

IS IT POSSIBLE THAT FOOD MADE KU SUNG GROW TALLER:

            Yes   No

WHAT FIVE NUTRIENTS MADE HER BONES GROW?

1. _____

2. _____

3. _____

4. _____

5. _____

WHAT FOODS IN KU SUNG'S AMERICAN DIET HAVE THESE NUTRIENTS?

Nutrient 1. _____

_____

Nutrient 2. _____

_____

Nutrient 3. _____

_____

Nutrient 4. _____

_____

Nutrient 5. _____

_____

YOUR SKIN

Your complexion is probably very important to you. A clean and clear face makes you look attractive to yourself and to others. The proper care of your skin involves many things. Cleanliness, plenty of sleep, and a good diet are three things that are needed for proper skin care.

Let us talk about the kind of diet that makes your skin healthy. All nutrients are important for healthy skin, but two nutrients are very important. These two nutrients are vitamins A and C. Each of these vitamins has a different job in skin care.

Vitamin A is needed by your body to replace the loss of skin cells. Every day you lose tiny bits of skin (skin cells) by rubbing and washing. Vitamin A helps the body to make new, healthy skin cells. Just remember that too much Vitamin A is just as bad as too little!

Vitamin C is needed for wound healing. This vitamin helps your body to repair scratches and bruises. Your body needs just the right amount of Vitamin C to keep your skin healthy.

Along with eating the proper foods, you need to keep your skin clean and to get plenty of sleep. If you do these things, your skin will probably stay clear.

FOODS FOR HEALTHY SKIN

Put an "A" in front of the foods that have Vitamin A. Put a "C" in front of the foods that have Vitamin C.

_____ limes	_____ spinach
_____ strawberries	_____ fresh lemonade
_____ apricots	_____ peaches
_____ squash	_____ white grapefruit
_____ oranges	_____ carrots
_____ broccoli	_____ turnip greens

YOUR SMILE

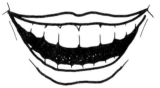

"Come on, dearie, let us see that great big *smile!*"
Think of how many times someone has asked you to smile.
Think of how many times other people see you smile.
Wouldn't it be great to have the most beautiful smile of all? The most obvious thing about your smile is your teeth. Strong, straight, and shining teeth are a very important part of a beautiful smile. Healthy teeth depend on three things:

1. Family background: Healthy teeth can be inherited from other family members (parents, grandparents).

2. Proper care: Teeth need regular brushing, flossing, and dental checkups to stay healthy and clean.

3. Nutritious diet: Many nutrients influence the strength of your teeth.

These three things—family background, proper care, a nutritious diet—determine how healthy your teeth will be.

Four nutrients that are very important for a healthy smile are Vitamin D, calcium, fluorine, and Vitamin C. Let us take a closer look at calcium and Vitamin C. Calcium helps teeth to stay healthy. Calcium and Vitamin C do other things for your body besides helping your teeth. We have talked about some other roles of calcium and Vitamin C.

NAME ONE OTHER ROLE OF CALCIUM: _____

NAME TWO OTHER ROLES OF VITAMIN C: _____

_____

We have also talked about where you can find these two nutrients.

MATCH THE FOODS WITH THE NUTRIENTS:

Tomato	Pudding	Cantaloupe	Orange
Grapefruit	Strawberries	Yogurt	
Cheese	Milk	Ice cream	

CALCIUM: _____

_____

_____

_____

_____

VITAMIN C: _____

_____

_____

_____

_____

YOUR EYES

Eyes are often the meeting place for two people. Your eyes say something when words cannot. Eyes are an important part of life.

Some people in the world are blind. Their eyes can no longer be used to see or to meet people. Much of the blindness in the world is due to a simple thing. Many people become blind because they do not have enough Vitamin A in their diet. A very small amount of Vitamin A could prevent this type of blindness. Some people do not know what foods to eat to prevent this blindness.

Do you know what foods to eat to prevent Vitamin A-deficiency blindness? If you have answered *no* to this question, read on. Remember, we have already talked about foods that have Vitamin A when we discussed bones and skin. Fill in the crossword puzzle on Sheet 2-11. It will help you to remember which foods contain Vitamin A.

Total blindness is not the only problem you may have when you are lacking Vitamin A. If you do not have enough Vitamin A, your eyes may have difficulty in dim light. Did you ever walk into a dark movie theater after being in the bright sun? Did it take you a long time or a short time to adjust to the dim light? If you have enough Vitamin A, this adjustment should take place fairly quickly. Without enough Vitamin A, it may take a longer time.

You may be starting to realize that this small nutrient, Vitamin A, is very important to the health of your eyes. You need just the right amount of Vitamin A to help you see well. And all it takes is eating a little bit of Vitamin A.

WHERE IS THE VITAMIN A?

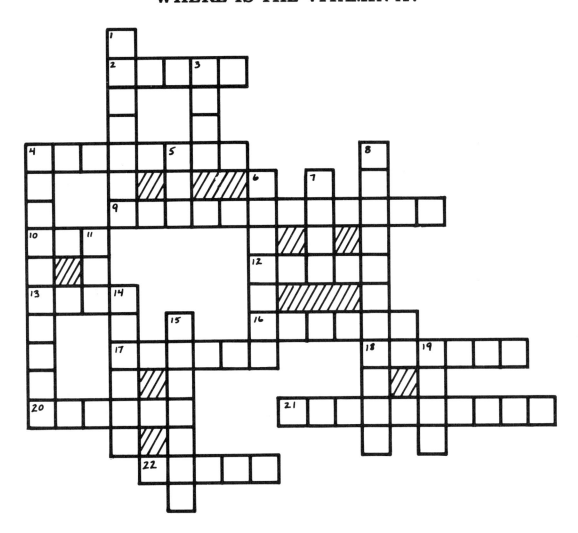

DOWN:

1. A dark-orange fruit that may be dried, canned, or fresh.
3. To communicate with by telephone.
4. Leafy greens whose red roots are also eaten as vegetables.
5. Used to row a boat.
6. A leafy, green vegetable. (Hint: Popeye loves this vegetable.)
7. "I just missed the bus. What a _____!"
8. A bright-orange vegetable that grows underground. (Hint: It is a relative of the potato.)
11. A loosely woven fabric made from string used to trap or catch.
14. Opposite of brother.
15. A Halloween vegetable.
19. A dark-green, curly-leaved vegetable. (Hint: This vegetable rhymes with mail.)

ACROSS:

2. A yellowish pink fruit with a soft skin and large pit.
4. A dark-green vegetable that grows in florets.
9. Leafy greens whose purple and white roots are also eaten as vegetables.
10. A song, "_____ Little Indians."
12. Opposite of day.
13. Mice, squirrels, and _____ are rodents.
16. A dark-orange vegetable that grows underground. (Hint: Rabbits are known to cherish this vegetable.)
17. A variety of gourdlike vegetables. (Hint: This vegetable is also the name of a sport.)
18. Subway _____ are used instead of coins.
20. When someone takes an oath, they end by saying "_____ _____ me, God."
21. A light-orange melon.
22. An organ meat.

YOUR NERVES

Your nervous system is like a series of electrical currents passing through all parts of your body. Nerves control your muscle movements, your coordination, your memory, and your moods. Imagine what life would be like with unhealthy nerves. You might experience some or all of the following if your nerves were unhealthy: irritability, weakness of muscles, fatigue, moodiness, excitability, or memory loss.

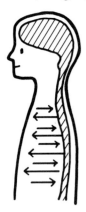

Believe it or not, what you eat affects your nerves. However, do not be fooled into thinking that a nutritious diet will cure all of your problems. Even the healthiest people will feel tired, moody, or irritable at times. What you eat can make a difference in how often you feel tired or irritable, however.

The B vitamins are one group of nutrients that affects your nerves. The important B vitamins are thiamin, riboflavin, and niacin. These three B vitamins are found in foods from the Meat-Poultry-Fish-Beans group and in foods from the Bread-Cereal group. In addition, riboflavin is also found in foods from the Milk-Cheese group.

The mineral calcium is also important to healthy nerves. The Milk-Cheese group is a rich source of calcium.

In summary, foods from the Meat-Poultry-Fish-Beans group, the Milk-Cheese group, and the Bread-Cereal group all contain nutrients that help make healthy nerves.

PLACE AN "X" NEXT TO THE FOODS THAT HELP YOU HAVE HEALTHY NERVES:

_____ tomatoes	_____ apricots
_____ meat	_____ dried beans and peas
_____ cereal	_____ oranges
_____ bread	_____ milk
_____ squash	_____ carrots
_____ cheese	_____ grapefruit
_____ eggs	_____ rice

YOUR BLOOD

Have you ever imagined what you would be like if you did not have any blood? Think about it . . .

Think about your body as a country, and think about your blood as the water in the rivers of the country. The water transports boats and barges that carry goods to people and remove their wastes. The water brings life to the towns and to the country. Your blood is like the river; it carries goods (nutrients and oxygen) to people (your organs and other body parts), and it removes their wastes (your body wastes).

Blood makes up a large part of your body, just as the oceans, lakes, and rivers make up a large part of the world. Water is the major ingredient in blood (93 percent), so you can see that your body contains a lot of water. In fact, water makes up about 60 percent of your body weight. If you weigh 100 pounds, then almost 60 of those pounds are water!

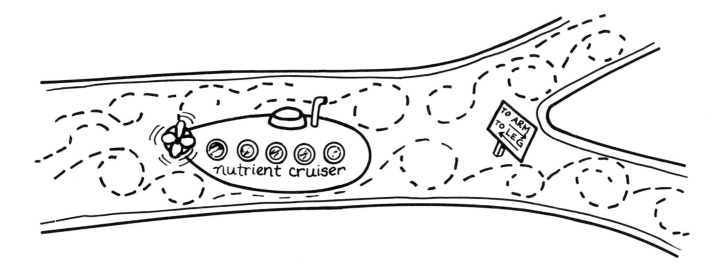

Water is not the only nutrient needed to make blood. Your blood needs certain other nutrients in order for it to work properly. Blood needs iron to carry oxygen from your lungs to all other parts of your body. Blood needs protein to build red blood cells. Vitamin C is also needed to help strengthen your blood vessels, which carry the blood.

For healthy blood, you need nutrients from these foods:

Water   Many foods and beverages

Iron   *Meat-Poultry-Fish-Beans group:* Meat, fish, poultry, dried beans and peas, seeds
           Bread-Cereal group: Whole-grain or enriched breads, rolls, cereals, rice, noodles, crackers

Protein   *Meat-Poultry-Fish-Beans group:* Meat, fish, poultry, eggs, dried beans and peas, nuts, seeds
           Milk-Cheese group: Milk, yogurt, cheese

Vitamin C *Citrus fruits:* Oranges, grapefruits, lemons, limes
           Other fruits and vegetables: Strawberries, cantaloupe, tomatoes, spinach, turnip greens, broccoli

---

Unscramble these words (Hint: They are all foods that help build blood and blood vessels):

LORLS _____   GEGS _____

SAPE _____   SHIF _____

STUN _____   NABES _____

KILM _____   EDESS _____

ATMOESTO _____   OLTRYUP _____

CROLOCIB _____   SLODONE _____

RETAW _____   REEGEVABS _____

SUMMARY

Now you have learned all you need to know about nutrition for keeping your body healthy. Right or wrong? If you answered "wrong," you are right! You have learned just a few important facts about how specific parts of your body work. You have learned that:

1. Vitamin A is important for healthy bones, skin, and eyes.
2. Vitamin D helps bones use calcium and become hard.
3. Vitamin E helps keep cell walls strong and healthy.
4. Vitamin K is needed for the clotting of blood.
5. Vitamin C is important for healthy bones and skin, as well as for healthy blood vessels.
6. The B vitamins (thiamin, riboflavin, niacin) help to keep nerves healthy.
7. Calcium and phosphorous are used to make bones and teeth strong.
8. Iron is important in the blood for it helps to carry oxygen throughout your body.
9. Zinc is important in many body functions using enzymes.
10. Fluorine strengthens teeth and bones.
11. Water is important for the blood, which carries nutrients to and wastes from your body's cells.

If you can't remember all of these specifics, try remembering this: Iron CaPAC. The term *Iron CaPAC* stands for some of the most important nutrients you have studied. If you remember these nutrients—iron, calcium, protein, Vitamin A, Vitamin C—you will be well on your way to becoming a nutrition expert!

Remember that in your study of nutrition, you have also learned about which foods you can eat to supply your body with all of the nutrients it needs. You have not yet learned about the fascinating relationships among all of the nutrients. You have not yet learned about the other forty or so nutrients, such as sodium, selenium, and biotin. Every day there are new discoveries being made in nutrition. And every day there is something new to learn!

WORD SEARCH ONE

Directions: The names of three nutrients are hidden in this puzzle. They are the *Ca*, the *A*, and the *C* in Iron CaPAC. Surrounding each nutrient are the names of foods containing that nutrient. The names may go up, down, or diagonally, and some names may be spelled backward and some names may be spelled forward. How many can you find? Draw a box around each nutrient and a circle around each of its food sources.

```
                                        E
                                    V   P
                                S   T   U
                            L   U   A   O
                        F   W   P   N   L
                    O   S   A   S   G   A
                M   O   X   T   N   E   T
            I   S   T   C   E   K   R   N
        B   R   E   A   O   R   G   I   A
        K   O   V   I   T   A   M   I   N   C
    C   M   B   V   R   O   V   E   A   E   A
E   X   E   I   N   R   P   N   L   N   T   R
D   I   E   T   R   S   E   S   A   O   T   M   O
L   H   L   H   P   Q   A   B   S   A   N   A   H   R
I   J   C   C   U   N   C   W   L   S   O   R   D   A
V   I   T   A   M   I   N   A   N   U   S   O   I   N
E   L   S   N   E   K   K   R   R   A   Z   S   L   G
R   H   R   I   G   P   A   T   A   R   E   S   T   E
    P   P   P   M   M   R   S   M   P   O   A   U   K
        N   S   A   U   K   A   L   A   J   T   L   M   Z   E   R   L   F   E
            H   H   P   L   E   R   R   E   M   S   L   I   K   S   A   S   L
                O   R   N   T   W   E   A   A   P   U   K   R   N   E   T   Y
                    V   A   S   Q   R   B   E   A   N   S   L   E   S   O   K
                        Z   E   N   Y   K   R   N   I   H   H   I   G   V   B
                            A   S   E   I   C   A   L   C   I   U   M   R   A
                                T   I   S   E   R   O   T   R   S   E   C
                                    E   T   C   D   C   T   V   E   P
                                        C   I   A   C   W   A   O
                                            U   N   O   N   J
                                                Y   R   R
                                                    B
```

WORD SEARCH TWO

Directions: This word maze has the names of the two remaining Iron CaPAC nutrients and the names of the foods that contain those nutrients. The names of the nutrients and of their food sources go up, down, and diagonally; and as in Word Search One, some names may be spelled backward, and some names may be spelled forward. How many names can you find? Draw a box around each nutrient and a circle around each of its food sources.

```
S  P  J  A  E  B  G  M  O  W  R
Q  U  L  R  Y  L  O  I  U  V  H  X
E  Z  H  A  B  U  S  N  A  E  B  O  E
A  P  C  N  R  E  A  N  L  O  I  N  L  D
V  T  A  O  E  B  Q  P  A  A  S  I  A  E  Y
O  R  N  G  V  E  P  S  H  L  T  C  P  E  W  L
C  H  I  L  I  R  O  N  O  B  U  V  J  I  W  H  G
A  S  P  K  L  R  E  R  I  N  C  U  F  R  N  E  P
D  O  S  D  A  I  K  E  N  C  A  R  H  B  I  K  E  A  G
O  A  Y  J  H  E  E  R  M  E  E  T  U  I  E  Y  S  E  T
F  B  A  U  B  S  R  G  E  O  P  I  L  V  C  E  T  N  U
   O  H  A  M  B  U  R  G  E  R  E  E  R  S  K  E  A  R
      M  E  C  C  S  O  I  L  O  S  G  J  L  R  E  N  P
         E  A  M  H  S  S  O  T  G  U  I  A  U  W  N
            A  O  T  E  T  N  E  F  M  D  E  T  I
               L  H  R  E  U  I  H  E  W  V  I
                  X  I  J  S  N  A  S  I  L
                     A  H  H  E  E  I  K
```

IRON CaPAC ANAGRAMS

Directions: Can you unscramble the following words? They all have something to do with Iron CaPAC. In the space next to each anagram, write the word. Next to that, write the Iron CaPAC nutrients that go with it (Iron, Ca, Pro, A, C). Place a star in the space when the word is a *nutrient*. If you cannot unscamble a word, see the list of choices that are upside down at the bottom of the page.

	Unscrambled Word	Iron CaPAC Nutrients
oofd		
ntutrine		
laccmui		
nior		
noitirtun		
wgrhto		
xneyog		
obold		
eniprto		
stuise		
octl		
hetet		
sboen		
casbirco daic		
A tamiinv		
yenreg		
veenrs		
praeir		
luibd		
kins		
ctnfioien		
smug		
yees		
neahlig		

Choices

energy	nutrient	
clot	nerves	Vitamin A
calcium	iron	tissue
build	infection	teeth
bones	healing	skin
blood	gums	repair
ascorbic acid	growth	protein
food	oxygen	
eyes	nutrition	

QUIZ
NUTRITION OVERVIEW: VITAMINS, MINERALS, AND WATER

Directions: Use the questions on Quiz Sheet 2-2 to help you fill in the answers to this crossword puzzle, which covers information you have learned in Units 1 and 2.

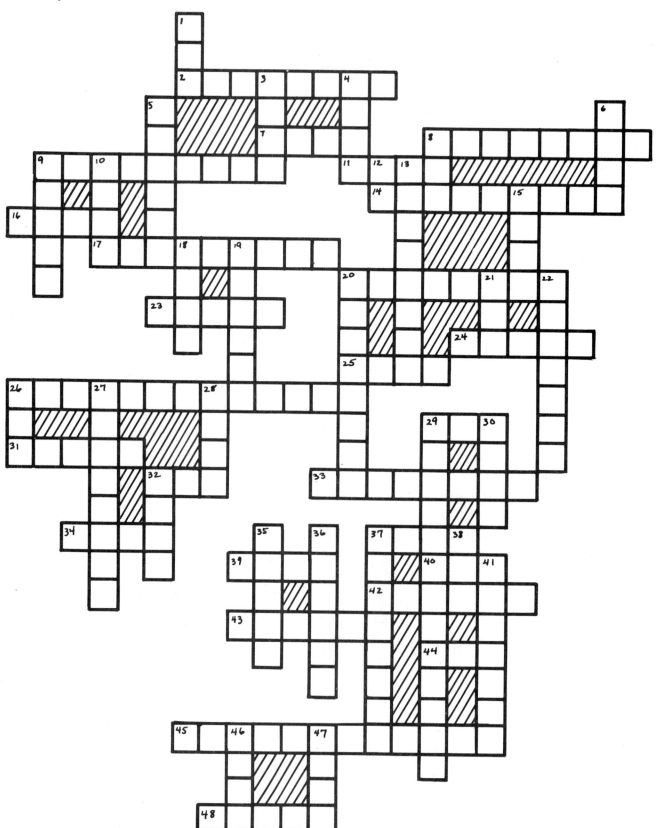

ACROSS:

2. The nutrient group that helps regulate body functions (Ex.: iron and calcium).
7. The organs of hearing.
8. _____, or whole-grain breads and cereals, are good sources of iron.
9. A group of nutrients needed to keep nerves healthy; includes thiamin, riboflavin, and niacin.
11. An upholstered couch.
14. The study of how your body uses food to make you grow, give you energy, and keep you healthy.
16. A toy that can be reeled up and down on a string; also the idea of losing weight, gaining it back, and losing it again.
17. Materials found in food having specific functions in keeping your body healthy; they usually cannot be made by your body (Ex.: proteins, fats, water).
20. The nutrient found in citrus fruits that is important for healthy bones, skin, and blood vessels.
23. The part of your body that makes you tall or short; it makes up your skeleton.
24. The little units that together form your body.
25. A common skin disease among teenagers and young adults.
26. The system of electrical currents passing through all parts of your body.
29. Foods can be packaged in a box, bag, or _____.
31. Calcium is important in _____ formation.
32. Enjoyment or pleasure.
33. The units that measure food energy.
34. A meal plan for eating and drinking.
37. Farmers do this to their fields with tractors.
39. To receive.
40. To get on base in baseball you need a _____.
42. Part of the air that is breathed into the lungs and carried by the blood to all body parts.
43. Units of measurement for body size in pounds or kilograms.
44. Any one of the 12 pairs of arched bones in the human skeleton.
45. Channels that carry blood.
48. The color of leafy vegetables that are high in iron.

DOWN:

1. The salted or smoked hind leg of a hog.
3. The part of your face with which you see.
4. You need to eat _____ calories than you use if you want to lose weight.
5. A legume (or nut) commonly made into a butter for spreading on sandwiches.
6. A legume that is not a pea or a nut.
8. To put food into the mouth, chew it, and swallow.
9. A liquid in your body made of 93% water; it carries oxygen and nutrients to your organs and other body parts, and removes their wastes.
10. A mineral important in the blood; it carries oxygen from the lungs to all body parts.
12. The surface of (Ex.: a scar _____ my body).
13. A job or action.
15. Having little flesh or fat.
18. The part of a vegetable that grows underground.
19. The ability to work; it gives your body the ability to breathe, to digest your food, to move your muscles, and to do all kinds of other activities.
20. The nutrient important in bones, skin, and eyes; it is found in dark-yellow and in orange fruits and vegetables.
21. Frozen water.
22. The mineral important in building bones, teeth, and keeping nerves healthy; it is found in milk.
26. A plant protein source (Ex.: pecans).
27. The nutrient group that helps to regulate body functions and operations.
28. The material covering the outside of your body.
29. A nutrient group that gives you energy.
30. The body's requirement for nutrients.
32. Another nutrient group that gives you energy.
35. A nutrient that makes up about 60% of the body's total weight.
36. The unit of measurement for body size, in feet and inches, or in meters and centimeters.
37. The nutrient group that rebuilds cells and tissues; it also gives you energy.
38. You can wear this if you lose your hair.
41. The small porous sacks that contain leaves or herbs for brewing.
46. A smell, fragrance, or aroma.
47. Any blood vessel that carries blood back to the heart.

Unit 3: RDA Doorway to Good Health

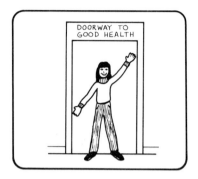

CONCEPTS

–It is recommended that healthy people take in a certain amount of each of the Iron CaPAC nutrients each day. These recommended amounts are called *Recommended Dietary Allowances* or RDAs.

OBJECTIVES

–Given the materials needed and using the concepts of *average need* and of the *safety factor*, the student will conduct an experiment to determine the height needed for a doorway that would (1) accommodate all the students in the classroom (sample) and (2) accommodate most students in their age range (population).

TEACHER'S UNIT INTRODUCTION

This unit introduces the *Recommended Dietary Allowances* (see Chart A). The term Recommended Dietary Allowances (RDA) refers to the recommended amounts of Iron CaPAC and other nutrients that should be consumed each day to promote good health. A classroom experiment that uses methods similar to some of those used by scientists to decide RDA values will show students how RDA values are determined.

The RDAs, which were first published in 1943, provide standards to serve as a goal for good nutrition. They are based on scientific evidence and are revised about every five years. The RDAs can be useful guides for

1. Evaluating the nutritional intake of populations or groups
2. Interpreting information about the composition of food
3. Establishing food assistance programs and nutrition education programs
4. Establishing guidelines for nutritional labeling of foods

There are several limitations of the RDAs that should be remembered if the RDAs are to be used properly. First, the RDAs are recommendations and not requirements. Our nutrient needs depend on our age, sex, body size, physical state, and genetic makeup. How active we are, and the environment we live in, can also affect nutrient needs. Illness and disease can change nutrient requirements. It is important to remember that the RDAs apply only to healthy people.

Our nutrient needs depend on several factors that can change, so it is impossible to list a single standard for all individuals. This means that the RDAs are dietary guidelines, not absolute values, for any one individual.

In Unit 3 students will design and run an experiment to find the height needed for a doorway tall enough to accommodate most people. Discussion of the results will establish the need for an average requirement that includes the addition of a safety factor to bring the average value up high enough to meet the needs of most of the population.

This unit encourages the use of the metric system for measuring the height of students. If a meterstick is not readily available, use a ruler with centimeters marked on one side.

This unit contains sophisticated concepts. It is important to remember, however, that because our experiment uses only one variable, it may result in an oversimplification of a true experimental situation, which involves many variables.

Unit 4, "RDA Meterstick to Good Nutrition," expands the concepts presented in this unit.

BASIC ACTIVITY

Time Needed: Three class periods

Materials Needed: Sheets 3-1 through 3-2: "RDA Doorway to Good Health"
Chart A: "Recommended Dietary Allowances"
Measuring tape *or* meterstick
Optional: cardboard, scissors *or* X-acto knife, tape *or* wire, marker
Optional: cassette tape recorder and blank tape
Quiz Sheet 3-1

Class Period 1

1. Before proceeding with Sheets 3-1 through 3-2, which describe the experimental process, allow students to discuss the different ways they might go about determining the RDAs for nutrients. Allow the different proposals to be criticized but emphasize that there is no one "right" way.

2. Distribute Sheets 3-1 through 3-2.

3. Discuss the size of the doorway and how it should be constructed. When deciding how large to make the doorway, some students may not understand why we want to make the doorway (and the nutrient RDA values) high enough to accommodate all individuals but still small enough to prohibit the wasting of doorway material (and nutrients). Try to explain the wastefulness and uselessness of making something too big. This concept is true for most things in the world today. There is also the possibility that consuming too much of a nutrient may be harmful. This possibility exists and is one that does concern nutritionists.

Class Period 2

1. The impact of this unit will be greater if students actually construct an RDA DOORWAY TO GOOD HEALTH. Cardboard from a large appliance box would be the best material for constructing a door frame. You could construct the doorway around the existing door frame of your room, or you could make it freestanding. To keep it upright, the doorway will require either masking tape to attach it to a door frame or else thin wire to suspend a freestanding doorway from the ceiling or from a light fixture. With a marker, print the height and name of each student along the side of the doorway, with the height of the tallest student and the safety factor clearly indicated.

2. Once the doorway is complete, compare the procedure for building the doorway with the procedure for determining the RDA for nutrients. Perhaps some students will have difficulty relating the height of the RDA DOORWAY TO GOOD HEALTH to the procedure for its determination. The former is the height of a doorway, something we can see and easily determine; the latter refers to the minute amounts of various nutrients believed to be needed by the body.

Class Period 3

1. Write the table below on the chalkboard.

<u>Recommended Dietary Allowances*</u>

	Iron	Calcium	Protein	Vitamin A	Vitamin C
Children, 7–10 yrs.	10 mg.	800 mg.	34 g.	3500 IU	45 mg.
Boys, 11–14 yrs.	18 mg.	1200 mg.	45 g.	5000 IU	50 mg.
Girls, 11–14 yrs.	18 mg.	1200 mg.	46 g.	4000 IU	50 mg.
*1980 edition					

2. Ask students to recall the RDA DOORWAY TO GOOD HEALTH that they constructed. Then pose questions such as the ones below to stimulate students' thoughts.

a. "Why is our doorway to health so tall?" Allow time for students to respond briefly. Accept the answers as they are given. This question is the first in a sequence of questions.

b. Then ask: "What do the letters *RDA* stand for?" (*Answer:* Recommended Dietary Allowance)

c. "Since the first letter of *RDA* is *R*, why aren't the RDAs called *Required* Dietary Allowances?" (The answer to this question might go something like this: "We are all pretty much alike, but not *exactly* alike. Consequently, scientists cannot find *one exact value* for a nutrient that will be just the amount that every one *requires*. Instead, scientists determine our average nutrient needs and add to that a *safety factor.* The safety factor raises the overall value so that the RDAs take care of practically all of us who have needs that are greater than average.")

3. Next to the classroom "RDA DOORWAY TO GOOD HEALTH" write the following words using large letters:

WHY IS OUR "RDA DOORWAY TO GOOD HEALTH" SO TALL?

4. Ask students to compose a short essay entitled "Why Our RDA Doorway to Good Health Is So Tall." Be sure students include enough information about RDAs in their essays so that a student or a teacher from another class could learn some basic facts about RDAs from their essays. To accomplish this, you may want to remind students to explain:

a. What RDAs are

b. Who develops them

c. How they're developed

Let students know that you will be evaluating their essays for clarity of expression and completeness of information.

5. You may want to record on tape the essay that best meets the criteria given above. The recording and the doorway may be shared with other classes. If you decide to record, you may want to ask the student who wrote the essay to read it into the cassette tape recorder.

6. Under the question "Why is our doorway to good health so tall?" use large letters to add:

LISTEN TO THE TAPE RECORDER TO FIND OUT. WHEN YOU ARE THROUGH LISTENING, PLEASE REWIND THE TAPE.

7. Place a tape recorder and the directions for using it on a table or chair under the question.

8. **Evaluation:** Distribute Quiz Sheet 3-1 and have students complete it independently. Discuss the answers as a class.

RDA DOORWAY TO GOOD HEALTH

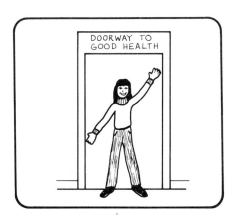

Do you know what an experiment is? You may have a very funny idea of what one is, but do not be concerned if you are not sure. An *experiment* is a formal and controlled procedure used to answer a question. For example, you might want to know: How many of my fellow classmates are left-handed? This would be your question. One way of answering your question would be to ask every one in the class to write his or her name. You could watch them and count those who use their left hand.

Some experiments are simple, like counting the number of left-handed students in a classroom, and others are complicated. Before determining the *Recommended Dietary Allowances,* scientists review experiments that might help them decide the correct amounts of Iron CaPAC, for example, that all of us need. Enough experiments may not have been conducted to justify a recommendation. Sometimes the answers are just not clear. but nutrition scientists make the best recommendations they can. An RDA may also be changed, from time to time, when new results from experiments become available.

To help you understand the process of setting an RDA, we will conduct an experiment. This experiment is similar to, but much simpler than, the ones actually used by scientists.

Pretend that you and your classmates want to build an "RDA Doorway to Good Health" that is only for the students in your class. Pretend that the materials for making the doorway are expensive—so you want to make it just big enough for the students in your own class.

How would you do this? Talk it over with your classmates and share your ideas. There are several good ways to construct the doorway. However, this lesson will show you one way that a scientist might use for selecting the correct height of the doorway. As you read through this method, think of ways in which it is similar to the method you would have used.

First, measure in centimeters the height of each student in the class. Your teacher will pair you with another student for you to measure. You may want to write every student's name and height on the chalkboard. Then determine the following:

What is the height of the tallest student?	_____ cm.
What is the height of the shortest student?	_____ cm.
What is the average height of all students in your class?	_____ cm.

The doorway should be at least as tall as the average height of the class. Then, to be sure that the doorway will be high enough for each person in your class, you must add a *safety factor.* How large should this safety factor be? Nutrition scientists figure safety factors in very special and sometimes complicated ways. Decide on a safety factor to be added to your class height average and be ready to explain the reasons why you chose this particular safety factor.

THE AVERAGE HEIGHT OF THE CLASS IS   _____ cm.

THE SAFETY FACTOR IS   _____ cm.

THE HEIGHT OF OUR RDA DOORWAY TO GOOD HEALTH IS   _____ cm.

REASONS FOR CHOOSING THIS SAFETY FACTOR: _____

_____

Remember that this RDA Doorway to Good Health is only for students in your own class. Your class is only a small part of all of the classes at your grade level. A scientist would say that your class is a *sample* of all students at your grade level. Those in the sample should be as much like those in the whole group as possible, but, of course, the number of people in the sample is much less than the number of people in the whole group.

Imagine that you were able to have all of the students at your grade level in your school, or in your school district, pass through your RDA Doorway to Good Health. What would happen? Would any of them bump their heads? We could not be sure unless we tried it, but, very likely, most students would pass through without any problem. However, it is also likely that a few students at your grade level would bump their heads.

COULD THE TALLEST MAN IN THE WORLD HAVE WALKED THROUGH YOUR DOORWAY TO GOOD HEALTH WITHOUT DUCKING WHEN HE WAS YOUR AGE? _____
(Check a book like the *Guiness Book of World Records* to see how tall the tallest man was at your age. You will probably have to change his height from inches to centimeters. If you do not have this book, pretend that at age 10 he was 190 centimeters tall. At age 11, he was 195 centimeters tall. At age 12, he was 205 centimeters tall. At age 13, he was 215 centimeters tall. And, by age 14, he was 220 centimeters tall.)

As you can see, your doorway is higher than necessary for most of your classmates. Probably even the tallest person in your class can walk through without stooping! Your doorway is not, however, high enough for the tallest man when he was your age.

Just as the doorway is higher than necessary for most of your classmates, the RDAs for nutrients are higher than the actual requirements of most people. For this reason, it is important to remember that the RDAs are meant as guides only. Not everyone needs that much of each nutrient. To be sure that *most* people will receive the amounts of nutrients they need, the RDA includes a safety factor. Nutrition scientists add the safety factor to the average requirement of the group to give us the Recommended Dietary Allowances for nutrients.

This is not an easy job for nutrition scientists. They must be very careful when they decide on an RDA for a nutrient. The RDA must be high enough to cover the needs of *most* people, but small enough so that no one is harmed by this amount. To be sure they have chosen the RDA wisely, nutrition scientists recheck their work against the results of the latest experiments about every five years.

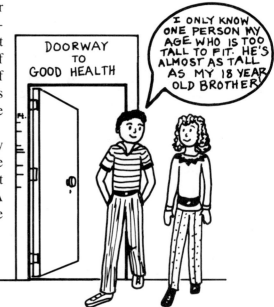

QUIZ
RDA DOORWAY TO GOOD HEALTH

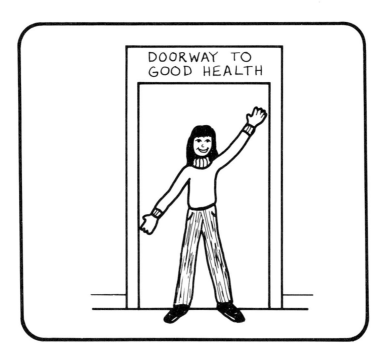

_____ 1. RDA means:
   a. Recommended Dietary Allowance
   b. Recommended Daily Allowances
   c. Required Dietary Allowance
   d. Required Daily Account

_____ 2. Scientists have done experiments on five individuals. Consider their results or data.

Name	Amount of Vitamin C required daily
Joshua	30 mg.
Susan	28 mg.
Jennifer	45 mg.
Billy	24 mg.
Joanne	18 mg.

What is the average requirement of this group of individuals for Vitamin C?
   a. 19 mg.
   b. 25 mg.
   c. 29 mg.
   d. 50 mg.

_____ 3. Scientists add a "safety factor" when they determine the RDAs for nutrients. What is the "safety factor"?
   a. A substance added to preserve the nutrients
   b. An amount added to the average nutrient requirement of a group of people
   c. An amount added to the highest nutrient requrement of a group of people
   d. An amount added to the lowest nutrient requirement of a group of people

Unit 4: RDA Meterstick to Good Nutrition

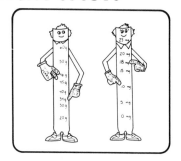

CONCEPTS

–Knowing the kinds and amounts of nutrients supplied by a food helps us determine the nutritional quality of that food.

–Information on the nutritional quality of foods can be found in a food composition table where the iron, calcium, and Vitamin C content are given in milligrams, the protein content is given in grams, and the Vitamin A content is given in International Units (IUs).

OBJECTIVES

–Using the Energy and Iron CaPAC Food Composition Table and the Key Nutrients in Food Chart, students will

1. Determine the number and amount of Iron CaPAC nutrients supplied by several foods

2. Relate a food's nutrient contribution to the Recommended Dietary Allowances

TEACHER'S UNIT INTRODUCTION

Some foods contain significantly greater amounts of Iron CaPAC nutrients than other foods. Foods also differ from one another in the amount of calories they each supply. Two or more foods that provide similar kinds and amounts of Iron CaPAC nutrients can differ widely in their caloric content.

In Unit 3, "RDA Doorway to Good Health," you learned that there are recommended amounts of the Iron CaPAC and other nutrients that should be consumed on a daily basis to promote good health. These are the *Recommended Dietary Allowances* (RDAs).

In assessing the nutritional quality of food, it is important to consider

1. The caloric value of the food

2. The number (variety) of individual essential nutrients present

3. The level at which the essential nutrients are present in comparison to the Recommended Dietary Allowances (RDAs)

For example, consider a one-cup serving, each, of skim milk, whole milk, and chocolate milk. All three provide similar amounts of essential nutrients and are considered to be good sources of protein and calcium, supplying between 20 percent and 25 percent of an eleven to fourteen year old's RDAs for protein and calcium, respectively. Yet their caloric contribution, per cup, differs drastically:

Chocolate milk (2% butterfat). . . . . .180 calories

White whole milk . . . . .160 calories

White skim milk . . . . 85 calories

Thus, calorie per calorie, skim milk gives the most nutrition—that is, it has the highest nutritional quality.

48

Units 8 and 9 in this kit expand on the concept of nutritional quality. In these units, students will compare the nutrient and calorie levels (written as percentages of the U.S. RDAs) in foods against standards to determine if the foods can be classified as being "nutrient dense."

It is the purpose of the activities in this unit to illustrate that

1. The kinds and amounts of essential nutrients a food supplies can be found in tables of food composition.
2. Some foods contain a greater variety and amount of essential nutrients than other foods (the focus is on Iron CaPAC).
3. The RDAs can be used to help assess the nutrient contribution of specific foods to the daily diet.

Throughout this lesson, students should be discouraged from labeling foods as "good" or "bad." Instead, they should be helped to look at the foods and at their nutrient values objectively, and as each contributes to the day's diet.

BASIC ACTIVITY

Time Needed: One class period

Materials Needed: Tables 4-1 through 4-2: "Energy and Iron CaPAC Food Composition Table"
Sheets 4-1 through 4-6: "Tables as Tools" (also used for Unit 5)
Chart C: "Key Nutrients in Food"
Quiz Sheet 4-1

1. Distribute Tables 4-1 through 4-2, "Energy and Iron CaPAC Food Composition Table," and provide an introduction, if necessary, including the units of measure used for the different nutrients.

2. Distribute Sheets 4-1 through 4-6, "Tables as Tools," and have the students complete items 1 through 5. Note that when the students choose six foods from Tables 4-1 through 4-2 that are highest in each of the Iron CaPAC nutrients, many other nutritious foods will be left off the list. Also note that the comparison of nutrient levels in one food with those in another will convey the idea of the relative nutritional values of foods, but it will not allow students to view the nutritional value as compared to a standard. Therefore, any discussion about the nutritional value of foods will be more open to interpretation than if a standard were used.

3. Have the students complete the remaining items (6 through 15) of "Tables as Tools." You may wish to run through an example for some or all of these items; you may wish to use different foods than any of those given. You may also wish to review the concept of Recommended Dietary Allowances. Alternatively, you may have students complete the remaining items as a homework assignment.

4. While completing the questions, students may inquire as to why there are age and sex differences in the RDAs. A simplistic answer to this would be that both body weight and growth rate influence the need for nutrients. Eleven through fourteen year olds are usually larger than seven through ten year olds, and thus it is recommended that eleven through fourteen year olds consume greater amounts of most essential nutrients than seven through ten year olds. In addition, eleven- through fourteen-year-old boys are often a little larger (and growing a little faster) than girls of the same age. It is thus recommended that eleven- through fourteen-year-old boys consume greater amounts of some of the essential nutrients than girls of this age.

Evaluation: Distribute Quiz Sheet 4-1 and have students complete it.

ENERGY AND IRON CaPAC FOOD COMPOSITION TABLE

Food and Serving Size	Weight	Energy	Iron	Ca	P	A	C
	g	cal	mg	mg	g	IU	mg
Apple, fresh—1	138	80	0.1	10	*	125	6
Apple pie—1/7 of 9" diameter	135	400	1.0	11	3	175	3
Applesauce, sweetened—1/2 cup	128	115	1.3	10	*	51	1
Apricots, fresh—3	108	55	0.6	5	*	2,890	11
Avocado—1/2	114	190	0.6	11	2	330	16
Banana—1	119	100	0.7	12	1	230	12
Beef pot pie—4 1/4" diameter	227	560	4.1	32	23	1,860	7
Beet greens, cooked—1/2 cup	73	15	1.4	72	1	3,697	11
Beets, cooked—1/2 cup	85	30	0.4	12	1	20	5
Biscuit—1, 2 1/2" diameter	40	155	0.7	47	3	T	T
Blueberries, fresh—1/2 cup	73	45	0.7	11	*	72	10
Bologna—1 slice, 1 ounce	28	85	0.5	T	3	0	0
Bread, enriched:							
cracked-wheat—1 slice	25	65	0.3	22	2	T	T
rye (light)—1 slice	25	60	0.4	19	2	0	0
white—1 slice	25	70	0.6	21	2	T	T
whole-wheat—1 slice	23	55	0.5	23	3	T	T
Broccoli, cooked—1/2 cup	78	20	0.6	68	2	1,937	70
Cabbage, cooked—1/2 cup	73	15	0.2	32	1	94	24
Cantaloupe—1/4, 5" diameter	133	40	0.5	19	1	4,505	44
Carrot, raw—1 medium	81	35	0.6	30	1	8,910	6
Cauliflower, cooked—1/2 cup	68	15	0.5	14	2	40	37
Cheese, American—1 slice, 1 ounce	28	95	0.2	163	6	260	0
Chicken[a]—1/2 breast	111	245	1.2	18	31	80	0
Chili con carne, w/beans—1 cup	230	305	4.3	82	19	150	0
Chocolate bar—1 ounce	28	150	0.3	65	2	80	T
Chocolate chip cookie—1	12	60	0.2	4	*	T	0
Corn, canned—1/2 cup	83	70	0.4	4	3	290	3
Corn grits, enriched—1/2 ounce dry (1/2 cup prepared)	123	60	0.4	1	2	73	0
Cupcake, yellow w/chocolate icing—1 average	46	185	0.4	20	2	209	T
Doughnut, cake, plain—1	42	165	0.6	17	2	30	T
Egg, plain—1	51	80	1.1	29	6	265	0
Fruit cocktail—1/2 cup	128	100	0.5	11	1	178	3
Gelatin (Jell-O)—1/2 cup	120	70	0	0	2	0	0
Gingerbread, homemade—1 piece	76	275	4.1	134	3	28	2
Grapefruit—1/2	98	40	0.4	16	*	78	37
Grapes, fresh—1/2 cup	80	55	0.3	10	*	80	3
Hamburger, no roll—1	85	245	2.7	10	21	34	0

*less than one gram protein
T means food contains only trace amount of this nutrient
[a]values for these foods are averages of several varieties, brands, cuts of meat, or methods of preparation

ENERGY AND IRON CaPAC FOOD COMPOSITION TABLE (continued)

Food and Serving Size	Weight	Energy	Iron	Ca	P	A	C
	g	cal	mg	mg	g	IU	mg
Ice cream, regular—2/3 cup	89	180	0.1	117	3	363	0
Lamb chop—2½ ounce	71	255	0.9	6	16	0	0
Lettuce, iceburg—½ cup	28	5	0.1	5	*	90	2
Liver, beef—3 ounce	85	150	7.5	9	22	45,390	23
Macaroni, cooked—½ cup	140	155	1.2	12	5	0	0
Macaroni and cheese, prepared from mix—¾ cup	156	290	1.6	114	9	560	0
Milk, fluid:							
chocolate, 2% butterfat—8 ounce	250	180	0.6	285	8	500**	2
skim—8 ounce	245	85	0.1	300	8	500**	2
whole—8 ounce	244	160	0.1	290	8	340	4
Oatmeal, cooked—½ cup	131	110	1.2	18	5	0	1
Ocean perch, breaded, fried—2½ ounce	70	160	0.9	23	13	T	T
Orange, fresh—1	131	65	0.5	54	1	260	65
Oysters, raw—6	90	60	4.8	84	8	276	0
Peach, fresh—1	100	40	0.5	9	*	1,330	7
Peanut butter—1 tablespoon	15	90	0.3	9	4	0	0
Pepper, green, raw—1	164	35	1.1	15	2	689	210
Pizza, with cheese—1/7 of 10" diameter	57	140	1.0	89	5	251	3
Plum, fresh—1	28	20	0.1	3	*	85	1
Popcorn, plain—1 cup	12	45	0.2	1	*	2	0
Pork chop—3 ounce	85	230	3.3	11	26	0	0
Potato:							
baked—1	156	145	1.1	14	4	T	31
chips—14	28	160	0.5	11	2	0	4
french fried—½ cup	55	150	0.7	8	2	T	12
Prunes—10 medium	96	240	4.0	50	2	1,540	T
Pumpkin pie—1/7 of 9" diameter	135	290	1.2	106	6	2,467	3
Raisins—¼ cup	42	125	0.9	23	1	7	T
Strawberries, whole—½ cup	75	30	0.7	16	1	45	44
Sweet potato, baked—1	146	205	1.3	58	3	11,826	32
Tapioca pudding—½ cup	116	150	1.2	77	2	19	1
Tomato, fresh—1 medium	123	30	0.6	16	1	1,107	28
Tuna, canned—½ cup	80	160	1.5	6	23	65	0
Turnip greens, cooked—½ cup	73	15	0.8	133	2	4,567	50
Turnips, cooked—½ cup	78	20	0.3	27	*	T	17
Veal roast—3 ounce	85	200	2.7	10	22	0	0
Watermelon, fresh—1 piece	426	140	0.8	84	3	1,596	42
Yogurt:							
skim milk—1 cup	227	125	0.2	452	13	16	2
whole milk—1 cup	227	140	0.1	216	8	280	1

*less than one gram protein
**fortified with Vitamin A
T means food contains only trace amount of this nutrient

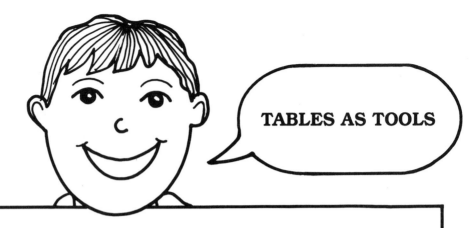

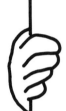

Today we are going to pull apart a table, but you won't need a saw or a screwdriver or even your own brute strength. Instead, you'll need a keen eye. We're going to pull apart and examine a nutrient table.

You have seen long lists of numbers in newspapers and magazines. Numbers can be confusing when you try to look at them all at once. But when you look at one or two numbers at a time, you can learn some interesting things about what those numbers represent. Look below and see for yourself!

1. Tables 4-1 through 4-2, "Energy and Iron CaPAC Food Composition Table," you will see a column labeled "Food and Serving Size." The foods in this list are in alphabetical order. Also in this table you will find columns for serving weight (in grams) and for energy (in calories). After these columns, you will see five columns of numbers. Each of these columns has a title at the top. Read across the last five column titles. What do they spell? _____

_____

2. That code should look familiar. What nutrients are represented by the code?

_____ _____

_____ _____ _____

3. a. Now look at the table and find the six foods that are highest in iron. On Sheet 4-2, "Nutritious Food Chart," list the name of each food and the amount of iron in it.

b. On the same chart list the six foods having the most calcium. Again, make sure to list the amounts of calcium in each food. (Notice that some of the high-calcium foods may already be in your list of high-iron foods. Be sure to include them in the calcium list anyway.)

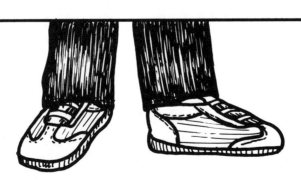

NUTRITIOUS FOOD CHART

Nutrient	Food	Nutrient Amount	Stars
Iron	_____ _____ _____ _____ _____ _____ _____	_____ _____ _____ _____ _____ _____ _____	
Calcium	_____ _____ _____ _____ _____ _____ _____	_____ _____ _____ _____ _____ _____ _____	
Protein	_____ _____ _____ _____ _____ _____ _____	_____ _____ _____ _____ _____ _____ _____	
Vitamin A	_____ _____ _____ _____ _____ _____	_____ _____ _____ _____ _____ _____	
Vitamin C	_____ _____ _____ _____ _____ _____ _____	_____ _____ _____ _____ _____ _____ _____	

    c. List the six foods that have the most protein. List the amount of protein in each food.

    d. List the six foods that have the most Vitamin A. List the amount of Vitamin A in each.

    e. List the six foods that have the most Vitamin C. List the amount of Vitamin C in each.

4. Next, put five stars beside the foods you listed on the chart that have all five key nutrients. If there are none, put four stars beside the foods that are listed for four nutrients, three stars beside foods listed for three nutrients, and two stars beside foods listed for two nutrients.

5. a. Which foods have two or more stars? _____

   _____

   b. What is special about these foods? _____

   _____

6. Using Tables 4-1 through 4-2: Energy and Iron CaPAC Food Composition Table, answer the following questions:

   a. How many milligrams of iron does 85 grams of hamburger contain? _____

   b. How many milligrams of calcium does one slice of American cheese contain? _____

   c. How many grams of protein does one egg contain?

   _____

   d. How many International Units of Vitamin A does one carrot contain? _____

   e. How many milligrams of Vitamin C does one tomato contain?

   _____

7. a. How many milligrams of iron do *you* need each day to meet the Recommended Dietary Allowance for iron? To find out, look at the iron meterstick here. _____

   b. Compare the amount of iron you need each day with the amount of iron in one 85-gram hamburger. If your only souce of iron today were hamburger, how many hamburgers would you need to eat?

   _____

   c. Draw a bar on the meterstick for iron as tall as the amount of iron in all those hamburgers you would have to eat.

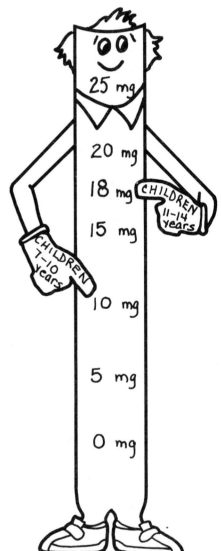

METERSTICK FOR CALCIUM

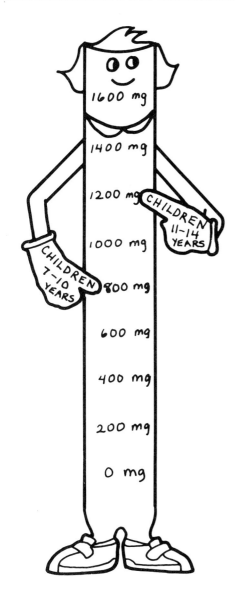

8. a. How many milligrams of calcium do *you* need each day to meet the Recommended Dietary Allowance for calcium? To find out, look at the calcium meterstick. _____

b. Compare the amount of calcium you need each day with the amount of calcium in one slice of American cheese. If your only source of calcium today were American cheese, how many slices of cheese would you need to eat? _____

c. Draw a bar on the meterstick for calcium as tall as the amount of calcium in all that cheese you would have to eat.

METERSTICK FOR PROTEIN

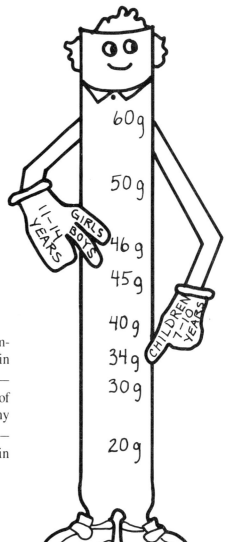

9. a. How many grams of protein do *you* need each day to meet the Recommended Dietary Allowances for protein? To find out, look at the protein meterstick. _____

b. Compare the amount of protein you need each day with the amount of protein in one egg. If your only source of protein today were eggs, how many eggs would you need to eat? _____

c. Draw a bar on the meterstick for protein as tall as the amount of protein in all those eggs you would have to eat.

METERSTICK FOR VITAMIN A

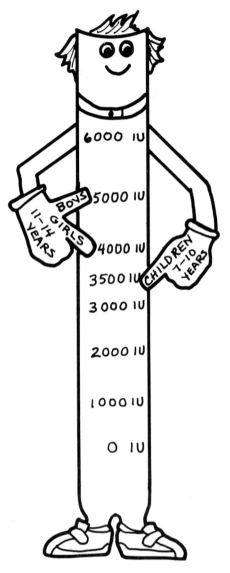

10. a. How many International Units of Vitaim A do *you* need each day to get the Recommended Dietary Allowance for Vitamin A? To find out, look at the Vitamin A meterstick. _____

b. Compare the amount of Vitamin A you need each day with the amount of Vitamin A in one carrot. If your only source of Vitamin A today were carrots, how many carrots would you need to eat?_____

c. Draw a bar on the meterstick for Vitamin A as tall as the amount of Vitamin A in all those carrots you would have to eat.

METERSTICK FOR VITAMIN C

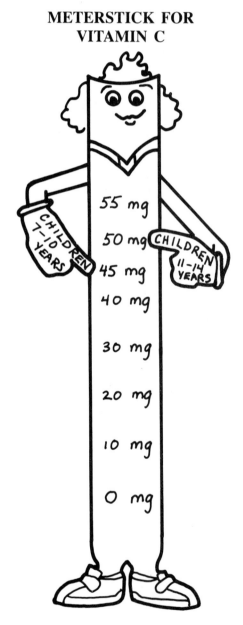

11. a. How many milligrams of Vitamin C do *you* need each day to meet the Recommended Dietary Allowance for Vitamin C? To find out, look at the Vitamin C meterstick.

_____

b. Compare the amount of Vitamin C you need each day with the amount of Vitamin C in one tomato. If your only source of Vitamin C today were tomatoes, how many tomatoes would you need to eat? ___

c. Draw a bar on the meterstick for Vitamin C as tall as the amount of Vitamin C in all those tomatoes you would have to eat.

12. a. Are these five foods—a hamburger, American cheese, an egg, a carrot, and a tomato—high in nutrients other than the one mentioned for each food? (Refer to Chart C, "Key Nutrients in Foods.") _____

   b. Name the other nutrients in which each food is high:

   Hamburger _____

   American cheese _____

   Egg _____

   Carrot _____

   Tomato _____

13. Of three snack foods—a doughnut, an apple, and one slice of American cheese—which snack is highest in the most Iron CaPAC nutrients? _____

14. Choose any after-school snack that is of high nutritional value. (Refer to Chart C and Tables 4-1 through 4-2.)

   a. What snack might you choose? _____

   b. How will you know if your snack is of high nutritional value? _____

15. Choose any dinner dessert that is of high nutritional value. (Refer to Chart C and Tables 4-1 through 4-2.)

   a. What dessert might you choose? _____

   b. How will you know if your dessert is of high nutritional value? _____

QUIZ
RDA METERSTICK TO GOOD NUTRITION

_____ 1. You can use a table of food composition to find out many things about a food. What is one thing you *could not* find out from looking up foods in this table?
a. How much a serving of a food weighed
b. How many calories were in the food
c. How many of the Iron CaPAC nutrients were in the food
d. The Recommended Dietary Allowance for the food

_____ 2. You looked up "Potato Chips" and "Baked Potato" in the table of food composition and you found:

Food	Serving Size	Weight g.	Energy cal	Iron mg.	Ca mg.	Protein g.	Vit A IU	Vit C mg.
Potato Chips	14	28	160	0.5	11	2	0	4
Baked Potato	1	156	145	1.1	14	4	T	31

T means food contains only a trace amount of this nutrient.

Based on the information given above, which statement below is true?
a. A baked potato is a good source of Vitamin A.
b. Fourteen potato chips contain more iron and protein than a baked potato.
c. A baked potato contains all of the Iron CaPAC nutrients but fourteen potato chips don't contain them all.
d. A baked potato has more iron and Vitamin C than fourteen potato chips.

_____ 3. Susan's Recommended Dietary Allowance for iron is 18 mgs. Today, Susan's only source of iron will be lima beans. If a cup of lima beans supplies 6 mgs. of iron, how many cups of lima beans would Susan have to eat to meet her RDA?
a. 2   c. 5
b. 3   d. 7

_____ 4. John's Recommended Dietary Allowance for Vitamin A is 5,000 IUs. Today, John's only source of Vitamin A was 2 eggs. If an egg has 265 IUs of Vitamin A, how much more Vitamin A would John have to eat to meet his RDA?
a. 1,000 IUs   c.   500 IUs
b. 4,470 IUs   d. 4,735 IUs

Unit 5: The Three Bs: Meeting Your RDAs

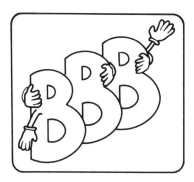

CONCEPTS

–The need for the three B vitamins (thiamin, riboflavin, and niacin) was determined by their deficiency diseases.

–A major function of thiamin, riboflavin, and niacin is to help release energy from food.

–Large amounts of the B vitamins are usually not found in single foods. The RDAs for the B vitamins are best met through eating a variety of certain foods.

OBJECTIVES

–Students will be able to identify

1. The names of the three B vitamins presented in this unit

2. The functions of thiamin, riboflavin, and niacin

3. Deficiency symptoms or diseases of each

4. Rich food sources of each

5. Food patterns that are most likely to meet the RDAs

TEACHER'S UNIT INTRODUCTION

Eight vitamins have been grouped together as the *Vitamin B complex:* thiamin (Vitamin B_1), riboflavin (Vitamin B_2), niacin, pyridoxine (Vitamin B_6), cobalamin (Vitamin B_{12}), folacin, pantothenic acid, and biotin. They are all water-soluble and function as cofactors (essential in helping enzymes to work) in specific reactions. For example:

1. Thiamin, riboflavin, niacin, pantothenic acid, and biotin are all involved in helping the body release energy from carbohydrates and fats. (Remember, the body cannot directly obtain energy from these vitamins. Energy is provided only from the fuel nutrients: carbohydrates, proteins, and fats.)

2. Folacin, cobalamin, and pyridoxine all help to build red blood cells.

3. Pyridoxine also helps in the breaking down of, and in the building of amino acids.

This unit focuses on thiamin, riboflavin, and niacin. These three B vitamins are micronutrients (as are all vitamins). They are needed only in small amounts. Chart A, "Recommended Dietary Allowances," and Sheets 5-6 through 5-7, "B Vitamins Worksheet," identify and compare actual amounts recommended. However, it is almost impossible to get the amounts we need each day of any one of these nutrients in single servings of a food. An exception to this would be superfortified foods such as breakfast cereals. To make sure we get an adequate daily intake of these nutrients, we need to eat a variety of foods every day. Chart C, "Key Nutrients in Food," identifies food sources of these nutrients. Table 5-1, "Mini Composition Table," gives information on the amounts of these nutrients in selected foods.

A *rich* food source of a nutrient supplies (per serving) one-fifth, or 20 percent, of the RDA level for that nutrient. A standard to use in determining if a food is nutritious is:

One serving of the food must provide 20 percent or more of the RDA for two or more nutrients. These nutrients are iron, calcium, protein, Vitamin A, Vitamin C, thiamin, riboflavin, and niacin.

It is important to remember that, while many foods will not meet this criterion, they may still supply valuable amounts of nutrients and thus are still of nutritional value.

You may be wondering about the adequacy of this standard, since only eight of the many essential nutrients have been considered. First, these eight essential nutrients include the vitamins and minerals scientists know the most about. Second, five of these eight nutrients are considered to be *indicator nutrients*. They are iron, calcium, protein, Vitamin A, and Vitamin C. The theory is that if you receive adequate amounts (amounts that meet your RDAs) of the indicator nutrients from foods in which these nutrients *naturally* occur, chances are your diet will also be supplying adequate amounts of other essential nutrients, including those that have not been established as essential. For example, consider whole milk, which is rich in protein and calcium. A cup of milk also supplies significant amounts of numerous other nutrients. For an eleven- to fourteen-year-old boy, a cup of milk provides 23 percent of the riboflavin, 19 percent of the phosphorus, 28 percent of the Vitamin B_{12}, 9 percent of the magnesium, and 5 percent of the thiamin that he needs according to the RDAs for his age group.

The theory specifies *naturally occurring* because some refined and fabricated foods will be good sources of the indicator nutrients if they are fortified with them. However, they may be lacking in other essential nutrients that would be supplied by choosing a diet of less refined and less fabricated foods.

In Unit 5, an introduction to nutrient standards and to the three B vitamins—thiamin, riboflavin, and niacin—is essential because subsequent units

1. Discuss, at length, the role of these B vitamins, of the Iron CaPAC nutrients, and of the concept of caloric energy and will teach a specific technique used to determine if a food is *nutritious*
2. Present the *nutrition label,* which includes data on these B vitamins

Because these B vitamins were discovered through their respective deficiency diseases, Unit 5 presents these diseases as a means for introducing the three nutrients and their respective bodily functions. Students will also become well acquainted, in this unit, with food sources of these nutrients.

For more information on the functions of these B vitamins and their deficiency diseases, see Chart C, "Key Nutrients in Food," and read the two stories, "The Case of the Wobbling Hens" and "The Case of the Volunteer Victims."

In Unit 9, "Determining Nutrient Density in Food," a more sophisticated standard is presented to ascertain whether or not a food can qualify as being *nutritious*. However, the term *nutrient dense* is used instead of *nutritious*. The concept of *nutrient density* contrasts the percent of the daily calorie needs supplied by a food with the percent U.S. RDA of each of the eight previously mentioned nutrients supplied by that food. The term *U.S. RDA* will be defined in detail in Unit 7, "RDA in the U.S.A."

This unit expands the number of nutrients that we will be considering in determining the nutritional quality of a food, so students are referred back to Sheets 4-1 through 4-6, "Tables as Tools" to determine if additional foods would qualify as being *nutritious*.

BASIC ACTIVITY

Time Needed: Two class periods

Materials Needed: Sheet 5-1: "B Vitamins Deficiency Chart"
Sheets 5-2 through 5-3: "The Case of the Volunteer Victims"
Sheets 5-4 through 5-5: "The Case of the Wobbling Hens"
Sheets 5-6 through 5-7: "B Vitamins Worksheet"
Sheets 4-1 through 4-6: "Tables as Tools"
Table 5-1: "Mini Composition Table"
Quiz Sheets 5-1 through 5-2

Class Period 1

1. As a means of introducing the names of the three B vitamins, ask students to name nutrients *other* than Iron CaPAC that they may have heard about or may have seen printed on food packages. Write responses on the board and then focus on thiamin, riboflavin, and niacin.

2. Ask students how they think these three B vitamins may have been discovered. List ideas on the board and save them for later reference.

3. Distribute Sheet 5-1, "B Vitamins Deficiency Chart" to all students. Distribute Sheets 5-2 through 5-3, "The Case of the Volunteer Victims" to one-half of the class; the other half receive Sheets 5-4 through 5-5, "The Case of the Wobbling Hens." Students should complete their readings and fill in all but the last column of Sheet 5-1 for the illness described in the story.

Note: Both of these readings are at the eighth-grade reading level. Depending on the abilities of your students, you may want them to read the stories aloud as a class.

4. Each student should share data with a classmate who has completed the opposite story in order for the student to complete his or her chart.

5. Review the ideas about how students thought the B vitamins were discovered. Erase ideas on the board that were incorrect. Point out that while no one had a story that talked about riboflavin, a lack of this vitamin can also lead to skin and eye problems.

6. Discuss with students some of the major functions of these B vitamins. Students should fill in the last column on the "B Vitamins Deficiency Chart," concluding that

   a. All three B vitamins help us to get the energy out of food; they help to break down fats and carbohydrates.

   b. Thiamin and niacin help keep the nervous system healthy.

   c. Riboflavin and niacin help keep the tongue and skin healthy.

Class Period 2

1. Referring back to Unit 4, "RDA Meterstick to Good Nutrition," review sheets 4-1 through 4-6, "Tables as Tools," with students. Review the method they used in determining the best food sources of each of the Iron CaPAC nutrients. (Students used a food composition table to identify which foods had the most of each.)

2. Ask students what other information, in addition to a food composition table, might be useful in determining if a food is a rich source of a nutrient.

3. Distribute Sheets 5-6 through 5-7, "B Vitamins Worksheet," and Table 5-1, "Mini Composition Table."

4. Explain that this exercise presents a way to use both the RDAs and a table of food composition to determine if a food is a *rich* source of a particular nutrient. The focus here is on the B vitamins.

5. Assign each student to each of the Iron CaPAC nutrients listed on Sheet 4-2, "Nutritious Food Chart." Ideally, four or five students will be assigned to each nutrient. Students will need to refer to Table 5-1, "Mini Composition Table" for the B vitamins and to Sheet 4-2 from Unit 4.

6. Have each student determine which of the six foods listed on Sheet 4-2 for his or her nutrient contains one-fifth or more of his or her RDA for any of the three B vitamins. Have students circle these foods and add one star for each B vitamin present at this level.

7. Have students report to you any foods that now qualify as being nutritious. Record these foods on the board, listing the B vitamins for which they are a rich source. The foods, and their respective nutrients, that should be listed on the board are:

Food	**Nutrients**
beans*	thiamin
beef pot pie*	thiamin, riboflavin, niacin
chicken breast	niacin
chicken liver	riboflavin, niacin
chicken pot pie*	thiamin, riboflavin, niacin
chili con carne*	niacin
hamburger	niacin
lamb chop*	niacin
liver, beef*	thiamin, riboflavin, niacin
macaroni and cheese*	thiamin
milk, chocolate	riboflavin
milk, skim	riboflavin
milk, whole	riboflavin
peas*	thiamin
pork chop*	thiamin, riboflavin, niacin
stuffed pepper	riboflavin, niacin
tuna	niacin
yogurt, skim	riboflavin
yogurt, whole	riboflavin

*Boys aged eleven to fourteen years will not report these foods as being rich enough in one or more of the B vitamins for their age group. As shown on the Answer Key to Sheets 5-6 through 5-7, "B Vitamins Worksheet," one-fifth of the RDAs for this age/sex group is slightly higher than the amount of B vitamins contained in these foods.

8. **Evaluation:** Distribute Quiz Sheets 5-1 through 5-2 and have students complete them independently. Discuss the answers as a class.

B VITAMINS DEFICIENCY CHART

ILLNESS	BEHAVIOR OF PERSONS WITH ILLNESS	APPEARANCE OF PERSONS WITH ILLNESS	DIET OF PERSONS WITH ILLNESS	MISSING NUTRIENTS	FUNCTIONS OF MISSING NUTRIENTS

THE CASE OF THE VOLUNTEER VICTIMS*

History holds a prominent place for people like Julius Caesar, Joan of Arc, and Napoleon. But who can name the countless thousands of "little" men and women who spread Caesar's power, won battles, and conquered Napoleon's empire? The achievements of one who is famous are made possible by innumerable acts of individual heroism by forgotten, unsung heroes. The science of nutrition has its unsung heroes also. Their collective deeds are remembered, but their individual names are long forgotten.

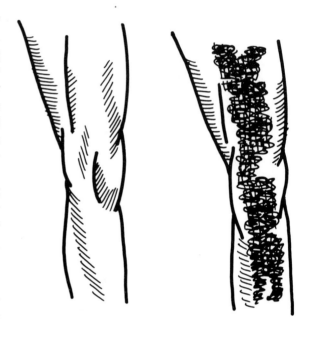

There is a disease called *pellagra* that was, and in many parts of the world still is, a serious threat to the health of society. The disease begins with a reddening of the skin, resembling sunburn, especially those parts of the body not covered by clothing. This redness develops later into dark, rough, red or brown blotches. The digestive system is weakened and there are symptoms that include indigestion, diarrhea, and soreness and irritation of the tongue. The body becomes very thin. In severe cases, the nervous system is disturbed. Insanity and death may result.

Pellagra is mentioned in medical writings dating back to at least 1735. It was described more than two hundred years ago by a court physician of Spain's King Phillip V named Don Gasper Casal. The Italian scientist Jujati wrote about the same disease in 1740. It was named by another Italian scientist, Frapoli, in 1771. In Italian, *pelle agra* means "rough skin." The disease was prevalent in many parts of Europe for 200 years. Pellagra developed in the United States around the time of the Civil War. It reached serious proportions in the South during the early 1900s.

In 1915, Dr. Joseph Goldberger of the United States Public Health Service was confronted with an epidemic of pellagra in the southern states. Over 10,000 Americans had died. After searching for two long years for the "germ" that caused pellagra, Goldberger had become convinced that the disease was *not* caused by a germ. In his investigations, Dr. Goldberger learned that at several southern hospitals many of the patients had the disease, but the doctors, nurses, and other hospital workers who handled the pellagra victims—and even slept in the wards with them—remained healthy! It seemed unlikely that the disease could be contagious. Then Dr. Goldberger made a valuable discovery. The staffs at the hospitals did not eat the same foods as the patients. In many cases, they ate a far richer and more varied diet.

Dr. Goldberger became convinced that a faulty diet was the cause of pellagra. He was able to wipe out the disease in a Mississippi orphanage by adding milk, meat, and eggs to the children's diets of corn pone, salt pork, hominy, and molasses.

© 1986 by The Center for Applied Research in Education, Inc.

---

*Courtesy, *The Great Vitamin Mystery.* Martin, M. National Dairy Council, Rosemont, IL 1968.

Dr. Goldberger then went to the governor of Mississippi to obtain permission to conduct an experiment on one of the state's prison farms. Twelve convicts volunteered to participate in the experiment in return for a promise of freedom from the governor if they survived!

Dr. Goldberger fed his subjects an experimental diet of cornmeal and grits, cornstarch, white flour, sweet potatoes, cane syrup and sugar, pork fat, and small amounts of greens, collards, and cabbage. These were the foods on which many poor southerners lived. After six months, six of the twelve had symptoms of pellagra. No one else on the prison farm did. These twelve men had taken quite a gamble to win their freedom and to advance medical science. Their names have been forgotten, but their deed is remembered.

In 1937, Dr. Conrad Elvehjem and associates at the University of Wisconsin demonstrated the effectiveness of *nicotinic acid* (niacin) in treating pellagra. Just thirty milligrams of the pure nicotinic acid cured a pellagra-stricken dog. Shortly thereafter, niacin was shown to be effective in curing pellagra in humans.

A question continued to perplex the scientests. It was discovered that milk did not contain much niacin, yet infants who lived on milk never got pellagra. Why was this, they wondered? Then it was discovered that people of all ages can manufacture their own niacin if their diets contain tryptophan, an amino acid that is abundant in animal protein such as that found in milk, poultry, and eggs.

Pellagra has not been wiped out completely. There are still some cases in the South, especially in the summer months, and most often among poor people. The disease is also found among people whose food intake is restricted or whose bodies fail to absorb or utilize nutrients. It is often associated with diseases such as alcoholism and certain liver disorders. There are also cases in other parts of the world where corn is the staple cereal, and the people are not able to get enough niacin in their diets.

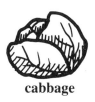
cabbage

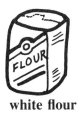
white flour

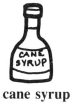
cane syrup

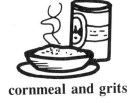
cornmeal and grits

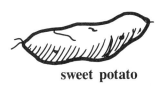
sweet potato

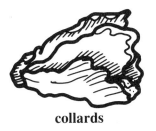
collards

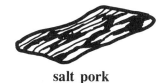
salt pork

THE CASE OF THE WOBBLING HENS*

How do you measure a hero? By the size or strength or age of the person? Perhaps you would agree that someone who saves the life of another is a hero. Suppose that someone saved not one life but thousands? That person would surely be classified as a hero! Christian Eijkman was just such a hero. So was Dr. K. Takaki, a high-ranking medical officer in the Japanese navy.

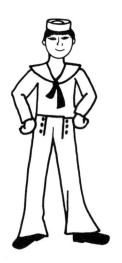

During the 1880s, the Japanese navy was attacked by a ruthless enemy. Silent and unseen, the killer slipped aboard ship and left its victims paralyzed and dying. This menace was no stranger to the peoples of Asia. For years this killer had been known by the name *beriberi*.

Beriberi is a serious disease of the nervous system, which was known in the Orient as early as 2600 B.C. The word "beriberi" means "I cannot." Victims of the disease cannot move easily and feet and legs become paralyzed. Leg and arm muscles wither and there may be swelling of the legs. Often the heart becomes enlarged. Extreme cases result in death.

In the early 1880s, beriberi was running rampant among the Japanese sailors. The fleet was kept at a strength of five thousand men, yet every year between one thousand and two thousand sailors were afflicted with the disease. Dr. Takaki decided to wage war against the dread killer.

Louis Pasteur and Robert Koch had, at that time, just proven the germ theory of disease. Medical people around the world then blamed microbes (germs) for all diseases. Yet the Japanese ships were new and clean. Dr. Takaki made even greater efforts to improve the sanitation aboard the ships. But beriberi raged on and the toll was rising.

Several questions perplexed the doctor. Why was beriberi more common in Oriental cities than it was in the villages? Why did it never occur on British ships? Why was it found only among rice-eating people? Takaki began to suspect that something was lacking in the rice diet of his people. In 1882, he was given permission to conduct an experiment.

In this experiment, two ships were equipped for a nine-month voyage over the same route through the South Seas. There were 276 men aboard each ship. One ship was supplied with the traditional rice diet of a Japanese sailor—clean white rice that had gone through the milling process. Aboard the other ship, sailors were fed the same diet that the British navy supplied to its men. These sailors received less rice and more whole-grain barley. Milk, meat, and vegetables were added to their diet.

Aboard the ship with the Oriental rice diet, there were 169 cases of beriberi and 25 men died. On the other vessel, there only 14 cases of the disease. It was discovered that all 14 men had refused to eat the British diet. They had smuggled aboard the food to which they were accustomed—rice!

Takaki was placed in charge of the diet of the Japanese navy. He added wheat and bread, meat, fish, vegetables, and milk, and decreased the intake of rice. Dr. Takaki was convinced that beriberi was a nutritional disease, but others at that time preferred to hold to the germ theory.

*Courtesy, *The Great Vitamin Mystery.* Martin, M. National Dairy Council, Rosemont, IL, 1968.

© 1986 by The Center for Applied Research in Education, Inc.

About this time, a Dutch physician named Christian Eijkman was working in a prison hospital on the crowded island of Java in the East Indies. Dr. Eijkman was also interested in finding a cure for beriberi. One thing in particular puzzled him about the disease. Wherever civilized Dutch rule had extended its influence, the incidence of beriberi was high. Yet in the uncivilized native villages where sanitation conditions were poor, the disease did not appear. Influenced by the work of Pasteur and Koch and their germ theory, Eijkman searched for the beriberi "germ." In fact, he thought he had found such a germ! He injected the germ into the bloodstreams of several chickens. After a few days, the chickens began to walk with a wobble, just like beriberi victims. The doctor thought for a while that he had isolated the cause of the disease, but he hadn't yet.

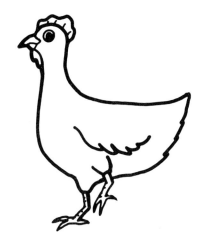

Soon Eijkman noticed that all of the chickens were wobbling when they walked, including those that had not received the injection. And then the chickens began to recover with no help from him, while the doctor's human patients continued to die. It was then that he made a vital discovery. A change had recently been ordered in the diet of the chickens. They had been switched from polished white rice to the cheaper brown, unmilled variety. This change in diet seemed to have brought about their recovery.

Thrilled with his disocvery, Dr. Eijkman set up an experiment. He fed white rice to one group of chickens and brown rice to another group. The chickens living on the milled white rice contracted beriberi. Those living on the unhusked brown rice remained healthy. When the ailing chickens were returned to a diet of brown rice, they were cured almost overnight. Dr. Eijkman had produced a vitamin deficiency disease in an animal and demonstrated its cure!

Dr. Eijkman wrote a report of his findings, but communications being poor, some time elapsed before his discovery was generally known. Several years later, members of the U.S. Army Medical Corps had still not read his report. As a result, a group of Americans unwittingly caused hundreds of deaths in the Philippines. Assigned to a prison hospital, they replaced the "dirty" brown rice with white polished rice. Shortly thereafter, the number of beriberi patients in the hospital rose sharply. After a few months there were even more cases and many people died. Then, one of the American doctors read Eijkman's report and the patients were returned to a diet of brown rice. Immediately the incidence of new beriberi cases dwindled. Clearly there was something in the brown husk of the rice kernel that prevented beriberi.

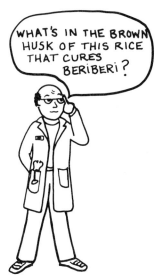

It was a Polish scientist, Casimir Funk, who named this mysterious substance. Working at the Lister Institute in London in 1911, he sifted through hundreds of pounds of rice outer coatings. Removing impurities, he ended up with about six ounces of white powder. A tiny portion of this powder could cure a pigeon suffering from beriberi. He called this substance a "vitamine"—a chemical substance vital to life. Funk had discovered an impure form of Vitamin B_1. The word "vitamine" was changed to "vitamin." Known for some time as Vitamin B, the antiberiberi substance was renamed Vitamin B_1 when it was discovered that there were other vitamins in the B family. Today Vitamin B_1 is known as thiamin.

Thiamin is very important in human diets. The best source of thiamin is pork. Other important sources of thiamin are other meats, fish, poultry and eggs, enriched or whole-grain bread or cereals, dried legumes such as peas and beans, potatoes, broccoli, and collards.

B VITAMINS WORKSHEET

To check your own intake of B vitamins, you first need to know what your RDAs are. Find your RDAs for thiamin, riboflavin, and niacin in this table:

	Children ages 7–10	Boys ages 11–14	Girls ages 11–14
Thiamin	1.2 mg.	1.4 mg.	1.1 mg.
Riboflavin	1.4 mg.	1.6 mg.	1.3 mg.
Niacin	16.0 mg.	18.0 mg.	15.0 mg.

Any food that has a value of at least one-fifth of your RDA for that nutrient can be considered as "rich" in that nutrient. First divide each of your RDAs by 5. List your values for "rich" sources of each B vitamin:

thiamin: _____   riboflavin: _____   niacin: _____

Now circle all of the values in Table 5-1, "Mini Composition Table," that indicate the foods that are rich in any of the three B vitamins.

Usually these three nutrients are considered together as the "B vitamins" or as part of the "Vitamin B Complex." Do any of the foods that you have circled have all three values?

YES   NO

You have just identified a problem. In the Iron CaPAC nutrients, you could find single common foods that had large amounts of one or two nutrients. Several foods were found to be rich sources of all three nutrients. But the B vitamins are harder to find in large quantities. Therefore, we have to rely almost totally on *combinations* of foods to supply our RDAs of the B vitamins. To see how combining foods works in supplying the RDAs, do these examples:

Example 1: Write the number of milligrams for each nutrient in oatmeal. Since you seldom eat oatmeal by itself, write the values for the nutrients in milk, too. Then add them together. What happens to the values when combined?

	Thiamin	Riboflavin	Niacin
oatmeal	_____	_____	_____
milk	_____	_____	_____
Total	_____	_____	_____

Example 2: Write the number of milligrams of each nutrient found in each of the following foods: a hamburger, french fries, and catsup. After you have finished this, find the total amount of each nutrient that has been consumed.

	Thiamin	Riboflavin	Niacin
Hamburger patty	____	____	____
2 Slices white bread	____	____	____
1 Serving french fries	____	____	____
2 Packets catsup	____	____	____
Total	____	____	____

Example 3: Now add a glass of whole milk to the foods in Example 2, but take out the french fries.

	Thiamin	Riboflavin	Niacin
Hamburger patty	____	____	____
2 Slices white bread	____	____	____
2 Packets catsup	____	____	____
1 Cup whole milk	____	____	____
Total	____	____	____

Do any of these combinations in Example 1, 2, and 3 reach one-fifth (20 percent) of your RDAs in all three nutrients? ____

Which ones? _____

Table 5-1

MINI COMPOSITION TABLE

Food and Serving Size	Weight g.	Thiamin mg.	Riboflavin mg.	Niacin mg.
Beans, navy, cooked—1 cup	190	.26	.14	1.4
Beef pot pie—4¼″ diameter	227	.25	.27	4.5
Bologna—1 slice, 1 ounce	28	.05	.06	.7
Bread, enriched:				
cracked-wheat—1 slice	25	.03	.02	.8
rye (light)—1 slice	25	.04	.02	.7
white—1 slice	28	.06	.05	.6
whole-wheat—1 slice	28	.06	.03	.6
Broccoli, cooked—½ cup	78	.07	.15	.6
Cantaloupe—¼, 5″ diameter	133	.05	.04	.8
Carrot, raw—1 medium	81	.05	.04	.5
Cheese, American—1 slice, 1 ounce	28	.01	.12	T
Chicken—½ breast	98	.07	.12	12.5
Chicken livers, chopped—1 cup	140	.20	2.44	6.2
Chicken pot pie—1 average	302	.34	.30	11.8
Chili con carne, with beans—1 cup	230	.07	.16	3.0
Cupcake, yellow with chocolate icing—1 average	46	.04	.05	.3
Doughnut, cake, plain—1	42	.07	.07	.5
Egg, plain—1	51	.05	.15	T
Hamburger, no roll—1	85	.08	.18	4.6
Ice cream, regular—⅔ cup	89	.03	.21	.1
Lamb chop—2½ ounce	71	.09	.16	3.5
Liver, beef—3 ounce	85	.22	3.56	14.0
Macaroni, cooked—½ cup	70	.10	.60	.8
Macaroni and cheese, prepared from mix—¾ cup	156	.27	.20	2.0
Milk:				
chocolate, 2% butterfat—8 ounce	250	.07	.40	.3
skim—8 ounce	245	.07	.34	.2
whole—8 ounce	244	.07	.39	.2
Oatmeal, cooked—½ cup	123	.10	.02	.1
Ocean perch, breaded, fried—2½ ounce	70	.07	.08	1.3
Oysters, raw—6	90	.12	.18	2.4
Papaya—¼ average	114	.02	.02	.2
Peanut butter—1 tbsp.	15	.02	.02	2.4
Peas, cooked—½ cup	80	.22	.09	1.8
Pepper, green, raw—1	164	.13	.13	.8
Pizza with cheese—⅐ of 10″ diameter	57	.10	.14	1.1
Pork chop—3 ounce	85	.96	.28	5.8
Potato:				
baked—1	156	.16	.06	2.6
chips—14	28	.06	.02	1.3
french fried—½ cup	55	.07	.04	1.7
Shrimp, cooked—½ cup	55	.01	.02	1.0
Strawberries, whole—½ cup	75	.02	.05	.4
Stuffed pepper, beef—1 average	185	.20	.33	3.6
Sweet potato, baked—1	146	.13	.10	1.0
Tomato catsup—1 tbsp.	15	.01	.01	.2
Tuna, canned—½ cup	80	.04	.10	9.5
Yogurt:				
skim milk—1 cup	227	.09	.52	.3
whole milk—1 cup	227	.05	.32	.2

QUIZ
THE THREE Bs: MEETING YOUR RDAs

_____ 1. What is thiamin?
   a. A mineral
   b. A C vitamin
   c. Vitamin B_1
   d. Vitamin A

_____ 2. What is pellagra?
   a. An illness caused by too much thiamin
   b. Vitamin B_3
   c. An illness caused by a deficiency of niacin
   d. Beriberi

_____ 3. Riboflavin and niacin are:
   a. Minerals
   b. B vitamins
   c. The same
   d. Not needed by the body

_____ 4. A major function of thimain, riboflavin, and niacin is:
   a. To prevent colds
   b. To cure arthritis
   c. To help our bodies release energy from food
   d. To become part of the bones and teeth

_____ 5. In which way is each of the B vitamins obtained most easily?
   a. You can eat anything you like, because all foods contain adequate amounts.
   b. Your total RDAs may be obtained from eating lots of certain foods.
   c. You should eat combinations of foods to get your total RDAs.
   d. Food does not contain these nutrients, so you should get them from your doctor.

_____ 6. A nutritious food:
   a. Is expensive
   b. Includes a food from one of the four food groups
   c. Includes lots of breads and cereal
   d. Is rich in two or more Iron CaPAC and B vitamin nutrients

_____ 7. Which food is a good source of thimain, riboflavin, and niacin?
   a. Liver
   b. Spinach
   c. Oranges
   d. Cheese

_____ 8. Which food is a good source of at least two of the B vitamins?
   a. Broccoli
   b. Macaroni and cheese
   c. Pork chop
   d. Chocolate milk shake

_____ 9. What is beriberi?
   a. An illness caused by a deficiency of thiamin
   b. Pellagra
   c. An illness caused by too much niacin
   d. Vitamin B_6

_____ 10. Knowing all that you do about the food sources of thiamin, riboflavin, and niacin, which choice would probably give you the most of all three of these nutrients?
   a. A chicken pot pie with a glass of milk
   b. An order of french fries
   c. A slice of cantaloupe with a scoop of ice cream
   d. A serving of macaroni and cheese

Unit 6: Your RDA for Energy

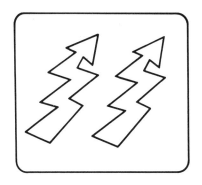

CONCEPTS

–The RDAs for energy (calories) do not have a *safety factor* added to them. They do not meet the needs of people who are quite physically active.

–People of different age/sex groups have different energy needs.

OBJECTIVES

–Students will be able to explain.

1. How the RDAs for energy differ from the RDAs for vitamins and mineral nutrients

2. How and why the RDAs for energy vary according to age and sex

TEACHER'S UNIT INTRODUCTION

Unlike the RDAs for protein, vitamins, and minerals, the RDAs for energy do not have a *margin of safety.* This means they are *not* set high enough to cover the energy needs of practically all healthy people in the United States. Individuals require different amounts of energy, which are largely based on their level of physical activity. Daily physical activity levels can range from sedentary to very active. The average person in the United States is considered to be *lightly active,* that is, engaged in light work or activity. The energy RDA for each age/sex group is set at the *average* need. If the energy RDA were set high enough to cover practically all healthy people, many would gain weight. Sample activities in four activity categories are as follows:

1. Sedentary
most seated activities (*examples:* office work, sewing, reading, driving, watching TV)
standing activities requiring little movement (*examples:* laboratory work, painting, lecturing in classroom)

2. Light
walking on level ground at an average pace
shop work (*examples:* mechanics, cabinet making)
restaurant work
light gardening
light housework (*examples:* sweeping, washing dishes and clothes)
mowing the lawn

3. Moderate
walking on level ground at a fairly fast pace
recreational cycling and swimming
shoveling snow
jogging
recreational canoeing and rowing

4. Heavy
walking extremely fast or uphill with a load
climbing steps or hills
cross-country skiing
running
handball
ditch digging
vigorous competition in sports (*examples:* basketball, swimming, football, cycling)

73

Take a moment to look at the energy RDAs for the various age/sex groups in Chart F, "Height/ Weight and Recommended Energy Intake." Quite astonishingly, you will discover that the RDA for the seven- to ten-year-old child is as high as that for a fifty-one- to seventy-five-year-old man and is higher than the RDAs for any of the female age groups (excluding pregnant and lactating women). You will also discover that the states of pregnancy and breast-feeding increase calorie needs. Thus, individuals who are in a state of growth have high calorie needs.

Another observation you can make from the energy RDAs is that males need more calories than females. This is because men are usually larger and have a greater amount of muscle than females. The greater the amount of muscle, the greater the number of calories required. Also, notice that when an individual is fully grown, his or her energy needs decrease with age. As adults grow older, their bodily processes slow down and they generally become less active.

In summary then, several factors that will influence energy needs are

1. Growth

2. Body size

3. Amount of muscle

4. Physical activity

In order to calculate nutrient densities (introduced in subsequent units) and to determine if a food can qualify as being nutrient-dense, a knowledge of individual energy (calorie) needs and the RDAs for energy are important. This unit will present information on factors influencing energy needs and the varying energy RDA values for the different age/sex groups. This unit assumes that students have a basic understanding of how the body uses energy and how energy is measured in calories.

This unit is also aimed at identifying some of the benefits of physical activity. It would be good to emphasize its role in weight control. Therefore, point out to students that the abundance of food in America oftentimes results in people eating more calories than they need. Regular exercise will help us to use up some of these unneeded calories and will help to keep us at a desirable weight.

When presenting the introductory information, it may be helpful to provide students with Chart A, "Recommended Dietary Allowances," and to write the activity categories on the board.

BASIC ACTIVITY

Time Needed: One class period

Materials Needed: Sheet 6-1: "Making Energy Recommendations"
Table 6-1: "Daily Recommended Energy Intakes for Persons of Different Ages"
Quiz Sheet 6-1

1. As a means of introducing the activity in Sheet 6-1, have students brainstorm factors that they believe influence how much energy (calories) an individual needs. If necessary, review the concept that energy is measured in calories. The brainstorming session should bring students to conclude that growth, body size, muscle mass, and physical activity all influence energy needs.

2. Ask students if they think energy RDAs might be different for people of different ages. Would energy RDAs be different for males and females?

3. List responses to Question 2 without judging them as correct or incorrect. To find the correct answers to these questions, have students complete Sheet 6-1, "Making Energy Recommendations," using Table 6-1, "Daily Recommended Energy Intakes for Persons of Different Ages."

4. Ask students to recall how the RDAs for the Iron CaPAC nutrients were set and postulate what might be the outcome of setting the RDAs for calories in the same way. Students should conclude that if the RDA were set high enough to meet the energy needs of practically all people within any RDA group, the average person would become fat.

5. Explain to students that the RDA for energy is set for the average individual. By *average* we mean a person who is of an average size and who gets an average amount of activity. Referring back to Unit 3, "RDA Doorway to Good Health," emphasize that the doorway for calories would be shorter than the one for nutrients and that, therefore, most people in the classroom would "bump their heads" while going through the calorie doorway. Students who are tall for their age would be likely to need more calories than the RDA for their age/sex group. Similarly, students who are very physically active would be likely to need more calories than the RDA for their respective age/sex group.

6. To further develop this concept, have students decide which of the following individuals would need more, less, or about the same amount, of calories as specified for his or her RDA. Conduct this activity in the form of a group discussion, and have students give justifications for their responses.

   a. A forty-year-old mail carrier of average weight and height who walks an all-day route. (*Answer:* More, because the average person is not as active as this, that is, the average adult male spends a good deal of his day sitting down or standing fairly still.)

   b. A twelve-year-old girl of average height and weight who walks to and from school each day (a trip of about two miles). After school, she helps with a few household chores and plays sports with friends outside. She does homework and watches a little television in the evening. (*Answer:* About the same, because this girl gets an average amount of activity every day.)

   c. A nine-year-old boy who is as tall as the average eleven or twelve year old and who gets an average amount of activity. (*Answer:* More, because he is bigger than the average person in his RDA age group.)

   d. A sixteen-year-old girl of average height and weight who is on the swim team and who practices swimming for two hours every day. (*Answer:* More, because swimming practice is a vigorous activity and the average girl does not get this much daily activity.)

   e. A twelve-year-old boy of average height and weight who gets little exercise at school and who reads or watches TV most of the time he is not in school. (*Answer:* Less, because the average twelve-year-old boy is more active than this. Have the class cite sample ways in which boys and girls can be more active than the average.)

7. If time permits, have the students make up their own descriptions of situations relating to energy needs and discuss them as a group.

8. **Evaluation:** Distribute Quiz Sheet 6-1 and have students complete it independently. Discuss the answers as a class.

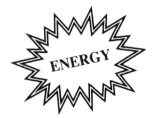

MAKING ENERGY RECOMMENDATIONS

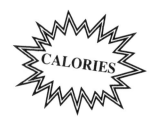

Directions: *Examine* Table 6-1, "Daily Recommended Energy Intakes for Persons of Different Ages," then answer these questions:

1. How many calories are recommended for a normal, healthy four-year-old child?

2. Looking farther down the chart, how many calories are recommended for a sixteen-year-old boy?

3. How many calories are recommended for a sixteen-year-old girl?

4. How many calories are recommended for a forty-five-year-old man?

5. How many calories should a forty-five-year-old woman have each day?

6. Are energy recommendations the same for men and women aged forty-five? _____ If not, what is the difference?

_____

7. What happens to energy recommendations after age fifty-one compared to ages twenty-three to fifty in both sexes?

_____

8. From Table 6-1, write two variables that affect energy recommendations:

  a. _____ b. _____

9. A seven-year-old child and a man over fifty-one have the same energy recommendations. How many calories are recommended?

10. Why is it recommended that a seven-year-old child have as many calories as a full-grown man who is certainly much

  taller and heavier? _____

_____

11. If you sat all day, would you need as many calories as the RDA amount? _____

  Why? _____

12. Would a construction worker who worked all day actively building need more calories than the RDA

  amount? _____ Why? _____

Table 6-1

DAILY RECOMMENDED ENERGY INTAKES
FOR PERSONS OF DIFFERENT AGES*

| | Age | Weight | | Height | | Energy |
	years	kg	lbs	cm	in	calories
Children						
	4–6	20	44	112	44	1,700
	7–10	28	62	132	52	2,400
Adolescents and Young Adults						
boys	11–14	45	99	157	62	2,700
	15–18	66	145	175	69	2,800
	19–22	70	154	177	70	2,900
girls	11–14	46	101	157	62	2,200
	15–18	55	120	163	64	2,100
	19–22	55	120	163	64	2,100
Adults						
men	23–50	70	154	178	70	2,700
	51–75	70	154	178	70	2,400
	76+	70	154	178	70	2,050
women	23–50	55	120	163	64	2,000
	51–75	55	120	163	64	1,800
	76+	55	120	163	64	1,600

*Adapted from *Recommended Dietary Allowances*, 1980. Washington, DC: National Academy Press, with permission.

QUIZ
YOUR RDA FOR ENERGY

_____ 1. How are the RDAs for calories different from the RDAs for protein, vitamins, and minerals?
    a. The RDAs for calories meet the needs of both healthy and unhealthy people
    b. The RDAs for calories are large enough to meet practically everyone's needs
    c. The RDAs for calories do not meet the needs of practically all healthy people
    d. For all people, there is just one RDA for calories

_____ 2. Which of the following boys would probably need more calories than the amount listed on an RDA chart?
    a. A boy who is smaller than other boys his age
    b. An active boy who is bigger than other boys his age
    c. A boy of average size for his age who exercises a little each day
    d. A boy who doesn't eat much

_____ 3. Why is the RDA for calories for a sixteen-year-old boy larger than for a fifty-five-year-old man?
    a. Sixteen-year-old boys are usually bigger than older men
    b. Sixteen-year-old boys eat more than adult men
    c. Older men usually get as much exercise as sixteen-year-old boys
    d. Sixteen-year-old boys are still growing but adult men are not

_____ 4. Why would an average teenage girl usually require less calories than an average adult man?
    a. Teenage girls get very little exercise
    b. Adult men have less muscle
    c. Adult men are bigger and have more muscle
    d. Teenage girls are more active than adult men

_____ 5. For each pair of individuals, place an "X" next to the one who requires more calories.
    a. _____ An average-size four-year-old girl
        _____ A large four-year-old boy
    b. _____ An eighteen-year-old boy who plays varsity basketball
        _____ An eighteen-year-old boy who plays chess
    c. _____ A girl who watches TV after school
        _____ A girl who takes a walk after school
    d. _____ A female wrestler
        _____ A male wrestler

Unit 7: RDA in the U.S.A.

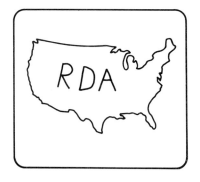

CONCEPT

–The U.S. RDA for each nutrient is usually the largest RDA found in all age/sex groups.

OBJECTIVE

–Students will be able to differentiate between the RDA and the U.S. RDA.

TEACHER'S UNIT INTRODUCTION

Strictly speaking, the U.S. Recommended Daily Allowances (U.S. RDAs) are amounts of proteins, vitamins, and minerals that are used as standards in nutrition labeling. They have replaced the Minimum Daily Requirement (MDR). The main purpose of this unit is to introduce the U.S. RDA.

The allowances for the U.S. RDA are based on the 1968 edition of the *Recommended Dietary Allowances* (RDA). The Food and Drug Administration of the United States government set up the U.S. RDAs in 1973. The U.S. RDAs were set up because new laws required food processors to provide information on the food label. The *U.S. RDA*, for most nutrients, is the highest RDA for all age/sex categories, excluding pregnant and breast-feeding women. In most cases, this is the RDA for fifteen- to eighteen-year-old males. The U.S. RDAs for calcium and phosphorus are set at one gram each because of their bulk, solubility, and the wide variability in age-based requirements. Remember that the RDAs include a safety factor (see Unit 3, "RDA Doorway to Good Health"), making them adequate for almost all healthy persons and more than adequate for most people. Consequently, a diet furnishing 100 percent of the U.S. RDA of a nutrient will also furnish the RDA of that nutrient for most people and more than the RDA for many people.

The U.S. RDAs are as follows:

Protein	45 g. or 65 g. (45 grams is the value used for foods containing high-quality protein. Usually this means protein of animal origin—for example, meat, fish, poultry, eggs, and milk products. The value used for foods of plant origin—that is, vegetables, legumes, nuts, seeds, breads, and cereals—is 65 grams.)
Vitamin A	5000 International Units (IUs)
Vitamin C	60 mg.
Thiamin	1.5 mg.
Riboflavin	1.7 mg.
Niacin	20 mg.
Calcium	1000 mg.
Iron	18 mg.

The U.S. RDAs list nutrient allowances for three other age categories. These, however, are for use with special groups of people. These groups are divided as follows:

1. infants (birth to 11 months)

2. children (one to four years)

3. pregnant and breast-feeding women

Allowances given for infants and children are used in the labeling of baby and junior foods. Most nutrient labels list the nutrient allowance for groups four years through adulthood. This category is the only group that will be presented in this unit in order to avoid confusion.

BASIC ACTIVITY

Time Needed: One class period

Materials Needed: Table 7-1: "The RDAs For Eight Nutrients"
Quiz Sheet 7-1

1. Write the words "United States Recommended Daily Allowance (U.S. RDA)" on the board. Ask students where they have seen this term before and what they think might be the difference between the *RDA* and the *U.S. RDA*. List responses on the board.

2. Distribute Table 7-1, "The RDAs for Eight Nutrients." To determine accurate answers to what the *U.S. RDA* is and to how it differs from the *RDA,* use the table to point out and discuss the following observations:

a. There is a U.S. RDA for each of the eight nutrients shown. Although there is an RDA for energy, there is no U.S. RDA for energy.

b. The U.S. RDAs can be used by all of the age/sex groups shown. How many groups are there? (*Answer:* twelve)

c. The U.S. RDA is used by all twelve groups. Do you suppose there is a separate U.S. RDA for each group or do they all share the same one? (*Answer:* They all share the same one.)

d. The U.S. RDA for each nutrient is usually the highest RDA found for all age/sex groups. (To illustrate this, students should find the highest value for the first five nutrients and enclose each one in a box. They should then connect the boxes with lines. Record students' findings on the board and label them the "U.S. RDA.")

e. An apple supplies six milligrams of Vitamin C. If you ate an apple, what percent of the U.S. RDA for Vitamin C would the apple give you? (*Answer:* $60 \div 6 = 10\%$). If your father ate this apple instead of you, what percent of the U.S. RDA for Vitamin C would he get? (*Answer:* the same) Why? (*Answer:* Because all of the age/sex groups shown on the worksheet have the same U.S. RDA.) For students having trouble comprehending the U.S. RDA concept, you may want to run through several other example problems. Select foods from the Energy and Iron CaPAC Food Composition Table used in Unit 4.

3. **Evaluation:** Distribute Quiz Sheet 7-1 and have students complete it independently. Discuss the answers as a class.

THE RDAs FOR EIGHT NUTRIENTS*

	Vitamin C (mg.)	Iron (mg.)	Thiamin (mg.)	Riboflavin (mg.)	Niacin (mg.)	Calcium (mg.)	Vitamin A (IU)	Protein (g.)
Children								
4–6 yrs	45	10	0.9	1.0	11	800	500	30
7–10 yrs.	45	10	1.2	1.4	16	800	700	34
Males								
11–14 yrs.	50	18	1.4	1.6	18	1,200	1,000	45
15–18 yrs.	60	18	1.4	1.7	18	1,200	1,000	56
19–22 yrs.	60	10	1.5	1.7	19	800	1,000	56
23–50 yrs.	60	10	1.4	1.6	18	800	1,000	56
51+ yrs.	60	10	1.2	1.4	16	800	1,000	56
Females								
11–14 yrs.	50	18	1.1	1.3	15	1,200	800	46
15–18 yrs.	60	18	1.1	1.3	14	1,200	800	46
19–22 yrs.	60	18	1.1	1.3	14	800	800	44
23–50 yrs.	60	18	1.0	1.2	13	800	800	44
51+ yrs.	60	10	1.0	1.2	13	800	800	44

*Adapted from *Recommended Dietary Allowances*, 1980. Washington, DC: National Academy Press, with permission.

QUIZ
RDA IN THE U.S.A.

_____ 1. The U.S. RDA is different from the RDA in what way?
  a. There is not a separate U.S. RDA value for each age/sex group.
  b. The U.S. RDAs do not list a value for iron and niacin.
  c. Each age/sex group has a separate U.S. RDA.
  d. The U.S. RDA does not deal with nutrients.

_____ 2. An orange is rich in Vitamin C. If your father and you both eat the same-sized orange, who will get more of the U.S. RDA for Vitamin C?
  a. You
  b. Your father
  c. Neither of you will get any
  d. Both of you will get the same

_____ 3. When you look at an RDA chart, you notice that the RDAs for thiamin are different. For children, the RDA is .9 milligrams (mg.); for teenage girls, it is 1.1 mg.; and for teenage boys, 1.4 mg. Which RDA is the most likely to be chosen for the U.S. RDA?
  a. The child's
  b. The teenage girl's
  c. The teenage boy's
  d. None of the above

Given the following information, solve problems 4 through 6.

RDA Table	Vitamin C (mg.)	Iron (mg.)
Children		
4–6 yrs.	45	10
7–10 yrs.	45	10
Males		
11–14 yrs.	50	18
15–18 yrs.	60	18
Females		
11–14 yrs.	50	18
15–18 yrs.	60	18

_____ 4. What is the *U.S. RDA* for iron?
  a. 10 mg.
  b. 18 mg.
  c. 60 mg.
  d. 100 mg.

_____ 5. Jason is 14 years old. He has just finished eating a watermelon wedge which has 30 mg. of Vitamin C. What percent of the *U.S. RDA* for Vitamin C did he meet by eating the watermelon? (Show your work.)
  a. 33 percent
  b. 50 percent
  c. 60 percent
  d. 66 percent

_____ 6. Sarah is 9 years old. She had some raisins containing 1 mg. of iron. What percent of *her* RDA did she meet by eating the raisins?
  a. .5 percent
  b. 5.5 percent
  c. 10 percent
  d. 12 percent

Unit 8: Identifying Nutrient-Rich Foods

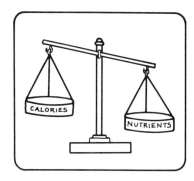

CONCEPT

–A food is said to be a rich source of a nutrient if each serving provides 20 percent or more of the U.S. RDA for that nutrient.

OBJECTIVE

–Using the U.S. RDA as a standard, students will be able to identify foods that are rich sources of each of the Iron CaPAC nutrients and of thiamin, riboflavin, and niacin as well.

TEACHER'S UNIT INTRODUCTION

In Unit 5, "The Three Bs: Meeting Your RDAs," you learned one method for identifying *rich food sources* of a given nutrient. A rich food source was defined as a food that supplies one-fifth of the individual's RDA for a given nutrient in one serving. A rich food source of a given nutrient can also be identified using the U.S. RDA. Any food in which one serving supplies 20 percent or more of the U.S. RDA for a nutrient is considered a rich source of that nutrient. This unit will help you practice identifying rich food sources of nutrients using the U.S. RDA. This unit also introduces you to Chart D, "Food Composition Table for Selected Nutrients." You will also be using Chart D in Unit 9.

Step four in the Basic Activity section asks students to recall and analyze a lunch they have consumed. It is best to do this activity in the afternoon, since students are more likely to be able to accurately recall a lunch they have just eaten than one consumed on the previous day. Additionally, you may wish to cue students in advance that they will be doing an activity in the afternoon that will require them to remember both the foods and amounts they will be eating for lunch that day. While not essential, you may also wish to have on hand a more comprehensive food composition table than the one provided in Chart D. Occasionally, a student will consume a food not listed in Chart D. Sources for additional comprehensive food tables are listed in the References/ Resources section located at the end of this kit.

BASIC ACTIVITY

Time Needed: Two class periods

Materials Needed: Chart D: "Food Composition Table for Selected Nutrients"
Sheet 8-1: "Food Recall Chart"
Quiz Sheet 8-1

Class Period 1

1. Briefly review with students the quantifiable method they used in Unit 5, "The Three Bs: Meeting Your RDAs," to identify rich food sources of thiamin, riboflavin, and niacin. Announce that rich food sources can also be identified using the U.S. RDAs. Any serving of food that supplies 20 percent (one-fifth) or more of the U.S. RDA for a given nutrient is a rich food source for that nutrient.

2. Distribute Chart D, "Food Composition Table for Selected Nutrients." Ask students why the table says "selected nutrients." Students should respond that there are many nutrients our bodies need in addition to the eight listed. However, these eight are the ones scientists know the most about in terms of how much we need. It is also believed that if we meet our RDAs for these eight nutrients, we will also be getting the correct amount of the other nutrients. An exception to this rule occurs when the diet is composed mainly of refined or fabricated foods that have been fortified.

3. Describe how to use the table to find rich food sources of selected nutrients. Students should practice using the table by identifying one or more rich food source for each of the eight selected nutrients. Discuss students' findings and list on the board two or three rich foods sources for each nutrient. Specify the amount of food and the percent of the U.S. RDA supplied for each food listed.

4. To illustrate the applicability of this unit's information to each student's diet, have each student recall and record that day's lunch and use Chart D to determine how many rich food sources he or she has consumed at the meal. This portion of the activity should be conducted as follows:

   a. Distribute Sheet 8-1, "Food Recall Chart," and run through with students the process of recording a simple lunch. Emphasize the importance of writing down:

   - All foods and beverages consumed
   - The amounts of each (that is, cup, tablespoon, slice)
   - The way in which the food was prepared (that is, raw, boiled, baked, fried)
   - Any food that they added to the food (that is, margarine, sugar)

   b. Students should look up in Chart D each food or beverage they have consumed and should record the percent of the U.S. RDA supplied for each selected nutrient. Alert students that they may have to divide or multiply in order to arrive at the correct figures if they have consumed an amount of food different from that specified in the table. You may wish to run through sample conversions with them. Also, if a student cannot find a food he or she has consumed, he or she may consult a more comprehensive table or may substitute a food from the table that is most similar to the one consumed.

   c. Students should also total each nutrient column to derive a total percent consumed for each selected nutrient.

5. If necessary, have students complete Sheet 8-1 as a homework assignment or during a free class period.

Class Period 2

1. From the completed Sheet 8-1, take a poll to determine the number of students who have consumed a total of 20 percent or more of the U.S. RDA for one nutrient. Record the results on the board.

2. Repeat the poll to determine the number of students who have consumed a rich food source for each nutrient. Some foods on a student's Food Recall Chart may appear to qualify as rich in one or more selected nutrients because the student has consumed more than the amount listed in Chart D. If the amount of food specified in Chart D does not contain 20 percent or more of the nutrient, it *is not* a rich source of that nutrient.

3. You are likely to find that some students have consumed 20 percent or more of the U.S. RDA for one or more selected nutrients without having consumed a rich food source of that nutrient. Have one or more students falling into this category identify the foods that have made important (but not rich) contributions of selected nutrients. All students should locate the foods in the table and take note of the percent of the U.S. RDA that these foods have contributed.

4. Have students who have consumed "rich" sources identify these foods.

5. Conclude by saying that many foods can make an important contribution toward meeting the U.S. RDA for each selected nutrient. Significant contributions of a selected nutrient may be obtained by consuming

- a single "rich" food source

- a combination of foods that are not individually rich, but that do contribute the nutrient

6. Point out that foods which are and are not rich sources of selected nutrients provide varying amounts of calories; it is important not to consume excess calories in meeting our nutrient needs. The next unit will introduce a method to use in selecting foods that considers both the nutrient *and* the caloric values of foods.

7. **Evaluation:** Distribute Quiz Sheet 8-1 and have students complete it.

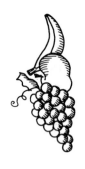
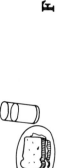

FOOD RECALL CHART

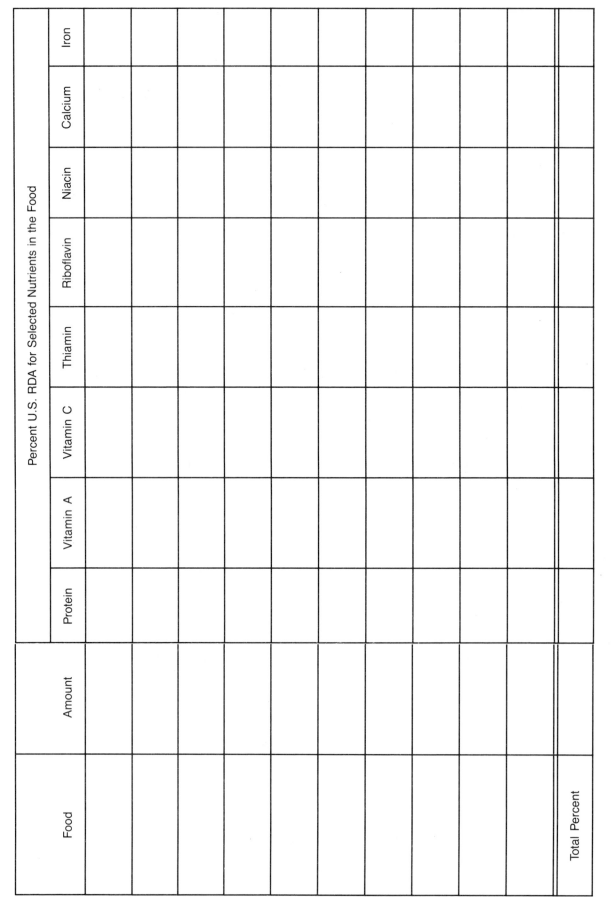

Percent U.S. RDA for Selected Nutrients in the Food

Food	Amount	Protein	Vitamin A	Vitamin C	Thiamin	Riboflavin	Niacin	Calcium	Iron
Total Percent									

QUIZ
IDENTIFYING NUTRIENT-RICH FOODS

_____ 1. A rich food source of a nutrient has to supply how much of the U.S. RDA per serving?
    a. Less than 20 percent, but more than 10 percent
    b. At least 25 percent
    c. 20 percent or more
    d. 30 percent

_____ 2. Susan has a choice of several vegetables that would contribute Vitamin A to her lunch:

    Two to three raw carrot strips, which supply 60 percent of the U.S. RDA
    Four cooked asparagus spears, which supply 10 percent of the U.S. RDA
    One baked sweet potato, which supplies 230 percent of the U.S. RDA
    One cup cooked broccoli, which supplies 80 percent of the U.S. RDA
Which of these vegetables would be considered a rich source of the vitamin?
    a. All of the foods
    b. Only the broccoli and the sweet potato
    c. Only the sweet potato
    d. All of the foods *except* the asparagus

_____ 3. Strawberries are a "rich" source of Vitamin C. The U.S. RDA for Vitamin C is 60 milligrams. In order to qualify as a "rich" source, one serving of strawberries must provide how much Vitamin C? Show your work.
    a. 3 milligrams   c. 12 milligrams
    b. 3 milligrams   d. 18 milligrams

    4. Using the Food Composition Table that follows, name at least one "rich" food source for each of the following nutrients:

a. Iron: _____   e. Vitamin C: _____

b. Calcium: _____   f. Thiamin: _____

c. Protein: _____   g. Riboflavin: _____

d. Vitamin A: _____   h. Niacin: _____

FOOD COMPOSITION TABLE

Percentages of U.S. RDA	Protein	Vitamin A	Vitamin C	Thiamin	Riboflavin	Niacin	Calcium	Iron
Asparagus—4 spears	2	10	25	6	6	4	2	2
Beans, dried—1 cup cooked	30	*	*	15	7.6	6	9	25
Bean sprouts—1 cup	6	*	15	8	8	4	2.1	6
Broccoli—1 cup	8	80	230	10	20	6	15	6
Celery—1 stalk	*	2.2	6	*	*	*	1.6	*
Chicken—3 ounce	45	2	*	2	10	40	*	8
Ice cream—1 cup	11	10.8	2	4	19.4	*	17.6	*
Peas—1 cup	15	15	60	30	10	20	4	15
Pizza with cheese— one-seventh of a pie	15	8	8	2	8	4	15	4
Pudding—1 cup	15	8.2	*	5.3	25	2	35	8

*None or less than 1 percent

Unit 9: Determining Nutrient Density in Food

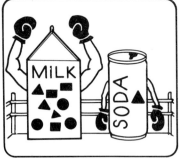

CONCEPTS

–For any given nutrient, the food with the highest nutrient density provides the greater amount of that nutrient, calorie per calorie.

–A food is classified as being *nutrient-dense* if it has nutrient densities for at least four nutrients equal to or greater than one.

–A food is also said to be *nutrient-dense* if it has nutrient densities for at least two nutrients equal to or greater than two.

OBJECTIVE

Using the data from the Food Composition Table for Selected Nutrients, students will be able to determine

1. The nutrient density of foods for specified nutrients
2. The best food sources of specified nutrients from a nutrient density standpoint

TEACHER'S UNIT INTRODUCTION

Up to this point, you have focused on the nutrient contributions of foods. A more complete method to use in determining the nutritional quality of a food is one that considers both its caloric and its nutrient contributions. This method enables you to determine the nutrient density of a food for any nutrient. The nutrient density of a food for a given nutrient is calculated by dividing the percent of the U.S. RDA of the nutrient by the percent of the daily calorie needs that a serving of the food provides:

$$\frac{\% \text{ U.S. RDA of nutrient supplied by the food}}{\% \text{ daily calorie needs supplied by the food}} = \text{nutrient density}$$

Remember that calorie needs vary according to age/sex group, and from individual to individual within each group. For purposes of this unit, one daily energy recommendation should be used in calculating the nutrient density. In this unit, we will use 2,500 calories. This is close to the RDA for energy of the average nine to fourteen year old.

Let's look at sample calculations of nutrient densities for two foods: green peas and peanut butter. Chart D, "Food Composition Table for Selected Nutrients," shows that one-half of a cup of fresh green peas (cooked) provides sixty calories and that a tablespoon of peanut butter provides ninety calories.

To calculate the percent of daily calories contributed by each food, perform the following calculations:

$$\frac{60 \text{ calories (in } \frac{1}{2} \text{ cup fresh cooked peas)}}{2{,}500 \text{ calories}} = .024 \times 100 = 2.4\%$$

$$\frac{90 \text{ calories (in one tablespoon peanut butter)}}{2{,}500 \text{ calories}} = .036 \times 100 = 3.6\%$$

These two figures—2.4 percent and 3.6 percent—are used in the denominators of the next set of calulations. We can look up the numerator (percent of U.S. RDA) for any of the eight nutrients given in Chart D and determine the nutrient density of the foods for each nutrient. Let's take protein, for example. The fresh cooked green peas supply 7 percent of the U.S. RDA and the peanut butter supplies 6 percent of the U.S. RDA. Therefore, the nutrient density for protein in green peas is greater than the nutrient density in the peanut butter—3 versus 2 respectively.

green peas		**peanut butter**	
$\dfrac{7\% \text{ U.S. RDA for Protein}}{2.4\% \text{ calorie needs}}$	$= 3$	$\dfrac{6\% \text{ U.S. RDA for Protein}}{3.6\% \text{ calorie needs}}$	$= 2$ (rounded)

If we continue with our calculations, we find that green peas have a higher nutrient density than peanut butter for all nutrients. We also find that, regardless of the serving size used, the nutrient densities will come out the same. Therefore, we do not need to specify serving size when stating the nutrient densities of a food.

The idea of nutrient density is important when planning diets in order to satisfy nutrient needs without exceeding calorie needs. If the nutrient density is less than 1 for a given nutrient, this tells us that the food is making a greater contribution toward energy needs than toward nutrient needs. Furthermore, if that particular food is the only dietary source of a given nutrient, you will have to exceed your calorie needs to satisfy the U.S. RDA for that nutrient.

A more complete way to look at this idea is to consider all of the foods in your daily diet. If your daily diet meets (without exceeding) your calorie needs, but contains only foods with a nutrient density of less than 1 for a given nutrient, the U.S. RDA for that nutrient will not be met on that day. Conversely, foods with a nutrient density greater than 1 for a given nutrient will make a greater contribution toward meeting the U.S. RDA for that nutrient than toward meeting daily calorie needs.

From a practical standpoint, diets that include a wide variety of foods have nutrient densities above, below, and approximately equal to 1. The important point to remember is that foods with higher nutrient densities give you more nutrients per calorie.

The nutrient density relationship can be portrayed through bar graphs. Bar graphs for cooked green peas and for peanut butter are included both within this unit and as a part of the Answer Key for this activity. The National Dairy Council publishes RDA Comparison Cards that give this same graphic representation for many foods. These comparison cards utilize the calorie value of 2,400 for children who are between seven and ten years old and for females who are from eleven to fourteen years old; they utilize the higher calorie value of 2,800 for males from eleven to fourteen years old.

In addition to Chart D, "Food Composition Table for Selected Nutrients," the calorie values and the percent of the U.S. RDA values can be found on food labels containing nutrition labeling information and on the National Dairy Council's food models. If you have a food for which no U.S. RDA percentages are available, you can determine the percentages, using a more comprehensive table of food composition (see the References/Resources section at the end of this kit) and the U.S. RDA values in Unit 7.

The concept of nutrient density is a relatively new idea. For the purposes of this unit, it is important to have students understand and remember the two criteria by which foods can be judged (see "Concepts").

The nutrient density approach offers advantages to the student. One benefit of this approach is that it is not necessary to take into account the serving sizes of various foods in order to judge the value of the foods. Using the equations presented in this kit, the student can quickly calculate the value of a food and compare it to a guideline.

Unfortunately, there are also some drawbacks to this approach. A few of the foods that we commonly think of us as "good" for us do not meet either of the criteria discussed at the beginning of this unit. Examples include apples, pears, raisins, and flounder. This does not mean that these foods are not nutritious. It simply means that when you consider the caloric contributions of foods, these foods do not make as significant a nutrient contribution to the daily diet as foods that meet one or both of these criteria. The nutrient density approach does not account for fiber, water, trace elements, or other substances that contribute to the value of food.

Up to this point, students have considered only the nutrient concentration of a food in determining how good a nutrient source a food may be. In fact, the last unit specified that a serving of food had to supply 20 percent or more of the U.S. RDA for a given nutrient in order to be considered a *rich* source of that nutrient. It is the purpose of this activity to teach students how to determine the nutrient density of foods and how to use this concept in choosing the food that provides, per calorie, the greatest amount of a given nutrient.

BASIC ACTIVITY

Time Needed: Two class periods

Materials Needed: Sheet 9-1: "U.S. RDA Bar Graph"
Chart D: "Food Composition Table for Selected Nutrients"
Quiz Sheets 9-1 through 9-2

Class Period 1

1. Challenge students with the following problem: *Suppose you have two or more foods and that a serving of each supplies the same amount of a certain nutrient. How can you determine which food will really be the "best" source of that nutrient?*

Use examples of a food in your challenge. For example, use a cup of whole milk, of skim milk, and of chocolate milk, each of which provides 20 percent of the U.S. RDA for protein. Accept responses until one student hints at the idea that the solution may involve considering the caloric value of the food. Place the caloric values of the foods you are considering on the board to illustrate that the food which supplies the least amount of calories would be the best source of the nutrient. This is true because you need to take in fewer calories to get the same amount of the nutrient. In other words, calorie per calorie, you get more of the nutrient. Further clarify this by converting the calorie figure into a percent of daily calorie needs supplied so that students can compare percents. The calculations for skim milk, whole milk, and chocolate milk are given here (rounded to the nearest whole percent):

Skim Milk $\quad \dfrac{85 \text{ calories/cup}}{2{,}500 \text{ calories}} = .034 \times 1000 = 3.4\% \ (3\%)$

Whole Milk $\quad \dfrac{160 \text{ calories/cup}}{2{,}500 \text{ calories}} = .064 \times 100 = 6.4\% \ (6\%)$

Chocolate Milk $\quad \dfrac{180 \text{ calories/cup}}{2{,}500 \text{ calories}} = .072 \times 100 = 7.2\% \ (7\%)$

Using Chart D, "Food Composition Table for Selected Nutrients," students should practice converting calorie values of foods into a percent of daily calorie needs supplied. For consistency, have all students use 2,500 as their daily calorie requirement.

2. On the board, write the U.S. RDA values for each nutrient (see Unit 7). Show students how the percent of calorie needs supplied and the percent of the U.S. RDA for a given nutrient can be graphed. Follow the format used in Sheet 9-1, "U.S. RDA Bar Graph." Work with those foods used in step 1.

Distribute two copies of Sheet 9-1, "U.S. RDA Bar Graph," to each student. Instruct students to prepare bar graphs for two different foods: a tablespoon of peanut butter and one-half of a cup of fresh green peas, cooked. Students should first calculate and graph the percent of daily calorie needs each food supplies. Next, the percent of the U.S. RDA for each of the eight nutrients specified should be graphed. Calorie and nutrient data can be found in Chart D, "Food Composition Table for Selected Nutrients." For each nutrient, students should determine which food gives the most nutrient value for the percent of calories supplied.

Note: Students should save their completed graphs for use in the "Advanced Activity."

4. Discuss student findings. Be sure to bring out the following points:

a. Rounded to the nearest percent, both foods supply similar amounts of daily calorie needs, that is, 4 percent and 2 percent respectively.

b. For the cooked peas, the percent of the U.S. RDA for each nutrient supplied is equal to, or greater than, the percent of daily calorie needs supplied.

c. The green peas are superior to peanut butter for each nutrient. From a calorie standpoint, the peas are clearly a better "bargain." However, the peanut butter does provide two nutrients (protein and niacin) in percent U.S. RDA amounts that are greater than the percent of daily calories supplied.

d. If you tried to meet your U.S. RDA for iron (or riboflavin or thiamin) by eating just peanut butter, you would have to eat more than twice as many calories as you need. Conversely, you would only have to eat two-thirds of your daily calorie allotment to meet the U.S. RDA for protein and one-third of your daily calorie allotment to meet the U.S. RDA for niacin.

e. Taking calories into consideration, the food that provides the greater amount of a nutrient, relative to the amount of calories supplied, is the best "bargain" (or the best source) for that nutrient.

Class Period 2

1. Introduce the concept of *nutrient density.* Illustrate the concept of density by drawing two equal-sized squares on the board and by placing a different number of dots within each square; the square with the most dots has the greater *density* of dots. The same kind of illustration can be done by placing an unequal number of toothpicks in two equal-sized containers.

2. Have students determine the nutrient density of fresh cooked peas and peanut butter for each of the eight nutrients graphed.

$$\text{Nutrient Density} = \frac{\%\ \text{U.S. RDA of nutrient supplied}}{\%\ \text{daily calorie needs supplied}}$$

Point out to students that the quotient is actually the ratio of the percent of the U.S. RDA of the nutrient, to the percent of daily calorie needs supplied. Thus, the larger the ratio, the greater the density. The food with the greater nutrient density is a better bargain (or better source) for that nutrient because it provides more of the nutrient calorie per calorie.

The nutrient densities for the nutrients in the peas and in the peanut butter are as follows:

	NUTRIENT DENSITY	
NUTRIENT	FRESH GREEN PEAS, COOKED	PEANUT BUTTER
Protein	4	2
Vitamin A	5	–
Vitamin C	14	–
Thiamin	8	<1
Riboflavin	3	<1
Niacin	5	3
Calcium	1	<1
Iron	4	<1

3. Proceed with the "Advanced Activity" below if you wish, or else use the quiz mentioned in step 4.

4. **Evaluation:** Distribute Quiz Sheets 9-1 through 9-2 and have students complete them. Some of the problems require calculations; ask students to show their work on the backs of the sheets for these. Discuss each answer and display the calculation for it on the chalkboard or on an overhead transparency.

ADVANCED ACTIVITY

Time Needed: One class period

Materials Needed: Sheet 9-1: "U.S. RDA Bar Graph" completed in the Basic Activity for green peas and peanut butter
Sheets 9-2 through 9-4: "Combining Nutrient Densities"
Chart D: "Food Composition Table for Selected Nutrients"
Quiz Sheets 9-1 through 9-2

1. Have students read and complete Sheets 9-2 through 9-4, "Combining Nutrient Densities." Because there are many nutrient density calculations to make, students should work in pairs and split the work whenever possible. For example, for questions 9 and 10, one student should take hamburger and the other dry beans. Note also that students will need to make reference to the U.S. RDA Bar Graphs completed in the Basic Activity.

2. Conduct a discussion following completion of Sheets 9-2 through 9-4. Emphasize that combining a variety of nutrient-dense foods will increase the overall nutritional quality of the daily diet. Also, encourage students to make the following considerations before consuming those foods that do not qualify as being nutrient dense:

   a. Does the food contain valuable amounts of any nutrient? If so, which nutrient and what are the nutrient densities?

   b. Can I combine this food with another food to make a nutritious combination?

   c. Is my day's total diet high in energy and low in nutrients? If so, would eating a nutrient-dense food be a better choice than this food?

3. **Evaluation:** Distribute Quiz Sheets 9-1 through 9-2 and have students complete them independently. Some of the problems require calculations; ask students to show their work for these on the backs of the sheets. Discuss each answer and display the calculation for it on the chalkboard or on an overhead transparency.

FOLLOW-UP ACTIVITIES

1. Complete Sheet 9-1, "U.S. RDA Bar Graph" for other foods listed in Chart D, "Food Composition Table for Selected Nutrients."

2. For specific nutrients, determine which foods will be better "bargains" than others (which foods have the greater nutrient density).

3. Use the National Dairy Council's RDA Comparison Cards to identify which foods provide the best "bargain" for specific nutrients.

U.S. RDA BAR GRAPH

Food: _____

Percent of
U.S.
RDA

60								
58								
56								
54								
52								
50								
48								
46								
44								
42								
40								
38								
36								
34								
32								
30								
28								
26								
24								
22								
20								
18								
16								
14								
12								
10								
8								
6								
4								
2								

Calories | Protein | Vitamin A | Vitamin C | Thiamin | Riboflavin | Niacin | Calcium | Iron

COMBINING NUTRIENT DENSITIES

In the activity on Sheet 9-1 you learned a very important skill: how to determine the nutrient density of a food for the Iron CaPAC nutrients as well as for thiamin, riboflavin, and niacin. In this activity, you will use nutrient densities to identify *nutrient-dense* foods.

A food is considered to be *nutrient-dense* if it meets one or both of the two criteria listed below:

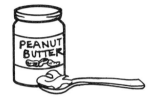

Criterion 1: The food has a nutrient density equal to or greater than *1* for at least *four* nutrients.

Criterion 2: The food has a nutrient density equal to or greater than *2* for at least *two* nutrients.

Think back to the peanut butter you analyzed on Sheet 9-1. Did it meet one of the two criteria above?

1. _____

If "yes," which one did it meet?

2. _____

What about the fresh cooked peas you analyzed on Sheet 9-1; which of the criteria did they meet?

3. _____

Both peanut butter and fresh peas can be considered as

4. _____

Most foods that come from the Basic Four Food Groups will meet one of the criteria for nutrient-dense foods. For example, let's take a look at the Meat-Poultry-Fish-Beans group. We've looked at one example already (peanut butter), which met one of the criteria. What about eggs, hamburger, and cooked dry beans? Using Chart D, "Food Composition Table for Selected Nutrients," determine whether these foods would qualify as being nutrient dense.

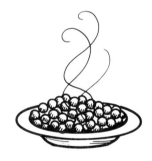

First, let's review the steps to follow using, for example, eggs:

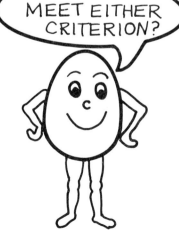

a. Look up *egg* in Chart D.

b. To determine the percentage of your daily energy needs supplied by one plain egg, calculate the following:

80 calories ÷ 2500 calories = .032

.032 × 100 = 3.2%

3.2% rounded to the nearest whole number = 3%

5. Using Chart D, determine if an egg supplies a nutrient density that is equal to or greater than 3 percent of the U.S. RDA for any of the eight nutrients, and write them here:

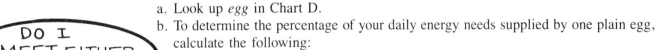

_____

6. Calculate the nutrient density for each of these nutrients by dividing the percent of the U.S. RDA, for each nutrient, by the percent of calorie needs supplied (rounded). For example, for protein, the calculation would be 14% ÷ 3% = 5. You do the rest and write your answers here:

_____

Does an egg meet both criterion 1 and criterion 2? 7. _____ Why?

8. _____

_____

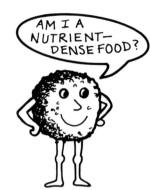

Now determine nutrient densities for hamburger and dry beans, cooked. Which criterion does hamburger meet?

9. _____ What about beans?

10. _____ If you examine vegetables, it will be hard to find one that does not qualify as being nutrient dense. Pick two from Chart D that you think may not qualify and report your findings here:

11. _____

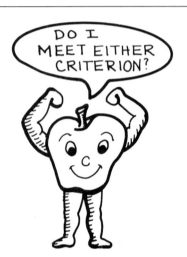

Check out the nutrient densities for an apple and a flounder (a type of fish). What did you discover?

12. _____

In the past, someone may have told you that these foods were "good" for you. Considering your answer to question 12, do you think an apple and flounder are "good" for you?

13. _____ Why? 14. _____

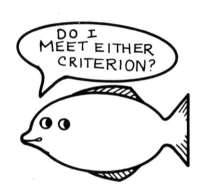

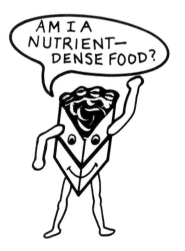

Now check out the nutrient densities for a piece of yellow cake with chocolate icing and for a slice of apple pie. What did you find?

15. _____

Do you eat foods like cake and pie because someone said they are good for you? I don't think so! Suppose all you ate one day was apple pie and cake with frosting. Also, suppose you ate enough of them to meet your daily calorie needs. You would not meet *any* of your nutrient needs for that day! In fact, you would have to eat *almost three times* your calorie needs to meet the U.S.

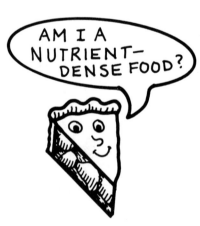

RDA for protein and *more than four times* your calorie needs to meet the U.S. RDA for iron! What other foods are similar to cake and pie in their nutrient contributions?

16. _____

Even though apples and flounder do not meet the criteria for being nutrient-dense foods, they do make valuable contributions of one or more nutrients to our diet. Thus these foods really are "good" for you, but they just don't make quite as good a nutrient contribution to the daily diet as foods that meet the criteria for nutrient-dense foods. Cake, pie, and other foods that are high in sugar and/or fat and low in nutrients do not make valuable nutrient contributions to our diet. They should be eaten only in small amounts and not too often.

QUIZ
DETERMINING NUTRIENT DENSITY IN FOOD

_____ 1. A cup of tomato juice supplies 12 percent of the U.S. RDA for iron and about 2 percent of the day's calorie needs. What is the nutrient density of the tomato juice for iron?
   a. 6
   b. .16
   c. .24
   d. 3

_____ 2. A cup of peas supplies 16 percent of the U.S. RDA for iron and 4 percent of the day's calorie needs. Comparing nutrient densities, which food provides the most iron per calorie—the tomato juice or the peas? (Refer to the answer you gave to question 1 for the nutrient density of tomato juice.)
   a. The peas
   b. The tomato juice
   c. Peas provide the same amount of iron, per calorie, as the tomato juice
   d. None of the above

_____ 3. One slice of a double-crusted apple pie supplies 400 calories and 5 percent of the U.S. RDA for Vitamin C. If you require 2,500 calories a day, what is the nutrient density of apple pie for Vitamin C?
   a. 1.0
   b. 0.3
   c. .5
   d. 3.0

_____ 4. If the nutrient density of an apple for Vitamin C is 3, which food provides the most Vitamin C per calorie, an apple or a slice of double-crusted apple pie? (Refer to the answer you gave to question 3 to help you determine the answer here.)
   a. The apple pie
   b. The apple
   c. The apple pie provides as much Vitamin C, per calorie, as the apple
   d. None of the above

_____ 5. Nutrient density bar graphs for ocean perch and prunes are shown here:

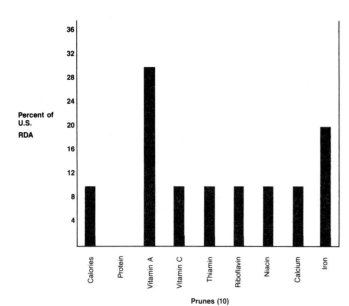

Prunes (10)

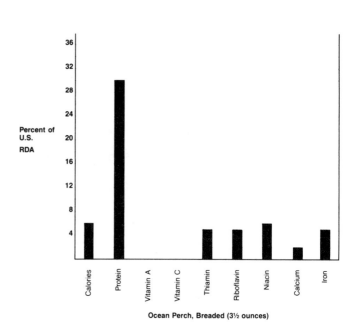

Ocean Perch, Breaded (3½ ounces)

Based on the information presented in these bar graphs:
a. Ocean perch would qualify as being a nutrient-dense food.
b. Prunes would not qualify as being a nutrient-dense food.
c. Neither food qualifies as being a nutrient-dense food.
d. Prunes would qualify as being a nutrient-dense food.

_____ 6. Look at the bar graph for ocean perch in question 3. If 2½ ounces of ocean perch supplied only 5 percent of the calorie needs, then:
a. The nutrient densities for protein and niacin would be lower.
b. Ocean perch would be a nutrient-dense food.
c. Ocean perch would not be a nutrient-dense food.
d. Ocean perch would have a nutrient density of at least 2 for two nutrients.

_____ 7. A nutrient-dense food must:
a. Have a nutrient density of 1 for two nutrients.
b. Have a nutrient density of 1 for four nutrients or 2 for two nutrients.
c. Have a nutrient density of 2 for four nutrients or 1 for five nutrients.
d. Be high in protein.

_____ 8. Grape juice has a nutrient density of 3 for Vitamin C, but less than 1 for the other seven nutrients. A pear has a nutrient density of 2.5 for Vitamin C, 1 for riboflavin, and less than 1 for the remaining six nutrients. Which would qualify as being a nutrient-dense food?
a. The pear
b. The grape juice
c. Neither
d. Both

SECTION II

DIET PLANNING

Unit 10: Eating Right, Feeling Well

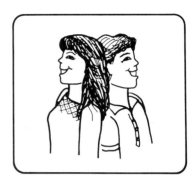

CONCEPT

–Nutrition affects the overall health of individuals, including their physical, mental, and emotional health.

OBJECTIVES

–Students will be able to identify human characteristics that signify good physical, mental, and emotional health.

–Students will be able to analyze the relationship between what they eat and how they feel (physically, mentally, and emotionally).

TEACHER'S UNIT INTRODUCTION

The first astonishing findings regarding the effects of food and nutrition on health appeared over 200 years ago. In 1750, Captain James Lind observed the beneficial effects of lime juice on a condition, later known as scurvy, that afflicts sailors on long sea voyages. He concluded that there was some substance in the food that cured the disease. This substance was identified, in 1907, as ascorbic acid and is commonly known as Vitamin C. Later, similar conclusions were reached regarding beriberi (a deficiency of thiamin) and pellagra (a deficiency of niacin). These nutrient-deficiency diseases demonstrate the effects of nutrition on the physical health of individuals. Deficiency diseases result in bleeding gums, dry skin, fatigue, shortness of breath, muscle cramps, aching bones, aching joints and muscles, loss of appetite, loss of muscle tone, cracked lips, inflamed tongue, and diarrhea. Deficiency diseases can also affect mental and emotional health. Such deficiencies can cause irritability, disorientation, depression, disorderly thinking, and confusion.

Nutritional excesses (overnutrition) are also associated with various disorders and diseases. Obesity is the result of continually eating more calories than are needed. Obese people have an increased risk of developing diabetes, stroke, kidney disease, high blood pressure, and heart disease. Too much refined sugar contributes to tooth decay. For some people, a high salt intake may lead to high blood pressure. Diets high in saturated fat and cholesterol may lead to heart disease or stroke in some people.

It is obvious that nutrition can affect physical health. But what about the effect of nutrition on the emotional and mental health of healthy people? There is quite a bit of evidence that food and nutrition affect your body every day. Stop and think about it. Have you ever felt light-headed or dizzy because you did not eat breakfast or because you did not eat all day? Did you ever experience a lack of concentration because you were hungry? Did you ever get a stomach cramp because you ate too much or because you ate the wrong kinds of food? Or did you ever become irritable or short-tempered because you were hungry? All of these examples indicate that nutrition has an effect on daily health, not only physically, but also mentally and emotionally.

Many educators are probably wondering: What is all this fuss about nutrition education? It may be interesting, but when it really comes down to brass tacks, is nutrition all that important? Discounting the strong biases of nutritionists (we know nutrition *must* be important!), this unit discusses the significant effects that nutrition has on the health of individuals and demonstrates the fact that nutrition affects not only physical health but also mental and emotional health.

This unit is designed to help students examine how food and nutrition affect their health. It is important to explore the concept of health prior to beginning this unit.

If the "Advanced Activity" is selected, students will need to begin filling out the worksheet one week in advance of the activity. Students should complete Sheet 10-2, "Food and Feelings Record," each day for one week.

BASIC ACTIVITY

Time Needed: One class period

Materials Needed: Sheet 10-1: "How Do You Feel?"
                     Quiz Sheet 10-1

1. Conduct a large-group discussion of the characteristics that indicate health. Begin by writing on the chalkboard three headings: *Physical, Mental,* and *Emotional.*

2. Have students list, under each heading, various traits that may be used to describe good health. The following list gives some examples:

Physical	**Mental**	**Emotional**
Normal weight	Attentive	Optimistic
Good posture	Working up to intellectual capacity	Patient
Shiny, smooth hair	Alert	Stable
Good color in skin	Interested in learning	Nonaggressive
Clear, bright eyes		Interested in living
Well-developed, firm muscles		
Sound teeth		
Firm, pink mouth and gums		

3. Distribute Sheet 10-1, "How Do You Feel?," and have students complete the sentence at the end of each description. Remind them that there are no right or wrong answers. They should complete the sentences by describing how they would really feel.

4. Begin a large-group discussion of students' answers on Sheet 10-1. Compare answers to see if each person might feel slightly different. Food and nutrition affect each person in a unique way. The most important point of this activity is to encourage students to notice the effect that food and nutrition have on their health and on how they feel.

5. Proceed with the "Advanced Activity" below if you wish, or else use the Quiz Sheet 10-1.

6. **Evaluation:** Distribute Quiz Sheet 10-1 and have the students answer the questions in short paragraph form. Discuss the answers in class and check to make sure the three components of good health are covered: physical, mental, and emotional.

ADVANCED ACTIVITY

Time Needed: Two class periods

Materials Needed: Sheet 10-2: "Food and Feelings Record" (Seven copies per student)
Quiz Sheet 10-1

Class Period 1

1. Distribute seven copies of Sheet 10-2, "Food and Feelings Record," to each student.
2. Ask the students to

a. Fill out one worksheet for each day of the week. This record should list *everything* they eat or drink during the given time period.

b. For each food, list in the appropriate columns:

- When it was eaten (time of day)
- Whether it was a meal or a snack
- A description of the food and of how much was eaten
- How hungry the student was before eating (extremely, somewhat, not at all)
- The number of minutes it took to eat the meal or snack
- Thoughts, emotions, and feelings, both before and after eating the food

c. At the bottom of the page ask students to describe their feelings at the end of the day. Were they tired? Irritated? Energetic? Comfortable? Depressed?

d. Discuss with students the effect of nutrition on physical, mental, and emotional feelings.

Class Period 2

1. After the prescribed number of days, bring students together for a large-group discussion.

a. Have them look at their food intake.

b. Have them label their feelings by placing

- A "P" next to the feelings that were physical
- An "M" next to those that were mental
- An "E" next to those that were emotional

c. Ask them to examine the relationship between the food they ate and the feelings they experienced afterward.

d. Have them notice also how the same foods might affect their feelings later in the day.

2. Encourage students to discuss their overall feelings for each day. Ask them how these feelings might relate to what they have eaten. Do they see any correlation between good and bad eating habits and good and bad feelings?

3. Conclude the activity by reminding students to be constantly aware of how food makes them feel, and remind them also that they should eat the foods that make them feel well.

4. **Evaluation:** Distribute Quiz Sheet 10-1 and have the students answer the questions in short paragraph form. Discuss the answers in class and check to make sure the three components of good health are covered: physical, mental, and emotional.

FOLLOW-UP ACTIVITIES

1. Have students role play people with various symptoms or signs of poor nutritional health. Have them also role play people with good nutritional health. Students in the audience may be asked to guess the specific symptom the role play is depicting.

2. Have students write short stories in which one person is eating a poor diet and the other person is trying to convince him or her to eat a better diet. Discussion between characters should involve some issues regarding symptoms of poor versus good nutritional health.

HOW DO YOU FEEL?

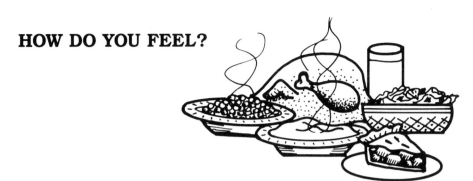

Directions: Write the ending to each sentence below in order to describe how you feel in each situation.

Imagine that . . .

You have just finished eating a Thanksgiving dinner of turkey, mashed potatoes, bread stuffing, gravy, baked corn pudding, cranberry salad, green beans, crescent butter-rolls, milk, pumpkin pie with whipped cream, and a few after-dinner mints.

I feel _____

Imagine that . . .

You are late for school. You have five minutes to catch the bus and you are not even dressed yet. You grab a doughnut on your way out the door. You have forgotten your lunch money (again) so you just buy a cola drink for lunch. Now you are sitting in class.

I feel _____

Imagine that . . .

You are visiting your grandmother (or aunt or best friend) and dinner includes most of your favorite foods. You eat the meal, totally enjoying each bite.

I feel _____

Imagine that . . .

You have recently been turned on to nutrition, and you have been eating all the foods you know are good for you—plenty of fresh fruits and vegetables, whole-grain breads and cereals, meat, poultry, fish, eggs, and milk—and everything seems to taste good, too! You have been getting plenty of exercise and enough sleep.

I feel _____

Imagine that . . .

You are at the carnival or circus. It is all so exciting! The people, the animals, the shows . . . and the *food*. You eat a little bit of whatever looks good to you—cotton candy, soft drinks, funnel cakes, ice cream, hot dogs, and french fries—you name it!

I feel _____

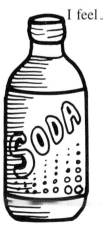

© 1986 by The Center for Applied Research in Education, Inc.

FOOD AND FEELINGS RECORD

Time of Day	Meal or Snack*	Food Eaten	Amount of Food Eaten	Hunger Rating**	Time Spent Eating	Feelings	
						Before	After

*Meal = M, Snack = S   **1 = Extremely hungry; 2 = Somewhat hungry; 3 = Not hungry at all

© 1996 by The Center for Applied Research in Education, Inc.

QUIZ
EATING RIGHT, FEELING WELL

The food you eat affects you. It affects your looks, the way you think, and the way you feel emotionally. In the boxes below, write two paragraphs. The first should describe "Health-Wise Sandy" who is in *good* nutritional health, and the second should describe "Health-Poor Terry" who is in *poor* nutritional health.

In each paragraph, remember to describe the three aspects of health (physical, mental, and emotional) in relation to nutrition.

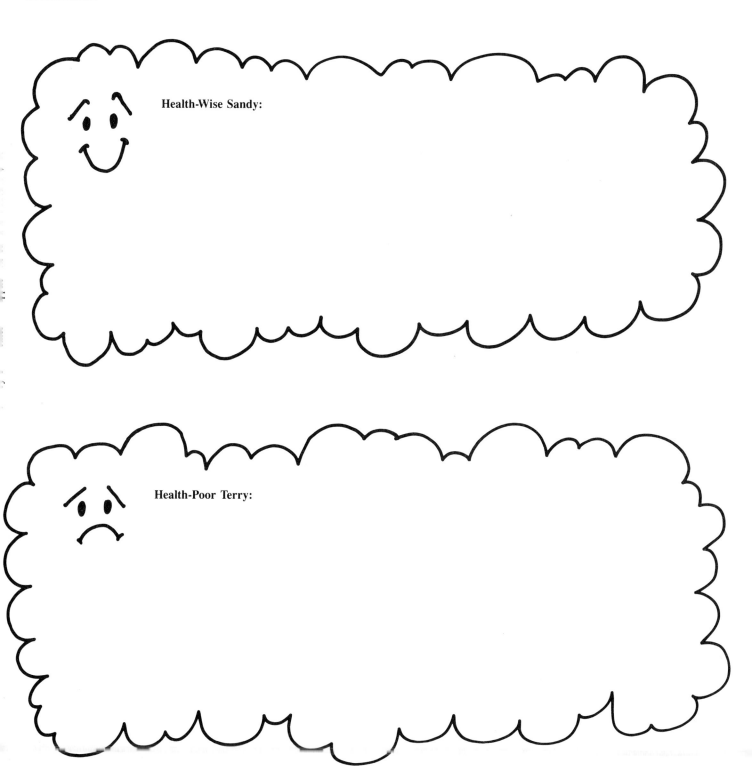

Health-Wise Sandy:

Health-Poor Terry:

Unit 11: How Do You Stack Up Nutritionally?

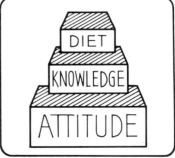

CONCEPTS

–Knowledge and attitudes about nutrition are equally important in affecting an individual's dietary habits.

–Nutrition attitudes, nutrition knowledge, and dietary habits can be measured using simple evaluation tools.

OBJECTIVES

–Students will be able to evaluate their dietary habits.

–Students will be able to evaluate their feelings, attitudes, and knowledge about foods and nutrition.

–Students will evaluate their current eating habits as well as their current health status.

TEACHER'S UNIT INTRODUCTION

Traditionally, *nutrition* has been the study of diet, nutrients, and food. It was hoped that if people learned more about a nutritious diet, they would begin to make changes in their habits. More and more, however, evidence has been growing that points out the weakness of this belief. Knowledge alone does not usually influence people enough to change their health habits. Knowledge, plus a positive attitude toward nutrition, however, will often help individuals to make better food choices. In order for individuals to improve their diet, and therefore their health, they need to know the facts and need to *want* to put what they know to work.

Nutritionists have developed evaluation tools to measure certain characteristics of individuals. Diet, being the most commonly examined item, may be measured in a variety of ways. One tool used to measure diet is the food frequency form. A sample of this form will be used in one of the activities in this unit and is fairly simple to complete. First, instruct students to check off one box for each food group in order to show the amount of food they usually consume in each category. Then score their food intake using the key. A score of 35 or above is adequate for good nutritional health. A lower score indicates a possible deficiency. Remember that this form is only one of the many tools needed to accurately diagnose a nutritional deficiency. Dietary surveys may indicate dietary inadequacies, but more sophisticated tests, such as blood tests and physical examinations, are necessary to diagnose an actual deficiency.

Evaluation of diets using the Daily Food Guide is another commonly used method. The amounts and types of foods eaten in a twenty-four-hour period are recorded and evaluated according to the recommended numbers of servings from several food groups. Chart B, "Daily Food Guide," will be discussed in later units.

A more complicated diet evaluation tool is the Nutrient Anaysis method. In *Nutrient Analysis,* all of the foods eaten by an individual, within a given amount of time, are recorded and analyzed using food composition tables. First, each food is found in the table; then, the amounts of various nutrients in that food are recorded on a worksheet, and finally, the amounts of each nutrient are totaled. The final result is a compilation of the total nutrients found in the food consumed. These totals can then be compared to the Recommended Dietary Allowance (RDA) for each nutrient. The results of this evaluation can be used to determine which nutrients are generally lacking in an individual's diet and which food habits need attention. A newer method of Nutrient Analysis is made possible through the use of the computer. Many software programs are available to analyze an individual's diet and to make recommendations for change (see the References/Resources section at the end of this kit).

Another area to measure is nutrition knowledge. It is important to discover how much individuals already know about nutrition so that you and they can decide what else they need to know to improve their diets.

Attitudes are another area to be measured. An attitude refers to how a person feels about something. Attitudes may be measured by completing a survey, during the course of which, the individual being surveyed is asked to agree or disagree with a series of statements. It is important to realize that there are no right or wrong answers and that, above all else, opinions should be given honestly.

A key step in nutrition education is to assess the nutrition knowledge, the nutrition-related attitudes, and the dietary habits of students. This assessment will provide an opportunity for the teacher, as well as for the students, to examine their ideas and habits regarding nutrition. The evaluation tools in this unit may be useful as a teaching strategy.

In the case of the attitude survey, "What Do You Think About Nutrition?" (Sheet 11-3) and "My Dietary Diary" (Sheet 11-6), you may want to ask students not to sign the sheets. Students may feel more inclined to record their true feelings about nutrition if they cannot be identified. If students answer the questions honestly, you will discover quite a bit about how they (as a group) feel toward nutrition. You will also be able to determine how much class time needs to be devoted to the development of positive attitudes toward nutrition. If the students already have positive attitudes, they are likely to be more receptive to the material you present.

You may also wish to be cautious about requiring names and participation on Sheets 11-7 through 11-8, "My One-And-Only Body." The students may feel shy and uncomfortable talking about their bodies. It is important, during this activity, that you discuss the variety of body shapes and sizes. At this age, students need to be reminded that they must accept their bodies in order to like themselves.

BASIC ACTIVITY

Time Needed: Two class periods

Materials Needed: Sheet 11-1: "Food Frequency Form"
Sheet 11-2: "Test Your Nutrition IQ"
Sheet 11-3: "What Do You Think About Nutrition?"
Sheet 11-4: "My Dietary Goals" *(optional)*
Quiz Sheet 11-1

Class Period 1

1. Introduce the activity by emphasizing the following points:

- Food habits are composed of individual food choices.

- Food habits are the types and amounts of foods that a person normally consumes.

- Food habits can be changed after individuals become conscious of them.

- Everyone has different food habits and feels differently about the relative importance of food.

2. Distribute Sheet 11-1, "Food Frequency Form," and have students complete it. Provide scoring information from the Answer Key at the back of this book. Place the scoring information on the chalkboard or on an overhead transparency. Have students score their own diets. Encourage discussion of their results by asking them the following questions:

- "What are your nutritional strengths? Weaknesses?"

- "What habits could you improve?"

- "What habits would you like to keep?"

3. Once students have completed this activity, begin a large-group discussion. Have students vote on the following questions, either by raising their hands, while you keep a tally on the chalkboard, or by noting their answers on paper.

   a. "How many of you enjoy eating fresh fruit?"

   b. "How many of you enjoy eating vegetables?"

   c. "How many of you enjoy drinking milk?"

   d. "How many of you enjoy drinking soft drinks?"

   e. "How many of you feel you eat too many sugary, rich foods (candy, cakes, cookies, soft drinks)?"

   f. "How many of you feel you do not eat enough fresh fruits and vegetables?"

   g. "How many of you would like to eat fewer calories? More calories?"

   h. "How many of you feel you weigh just the right amount? Too much? Too little?"

   i. "How many of you like to try new foods?"

   j. "How many of you would like to eat differently?"

Encourage a discussion of each question. Ask additional, similar questions if appropriate.

4. Have students complete Sheet 11-2, "Test Your Nutrition IQ." Emphasize the importance of being honest and reflective. After an adequate time interval, discuss the answers and have students score themselves. Refer to the Answer Key at the back of this book for annotated answers.

5. Have students complete Sheet 11-3, "What Do You Think About Nutrition?," and discuss the worksheet by encouraging students to share their attitudes and opinions with the class. Refer to the Answer Key for comments. For students who seem reluctant to share information in a large-group setting, begin discussion of the answers in small groups and then return to the large-group setting. This technique will help build students' confidence in expressing their attitudes. Have students retain all of their evaluation forms for later use.

Class Period 2

1. Have students complete Sheet 11-4, "My Dietary Goals." Discuss how to complete the Self-Contract. Tell students to

    a. Fill in their names.

    b. Fill in the goal number and description of the goal they would *most* like to reach.

    c. Fill in a target date for beginning work on the goal.

    d. Name the first step toward attaining the goal that they will take. For example, if they chose goal #5 ("I do not eat foods high in fat, such as fried or greasy foods") their specific first step might be to avoid eating french fries on their next visit to a fast food restaurant.

    e. Date and sign the contract along with at least one witness. (*Note:* Some students will not be ready or willing to take this step in changing their food habits. These students should be encouraged to pursue their personal goals.)

2. Proceed with the "Advanced Activity" if you wish, or else use Quiz Sheet 11-1.

3. **Evaluation:** Distribute Quiz Sheet 11-1 and have the students write short paragraphs for their answers. Discuss their paragraphs as a class.

ADVANCED ACTIVITY

Time Needed: Two class periods

Materials Needed: Sheet 11-5: "My Dietary Diary"
                            Sheets 11-6 through 11-7: "My One-And-Only Body"
                            Sheets 11-8 through 11-10: "Nutrition Super Sleuth"
                            Quiz Sheet 11-1

Class Period 1

1. Distribute Sheet 11-5, "My Dietary Diary," and ask the students to answer the following questions in the appropriate square. This sheet often evokes and encourages discussion.

SQUARE #	QUESTIONS
1	*My Favorite Foods as a Child:* "What foods did you like to eat the most when you were little? Are they the same now? Did you like foods such as mushrooms, eggs, garlic, onions, or red beets? Do your parents like these foods? Do they eat them?
2	*Foods I Would Not Want My Own Children to Eat:* "What foods would you *not* feed your baby (or your younger brother or sister, or your niece or nephew)? Would you feed him or her soft drinks, candy, cake, coffee, or beer? Why or why not?"
3	*Foods I Use to Celebrate:* "What foods do you eat on holidays? For example, what foods do you eat on your birthday? What foods do you use to reward yourself? For example, what foods do you eat after winning a ball game? Why are these foods chosen over other foods?"

4   *Foods I Use for Comfort When I Am Sad or Lonely:* "Do you ever eat for reasons other than hunger? Do you eat when you are sad or lonely? Do you eat if your best friend forgets to call you? Do you eat because you are bored with your homework? Do you eat because it is Saturday night and you don't have anything else to do? What foods do you eat when you have these feelings?"

5   *Foods My Body Needs:* "List foods you *think* are healthful or good for you. What foods do you need to stay alive and healthy?"

6   *Foods I Have Eaten in the Last Twenty-Four Hours:* "List all of the foods or drinks that you have consumed in the last twenty-four hours. Be sure to include gum, candy, snacks, tea or coffee, butter on your bread, and so on. Are these the kinds of foods you usually eat? Why or why not? How do these foods compare with the list in square #5 of foods your body needs?"

2. Discuss students' responses. Students learn about their own eating habits by hearing how similar or different they are from those of others. Try to share some of your thoughts about your own dietary habits with the students.

3. Discuss the students' answers in square #6 in detail. Describe how students might evaluate their own diets. Have them compare the answers in square #6 to those in square #5 to see if they are actually eating the foods *they* think they should be eating. Then give a simple description of two methods of rating diets—nutrient analysis and the procedure using the Daily Food Guide—that were described in the "Teacher's Introduction" to this unit.

Class Period 2

1. Using Sheets 11-6 through 11-7, "My One-And-Only Body," ask the students to assess their nutritional status by reviewing the following characteristics related to good health:

	Good Nutritional Status	**Poor Nutritional Status**
General	• Active, alert, good-natured, interested, attentive	• Listless, apathetic, inattentive, irritable, tired
Hair	• Shiny, smooth	• Dry, brittle, stiff, lack of shine
Skin	• Healthy glow	• Cracked, dry, flaky, pale
Eyes	• Clear, bright	• Dull eyes, swollen lids, circles underneath
Muscles	• Well-developed, firm	• Soft, flabby
Teeth	• Sound	• Decayed
Mouth	• Firm, pink	• Cracks in corners, pale
Gums	• Reddish pink, firm	• Soft, spongy, bright red
Digestion	• No complaints	• Constipated, frequently upset stomach
Posture	• Stands straight	• Stooping, slumping, protruding stomach
Health	• Excellent	• Susceptible to illness
Weight	• Normal	• Over- or underweight

2. Distribute Sheets 11-8 through 11-10, "Nutrition Super Sleuth." Have students read each case study and answer the questions following each one. Begin a large-group discussion of each case on the worksheets. Ask the students to write individual paragraphs describing their own diets, any dietary problems they have, and to propose solutions to their dietary problems.

3. **Evaluation:** Distribute Quiz Sheet 11-1 and have the students write short paragraphs as their answers. Discuss their paragraphs as a class.

FOLLOW-UP ACTIVITIES

1. Have students compose an "Eater's Bill of Rights" stating what rights individuals have in regard to their eating habits.

2. Prepare a bulletin board of unusual foods. Categorize them according to the Daily Food Guide.

3. Ask students to write a short story about good nutrition. The story should include at least two characters, one of whom may be the author. If the students are willing, have them share their stories with the rest of the class.

4. Use a "Dear Abby" format to ask students about food choices. Students may want to contribute questions in advance for this activity. An example might be:

Dear Abby,

My sister is on a strict vegetarian diet. Her favorite foods are soybeans and kidney beans; bulgur; millet, and other grains; peanut butter; leafy green vegetables, such as spinach and kale; and any other vegetable you can think of. It is my turn to plan and prepare the family dinners next week. How can I plan and prepare a meal for her that is nutritionally adequate and still make foods she likes and will eat? I am heading for a dietary disaster! Help!

Losing My Noodle, from Nebraska

5. Using their favorite food lists and working in small groups, have the students plan and prepare a nutritious party meal or snack. This activity will encourage students to compromise about selecting nutritious foods, as well as favorite foods.

6. Have students prepare a joint list of their favorite foods. Have them petition or ask the school food service supervisor to prepare some of these favorite foods for lunch, if he or she is not already doing so.

FOOD FREQUENCY FORM

Directions: Place a check mark in one box in each line that describes how often you eat from each particular food group.

Food Groups	Hardly Ever	Several Times Per Week	Once Daily	Two Times Per Day	Three or More Times Per Day
MILK, PUDDING, CUSTARD, YOGURT, CHEESE					
ANIMAL PROTEINS (beef, chicken, pork, fish, eggs)					
VEGETABLE PROTEINS (beans, nuts, peas)					
FRUIT or JUICE OF: orange, grapefruit, tangerine, strawberries, tomato, green pepper					
BROCCOLI, LIMA BEANS, SPINACH, LETTUCE, OTHER GREENS					
any other FRUIT or VEGETABLE					
any type of CEREAL, BREAD, ROLL, RICE, CRACKER, NOODLES, MACARONI, SPAGHETTI					

TOTAL SCORE = _____

TEST YOUR NUTRITION IQ

Directions: Place a "T" next to each sentence that is true and an "F" next to each sentence that is false.

_____ 1. Honey is more nutritious than sugar.

_____ 2. A medium potato has fewer calories than a large apple.

or

_____ 3. A kiss uses up 50 calories.

_____ 4. You do *not* need to eat a lot of meat to be a good athlete.

_____ 5. B vitamins help to keep your nerves healthy.

_____ 6. Potato chips are a good substitute for potatoes.

_____ 7. Taking large doses of Vitamin C is harmless.

_____ 8. Ingredients on food labels are listed in alphabetical order.

_____ 9. Large doses of Vitamin A will clear up acne.

_____ 10. Carbohydrates are fattening.

To calculate your nutrition IQ: 9–10 Correct answers—EXCELLENT
7–8 Correct answers—GOOD
6 Or fewer correct answers—POOR

WHAT DO YOU THINK ABOUT NUTRITION?

Directions: Check the box that tells how you feel about each statement. Remember: There are no right or wrong answers. Be honest!

	Strongly Agree	Agree	Do Not Know	Disagree	Strongly Disagree
1. Nutrition is not so important as long as I am eating a lot of food.					
2. I eat whatever I want and never think about it later.					
3. I feel best when I eat nutritious foods.					
4. I like to make my own decisions about what I eat, but often I eat what everybody else is eating.					
5. If I take a vitamin pill in the morning, I do not have to worry about what I eat.					
6. If I am not eating well, surely my health will suffer.					
7. The food I eat has nothing to do with the way I feel.					
8. I would really like to change my eating habits.					

MY DIETARY GOALS

Directions: Place a check mark in front of each sentence with which you agree. Be honest!

_____ 1. I eat many different kinds of foods.

_____ 2. I do not eat foods high in sugar, such as soft drinks, candy cookies, and cakes.

_____ 3. I do not eat salty foods, such as chips and pretzels.

_____ 4. I do not use the salt shaker at mealtimes.

_____ 5. I do not eat foods high in fat, such as fried or greasy foods.

_____ 6. I weigh just about the right amount. I am not underweight or overweight.

_____ 7. I eat only when I am hungry and eat until I am full. I never eat more than I need.

_____ 8. I eat plenty of fresh fruits and vegetables. I eat at least four servings of them every day.

_____ 9. I eat mostly whole-grain breads and cereals.

_____ 10. I eat cheese, yogurt, and ice cream or drink milk four times a day.

   If you have checked all of these sentences, your food habits probably need very few changes. If you have checked less than 5, you may be headed for trouble. Review the dietary goals above. Of the goals you did not check, decide which *one* you would most like to reach.

I would like to reach Goal # _____: _____
                                                        (describe)

My Dietary Goal Self-Contract

   I, _____ , would like to change my food habits.

The dietary goal I would like to reach is Goal # _____: _____
                                                                          (describe)

_____ .

I would like to begin working toward this goal on _____ . My first
                                                                          (date)

step on this day will be to _____
                                                (name specific first step you will take)

_____ .

_____   _____
         (your signature)   (signature of witness)

_____   _____
              (date)   (date)

MY DIETARY DIARY

1 My Favorite Foods as a Child:

2 Foods I Would Not Want My Own Children to Eat:

3 Foods I Use to Celebrate:

4 Foods I Use for Comfort When I Am Sad or Lonely:

5 Foods My Body Needs:

6 Foods I Have Eaten in the Last Twenty-Four Hours:

MY ONE-AND-ONLY BODY

My current height: _____ feet _____ inches

I am _____ short _____ medium _____ tall

My current weight: _____ pounds

I am _____ underweight _____ normal _____ overweight

Directions: Place a check mark along each line below to describe how you feel. If you check very close to the statement, it means the words describe you very well. If you check in the middle, it means you don't feel anything about the statement (are you *really* being honest?). Check anywhere you like along each line.

active, alert, good-natured, interested, attentive	listless, apathetic, inattentive, irritable, tired
shiny and smooth hair	dry, brittle, and stiff hair that lacks shine
healthy, glowing skin	cracked, dry, flaky, and pale skin
clear and bright eyes	dull eyes, swollen eyelids, circles underneath
firm, well-developed muscles	soft and flabby muscles
sound teeth	decayed teeth
firm, pink mouth	pale mouth with cracks in corners
firm, reddish-pink gums	soft, spongy, bright-red gums
no complaints with stomach	frequently constipated or frequently upset stomach
straight posture	stooping, slumping posture with protruding stomach
excellent health	susceptible to illness
normal weight	underweight or overweight

Directions: Answer each of the following questions. Be honest!

1. What part of your body do you feel the best about? Why?

2. What part of your body do you feel the worst about? Why?

3. How do you feel about your general appearance? Explain.

4. Do you get sick often? Explain.

5. Do you have enough energy to do everything you want to do? Explain.

6. What can you do to improve your health and increase your energy?

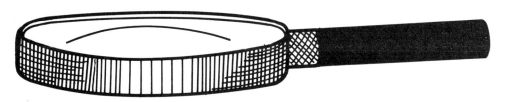

NUTRITION SUPER SLEUTH

Directions: Be a nutrition "Super Sleuth" and find the clues in each mystery case below that tell you whether or not each person has a dietary problem. Read each case and solve it by answering the questions.

THE CASE OF THE   John Delaney walks into your office dragging his feet and slowly slumps into the
MISSING LINK   chair facing you.

"What's wrong with you?" you ask.

"I thought *you* were supposed to give *me* the answer!" exclaims John. "That is why I am here, after all."

"Maybe if you tell me what you have been eating," you suggest, "we will be able to figure out what your problem is."

"Well," starts John, "I have recently become a vegetarian and have stopped eating red meat, chicken, fish, and eggs. I've heard that brown rice is a perfect food, so I have been eating only rice almost every day. I include some fruits and vegetables once in a while. What do you think my problem is?"

"This case will be easier than I thought!" you exclaim confidently.

1. Does John have a problem with his eating habits? _____ Yes _____ No

   a. If yes, what is his major problem? _____

   _____

   b. If yes, and if he still wants to remain a vegetarian, what is one solution to his problem? _____

   _____

2. How do you feel about John's diet? _____

   _____

3. Could *you* follow a vegetarian diet, providing that it was well-balanced and contained all the nutrients you needed? Why or why not? _____

   _____

   _____

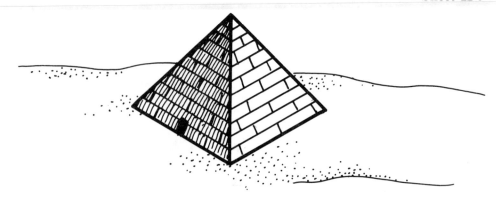

THE EGYPTIAN CONNECTION

The records of Abdel Touhami have recently been uncovered in the desert sands. Through a translator, you are able to discover his food habits, which are, as you might suspect, quite different from your own. From your research, you have made a sketch of the foods eaten in Abdel's lifetime: (1) homemade bread made with spelt (a type of red wheat) or corn; (2) ox flesh, goat meat, dog meat, turtles, snakes, crocodiles, barnacles, and snails; (3) many kinds of raw fish, either salted or dried in the sun; (4) quail and other small birds, served uncooked or roasted; (5) sweet wine made from barley; (6) olive and radish oil; (7) fresh fruits such as figs, apples, cherries, grapes, pomegranates, and watermelon; (8) lotus flowers of many colors; (9) beets, garlic, onions, artichokes, cabbage, watercress, leeks, and chickpeas; (10) fresh milk and cheeses.

1. Did Abdel have a problem with his eating habits? _____ Yes _____ No

   a. If yes, what was his major problem? _____
   _____

   b. If yes, what would be the solution to his problem? _____
   _____

2. How do you feel about Abdel's diet? _____
   _____

3. Could you eat Abdel's diet, provided that it was well-balanced and contained all of the nutrients you needed? Why or why not? _____
   _____
   _____

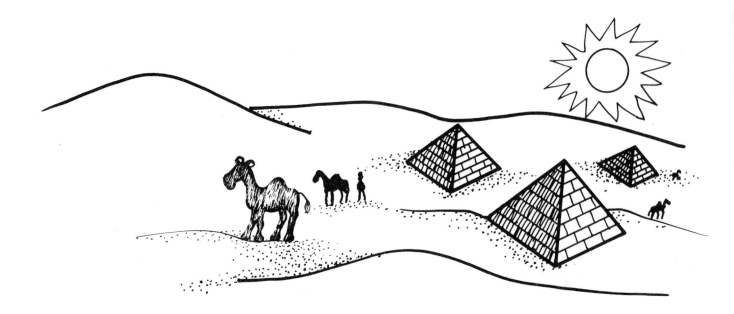

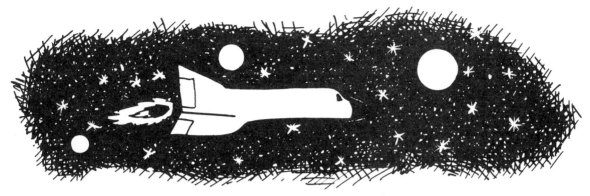

LOST IN SPACE!

"Michelle Miller—are you ready for liftoff?"

"5 – 4 – 3 – 2 – 1 – *Lift Off!*"

Michelle Miller and her crew have just taken off in *Orbitron-10*. Destination: *Skylab-26*. They have been preparing for this moment for months. Many hours have been spent getting equipment and supplies ready for the long journey. Food preparation has been carried out with care.

The menu is not notably different from the foods you might expect at home. Meat, poultry, eggs, fruit juices, puddings, and soups are among the food selections. The form in which the food is stored, however, is quite different from that at home. Most foods in space are dehydrated, thermostabilized, or frozen. Other foods, such as high-energy bars, are a formulated nutrient-fortified product derived from a concentrated food source. (The bars, by the way, are fortified with Vitamin C and iron.)

Michelle and her crew have now finished their first orbit around the earth and are preparing for a meal on board *Orbitron-10*. The menu will include fast-frozen meatballs with a gravy packet, dehydrated milk, and dehydrated vanilla pudding.

But wait! The spaceship is gaining speed uncontrollably! The equipment is going haywire! The controls are useless. The spaceship appears to be heading out of the earth's orbit toward regions unknown. Luckily, the spaceship is equipped with enough food, water, and supplies for over one year. Even though they are lost in space, they may be able to survive long enough to correct the malfunction and get back to earth.

1. Will Michelle have any problems with this diet over a year's time? _____ Yes _____ No

   a. If yes, what will be her major problem? _____

   _____

   b. If yes, what is the solution to her problem? _____

   _____

2. How do you feel about Michelle's diet? _____

   _____

3. Could you eat Michelle's diet, provided it was well-balanced and contained all of the nutrients you needed? Why or why not? _____

   _____

   _____

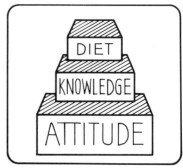

QUIZ
HOW DO YOU STACK UP NUTRITIONALLY?

Write a short paragraph in the space below describing your nutritional strengths and weaknesses. Answer the following questions in the paragraph:

1. How much do you know about nutrition? Do you know enough? Would you like to know more? What would you like to learn about?

2. How do you feel about nutrition? Do the foods you eat affect how you feel?

3. What are some of the foods you eat that are nutritious? What are some of the foods you eat that are not nutritious? Would you like to change what you eat? What changes would you like to make? Would these changes be difficult or easy for you to make?

_____
_____
_____
_____
_____
_____
_____
_____
_____
_____
_____
_____
_____
_____
_____
_____
_____

Unit 12: Start the Day Better with Breakfast

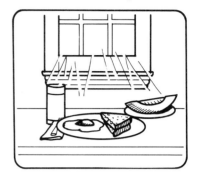

CONCEPTS

– Breakfast is an important meal of the day because it resupplies the body with energy and nutrients for the new day.

– Breakfast should supply approximately one-third of the Recommended Dietary Allowance (RDA) for energy and nutrients.

– Breakfast can be easy and quick to prepare.

– There are a number of typical nutritious breakfasts, but there is also a variety of other nutritious foods that we can eat at breakfast.

OBJECTIVES

– The students will be able to list the reasons why breakfast is important.

– Each student should be able to list various foods that could be served for breakfast. The suggested menus should provide one-third or more of the U.S. RDA for the Iron CaPAC nutrients.

– Students will prepare and consume a breakfast.

– Students will be able to evaluate the breakfast prepared in terms of cooking skills, time, cost, nutrition, and appeal.

TEACHER'S UNIT INTRODUCTION

People have different ideas about meals and snacks. Some people believe that the most efficient way for your body to use food is by supplying it with small amounts of food throughout the day. Six or seven small meals could be eaten and still provide your body with the nutrients and calories you need. Another pattern of meal planning is the traditional three square meals of breakfast, lunch, and dinner.

No matter which meal pattern you choose, the morning meal, or morning snack, still comes out on top as very important. Think of it this way—your body has been without food for nearly half a day. If your last meal or snack was at 9 P.M. and you awaken at 7 A.M., you have spent ten hours of your day foodless. This means that within the next fourteen hours you must eat enough nutrients and calories for the entire day. It is like having a drought for ten weeks, and then getting fourteen weeks of rain. The result? Flooding. In your body the same thing may happen. Hours of fasting relieved by hours of eating may cause your body to become overtaxed, which could lead to inefficient use of the nutrients eaten.

For some people, breakfast is not appealing because they are not hungry in the morning. There may be several reasons for this occurrence and there are many possible solutions. Often, the heaviest concentration of calories comes in the evening. Dinner and late night snacks may add up to more than half of the day's calories. Your body cannot use them all while you are asleep, and so the calories may linger and diminish your appetite in the morning. A possible solution is to cut back on your evening meal and snacks, allowing for a hearty breakfast and a more balanced spread of calories during the day.

A second reason for lack of hunger in the morning is that the body may not be entirely awake. The digestive system is still at rest and the appetite is low. A possible solution is to allow time for stretching or wake-up exercises or just to allow time, in general, for your body to awaken before mealtime.

Other excuses commonly given for missing breakfast include:

- Not enough time to eat breakfast
- Distinterest in foods frequently served at breakfast
- Longtime habit of skipping breakfast
- Cutting down on meals to control weight
- Parents working irregular hours so children must prepare own meals

There should be no excuse for missing breakfast. It can be a very simple meal (often with no cooking involved); it can be prepared and eaten in a few minutes; and it can consist of foods different from the typical fare for variety and for those who are watching their weight.

Breakfast can make an important contribution of nutrients as well as calories. Nutritionists recommend that approximately one-third of an individual's daily requirement of both calories and nutrients be provided at breakfast. In terms of food groups, this means at least one serving from the Milk-Cheese group, one serving from the Fruit-Vegetable group, one serving from the Bread-Cereal group, and possibly one serving from the Meat-Poultry-Fish-Beans group. Any of these (or similar) menus provide a good breakfast:

1 cup skim milk 1 slice whole-wheat toast with   2 Tbsp. peanut butter ½ cup tomato juice

1 slice pumpernickel bread with 1 ounce melted cheese and 1 slice tomato, browned on top ½ grapefruit

1 banana smoothie
  (½ cup orange juice, ½ cup yogurt, 1
  banana, and ½ cup milk blended)
1 bran muffin

1 scrambled egg 1 slice toast with melted cheese ½ cup orange juice

¾ cup cereal with milk and sliced peaches 1 cup hot chocolate

---

Before beginning this unit, take an informal survey to see how students feel about breakfast and whether or not they eat a nutritious breakfast on most mornings.

Notice your students' energy and concentration level as lunch time approaches. You may see that those students who generally eat a nutritious breakfast are better able to maintain their energy and concentration throughout the morning than are their classmates who do not eat breakfast.

Research studies have shown that children and adults who had eaten a nutritious breakfast exhibited improved physical and mental performance. Breakfast has also been shown to influence

- The amount and accuracy of work done in the later morning hours
- Weight control (because there is less tendency to overeat later in the day)
- The number of accidents at school and work

School personnel have noted irritability, lethargy, and restlessness in children who do not eat breakfast before leaving home.

BASIC ACTIVITY

Time Needed: Two class periods

Materials Needed: Sheet 12-1: "No-Breakfast Cue Cards"
Sheet 12-2: "Mix-and-Match Breakfast Menus"
Sheets 12-3 through 12-4: "Rate Your Breakfasts"
Quiz Sheets 12-1 through 12-2

Class Period 1

1. To introduce the importance of a nutritious breakfast, have students engage in a role-playing activity. Make one copy of Sheet 12-1, "No-Breakfast Cue Cards," which describes the possible symptoms of an individual who has missed breakfast:

> #1–A person with a headache
> #2–A person who is sleepy
> #3–A person who cannot concentrate
> #4–A person who has a stomachache
> #5–A person who is irritable, grumpy, or cranky
> #6–A person who is aggressive and gets into fights or arguments

2. Cut the sheet into six cards.

3. Have students role play the people described on the cue cards. Then ask the students to role play any other symptoms that they think might be caused by skipping breakfast.

4. Discuss the reasons why breakfast is important. In the discussion, emphasize the following ideas:

   a. If one meal is skipped, it is difficult to consume adequate nutrients and calories in the few remaining hours of the day.

   b. Eating a large meal late in the day to make up for missing breakfast is not a good idea because it overloads the system.

   c. Breakfast can increase attention span, improve learning, improve attitude, and make you feel better overall.

5. Distribute Sheet 12-2, "Mix-and-Match Breakfast Menus" and have the students use them as a note-keeping device. List on the chalkboard all of the foods students can think of that may be eaten at breakfast.

6. Have students categorize the foods under food group headings on the board. Elicit responses that cover as many different breakfast foods as possible. Suggest unique breakfast foods if students do not offer them.

7. Break the class into small groups, or pair students up, or have them work on an individual basis to select foods from each column to form three different breakfast menus.

8. Discuss the various breakfast menus. Vote for the favorite.

Class Period 2

1. Prepare the breakfast that was voted as the favorite during the last class. Also prepare an unusual breakfast.

2. Have the students describe and rate each breakfast on Sheets 12-3 through 12-4, "Rate Your Breakfasts." The last part of this activity asks students to write a paragraph comparing and contrasting the two breakfasts.

3. Proceed with the "Advanced Activity" if you wish, or use the quiz discussed in step 4.

4. **Evaluation:** Distribute Quiz Sheets 12-1 through 12-2 and have students complete them independently. Discuss the answers as a class.

ADVANCED ACTIVITY

Time Needed: One class period

Materials Needed: Chart D: "Food Composition Table for Selected Nutrients"
Quiz Sheets 12-1 through 12-2

1. Write the following breakfast menu on the chalkboard:

> 1 glass orange juice
> 2 scrambled eggs
> 2 slices whole-wheat toast
> 1 glass lowfat milk

2. Using the menu above as a reference point, ask students to answer the following questions concerning the importance of breakfast:

- Looking at the menu on the board, would you call this a breakfast, a lunch, or a dinner meal? (*Answer:* Breakfast)

- Would you say that this meal was nutritious? Why? (*Answer:* Yes, because it provides one-third of the U.S. RDA for each of the Iron CaPAC nutrients.)

- Do you think breakfast is an important meal? Why? (*Answer:* Yes, because breakfast provides the body with nutrients following a ten- to twelve-hour fast.)

- How many of you skipped breakfast this morning? (*Answers vary*)

- Why didn't you have breakfast? (*Answers vary*)

- Of those who had breakfast, what did you eat? (*Answers vary*)

3. Further discuss the topic of breakfast and its importance: Breakfast is an important meal that we should not miss. Often we get locked into the types of foods we think we should eat for breakfast, but any combination of foods can provide a nutritious breakfast if it provides a balance of nutrients.

4. Have each student create three breakfast menus using unconventional breakfast foods. Each menu should provide one-third or more of the U.S. RDA for Iron CaPAC nutrients. Students will need to use Chart D, "Food Composition Table for Selected Nutrients." Have the students give each menu a descriptive title—for example, "Old Faithful" for the traditional breakfast.

5. List the suggestions of the unconventional breakfast foods described below on the chalkboard for students who are in need of idea-starters.

- Scrambled eggs with vegetables (tomatoes, onions, green pepper)

- Eggs sprinkled with grated cheese

- French toast, waffles, or pancakes topped with peanut butter or cottage cheese

- Various fruit combinations

- Cheese cubes with fruit

- Split leftover rolls, biscuits, or muffins, and toast in oven with bacon, sausage, ham, and/or cheese on top

- Cottage cheese blended with pineapple spread on toast
- Tuna topped with melted cheese on toast
- Peanut butter and banana slices on toast
- English muffin pizza

6. When the menus are completed, display them on a bulletin board, bind them into a class book, or otherwise make them available to the entire class so that students can examine the diversity of food choices.

7. **Evaluation:** Distribute Quiz Sheets 12-1 through 12-2 and have students complete them independently. Discuss the answers as a class.

FOLLOW-UP ACTIVITIES

1. Have students research the kinds of breakfast foods people in other countries enjoy. If possible, prepare some of these breakfasts.

2. Have students investigate the school breakfast program: What is it? How does it help students improve their nutrition? If your school does not have such a program, why not?

3. Have students role play in pairs: One student does not want to eat breakfast, and the other student is trying to convince the first one to eat breakfast. After several minutes, have students reverse roles and, perhaps, also change partners.

NO-BREAKFAST CUE CARDS

1 Person with a headache

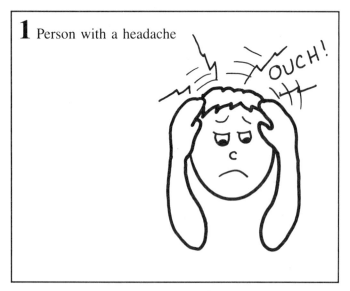

2 Person who is sleepy

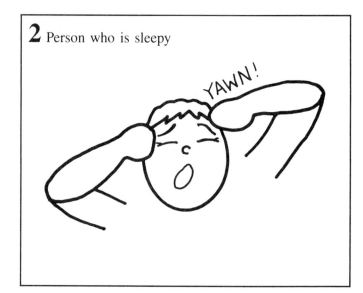

3 Person who cannot concentrate

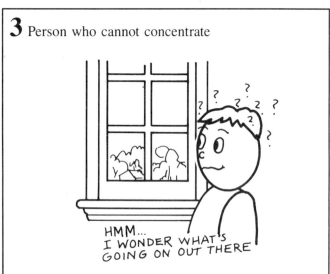

4 Person with stomachache

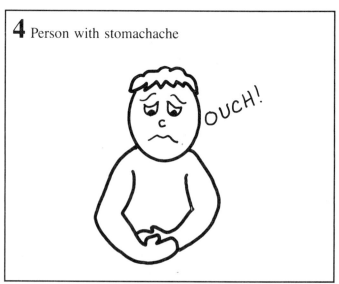

5 Person who is irritable, grumpy, or cranky

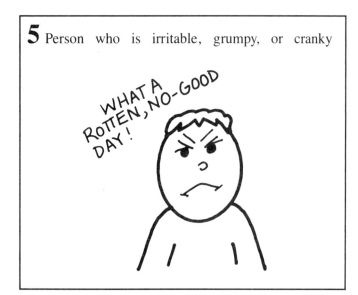

6 Person who is aggressive and gets into fights or arguments

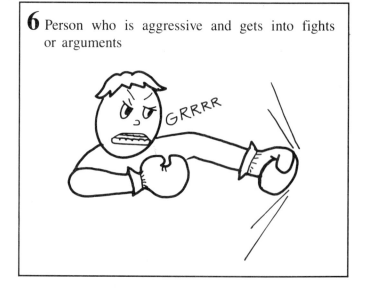

MIX-AND-MATCH BREAKFAST MENUS

Directions: List foods you would like to eat for breakfast under each of the following food group headings. Remember: For the best nutrition, select foods that provide a lot of nutrients for a few calories. Note that presweetened cereals are a less nutritious choice because they contain a lot of sugar (calories). Be creative with your food choices! Traditional breakfast foods (like orange juice, eggs, bacon, and toast) are not the only foods you can eat in the morning.

Milk- Cheese Group	Meat- Poultry- Fish-Beans Group	Fruit- Vegetable Group	Bread- Cereal Group	Fats- Sweets- Alcohol Group

A nutritious breakfast should include:
1 serving from the Milk-Cheese group
0–1 serving from the Meat-Poultry-Fish-Beans group
1 serving from the Fruit-Vegetable group
1 serving from the Bread-Cereal group

Directions: Plan three breakfast menus below using the correct number of servings from each of the food groups listed above. Use the breakfast items you have selected. No food may be used more than once.

Breakfast 1:	Breakfast 2:	Breakfast 3:

RATE YOUR BREAKFASTS

Directions: Answer the following questions about the two different breakfasts you prepared. List the breakfast menus here:

Favorite Breakfast	**Unusual Breakfast**
_____	_____
_____	_____
_____	_____
_____	_____
_____	_____
_____	_____

Nutrition:

1. Did this meal contain at least:

_____ 1 serving Milk-Cheese group

_____ 0–1 serving Meat-Poultry-Fish-Beans group

_____ 1 serving Fruit-Vegetable group

_____ 1 serving Bread-Cereal group

Appeal:

2. Describe the <u>textures</u> of the foods:

3. Describe the <u>colors</u> of the foods:

4. Describe the <u>temperatures</u> of the foods:

5. Describe the <u>flavors</u> of the foods:

_____ 1 serving Milk-Cheese group

_____ 0–1 serving Meat-Poultry-Fish-Beans group

_____ 1 serving Fruit-Vegetable group

_____ 1 serving Bread-Cereal group

| **Favorite Breakfast** | **Unusual Breakfast** |

6. Describe the <u>sizes</u> and <u>shapes</u> of the foods:

_____   _____

_____   _____

7. Describe whether or not you liked the meal. Why or why not?

_____   _____

_____   _____

_____   _____

Preparation Time:

8. How long did the meal take to prepare?

_____ minutes   _____ minutes

Preparation skills:

9. How difficult was the meal to prepare?

____ extremely   ____ average   ____ extremely   ____ average

____ somewhat   ____ easy   ____ somewhat   ____ easy

Cost:

10. How expensive was the meal?

____ extremely   ____ average   ____ extremely   ____ average

____ somewhat   ____ easy   ____ somewhat   ____ easy

11. Would you prepare this menu at home? Why or why not?

_____   _____

_____   _____

_____   _____

12. Compare and contrast the two breakfasts.

_____

_____

_____

_____

_____

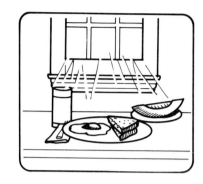

QUIZ
START THE DAY BETTER WITH BREAKFAST

1. Place a check mark beside each breakfast menu below that provides one-third of the recommended servings from the Daily Food Guide. For each breakfast that does *not* meet the requirements, write in menu changes to meet the requirements.

   a. _____ 1 slice whole-wheat toast
   ¾ cup cereal with milk

   b. _____ 1 cup hot chocolate
   ¾ cup oatmeal with
   apples and raisins

   c. _____ 2 slices leftover cheese pizza
   small glass of tomato juice
   1 glass of milk

   d. _____ melted cheese sandwich
   3 slices of tomato

   e. _____ 2 scrambled eggs
   small glass of orange juice
   1 pumpernickel muffin

   f. _____ ¾ cup refried beans
   2 tortillas
   1 glass of milk
   1 apple

2. Write one breakfast menu that meets the requirements for a nutritious breakfast.

3. List two reasons why breakfast is important:

   1. _____

   2. _____

4. Karen can't eat as much as her father. She usually has black coffee and dry toast. Does Karen eat a good breakfast?
   a. Yes, because she has reduced the calories.
   b. No, because girls should not drink coffee.
   c. No, because none of the Iron CaPAC nutrients are adequate.
   d. No, because good breakfasts include eggs.

_____ 5. Pat likes to have "one" food for breakfast. An example of "one" food is a bowl of whole-grain cereal in one cup of milk. On top is a mixture of raisins, prunes, and blueberries. Does Pat include good sources of Iron CaPAC in the "one" food?

    a. No, because there is no source of Vitamin C.

    b. No, because there is no source of iron.

    c. No, because there is no source of protein.

    d. Yes, because Iron CaPAC sources were used.

_____ 6. Ricco likes to make casseroles. One of his breakfast casseroles includes rice, beans, tomatoes, and asparagus tips, covered with melted cheese. Since he uses diced chili peppers, he drinks water to cool his mouth. Is this a nutritious breakfast?

    a. No, because there is no source of protein.

    b. No, because there is no source of Vitamin A.

    c. No, because there is no source of calcium.

    d. Yes, because Iron CaPAC sources were used.

_____ 7. Hank usually picks up his "breakfast" on the way to school. He starts with a glass of milk while he dresses and eats a tomato while heading for Sam's Sandwich Shop where he picks up a "quarter pound" hamburger. What can you say about this breakfast?

    a. It has met one-third of the U.S. RDA for each of the Iron CaPAC nutrients.

    b. It is inadequate because there aren't eggs, orange juice, or cereal.

    c. The tomato provides Vitamin A but not Vitamin C.

    d. The breakfast is too low in iron.

_____ 8. Karen's father was raised on a farm. He believes that everyone should have a good breakfast. He has the same type of breakfast every morning: meat, eggs, oatmeal, toast, and coffee with cream. Would you agree that this is a good breakfast?

    a. Yes, because it includes meat and cereal.

    b. No, because very little Vitamin C is provided.

    c. No, because foods supplying iron are missing.

    d. Yes, because it includes all the Iron CaPAC nutrients.

Unit 13: Your School Lunch

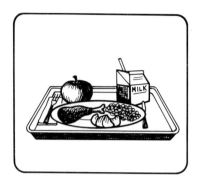

CONCEPTS

–Nutritious meals can be selected in most school cafeterias.

–The School Lunch Pattern includes milk, meat or meat alternate, vegetable and/or fruit, and bread or bread alternate.

OBJECTIVES

–Students will be able to select nutritious foods from school cafeteria menus.

–Students will be able to propose one idea for improving the school cafeteria lunch.

–Students will be able to recognize a School Lunch Pattern.

TEACHER'S UNIT INTRODUCTION

The National School Lunch Program was originally designed with two purposes: to solve the hunger problem among school-aged children and to make use of the excess food grown by U.S. farmers. Today, the lunch offered in schools participating in the National School Lunch Program must follow what is called a School Lunch Pattern. Serving sizes vary according to the age of the child being served. The following School Lunch Pattern is recommended for children nine years old and older:*

Milk	• Unflavored, fluid lowfat, skim, or buttermilk must be offered • Whole or flavored milk may be offered	½ pint
Meat or Meat Alternate	• Lean meat, poultry, or fish • Cheese • Large egg • Cooked dry beans or peas • Peanut butter (or an equivalent quantity of any combination of any of the above)	2–3 ounce 2–3 ounce 2–3 ounce 1-1½ cup 4–6 Tablespoons
Vegetable or Fruit	• Two or more servings of vegetable or fruit or both	¾ cup
Bread or Bread Alternate	• Must be enriched or whole grain • Bread alternates incude rice, macaroni, noodles, other pasta products, other cereal products, such as bulgur or corn grits, and products such as biscuits, rolls, or muffins	8–10 servings/week

*The smaller serving sizes apply to children nine to twelve years old; the larger serving sizes apply to children twelve years or older.

The school must operate the lunch program on a nonprofit basis, must serve meals at regular meal hours, must provide lunches free or at a reduced cost to those students unable to pay, and must serve meals that meet nutritional guidelines. In order to encourage schools to participate, the U.S. Department of Agriculture provides help in the form of surplus food and supplies, money, and technical advice.

The National School Lunch Program has the potential to teach students about food and nutrition in a direct and practical way. If properly operated, it gives students the opportunity to observe and participate in at least one nutritionally balanced meal each day. The idea that "you learn by doing" can be put into practice.

Many school lunch programs, however, do not meet these expectations. The lunches are planned and prepared according to traditional menus and ideas. For lack of better funding, schools are encouraged to use government surplus foods, such as lard, fruit in heavy syrup, and canned meats, that may be less nutritious or less palatable choices than other foods. Although some school lunch programs may be difficult, if not impossible, to change, students and parents should be encouraged to become active voices in developing their lunch program. This unit can serve as a focal point for a campaign to improve your school lunch program.

BASIC ACTIVITY

Time Needed: Two class periods

Materials Needed: Sheets 13-1 through 13-3: "Your School Lunch"
Copies of your school's lunch menus from the past week
Quiz Sheet 13-1

Class Period 1

1. Invite the school food service supervisor to visit the class and discuss the school lunch program. Make sure to give the supervisor a copy of Sheets 13-1 through 13-3, "Your School Lunch," beforehand so that the material presented during the discussion coincides with the material presented on the worksheets.

2. Have each student prepare at least one question to ask. The following is a list of possible questions that may help students who have trouble thinking of their own:

- What is the purpose of the School Lunch Program?
- Describe the School Lunch Pattern and give examples from our menus.
- Does the School Lunch Pattern provide good nutrition for the students?
- Does the atmosphere in the cafeteria promote good eating habits?
- Who plans the school lunch menu?
- When planning the menu, what kinds of things are taken into account (for example, the nutrition, taste, texture, color, sizes and shapes, and "saleability" of the foods)?
- Who controls the budget for the School Lunch Program?
- How much input into the Program comes from students, parents, teachers, and administrators?
- Would you like more, or less, input from any of these groups? Which ones?

- The U.S. Dietary Guidelines state that we should be eating less sugar, more fruits, vegetables, and whole grains, less salt, less fat, and fewer calories. Has the School Lunch Pattern changed since these goals were described?

- What factors influence "plate waste"? Is there a conscious effort to reduce plate waste?

- What do you think about prepackaged hot lunches for the school program?

- Is there any effort to use homemade items for the school program?

- What do you think about vegetarian lunches? Are there provisions in the School Lunch Pattern especially for vegetarian students?

3. Have the students take notes while the supervisor is speaking.

4. Have the students translate their notes into an outline form. They may then be able to use the outlines to help create ideas for improving the lunch program in your school.

Class Period 2

1. Have students read and complete Sheets 13-1 through 13-3, "Your School Lunch," using copies of your school's lunch menus from the previous week. Students may finish the worksheets as a homework assignment, if necessary.

2. Discuss Sheets 13-1 through 13-3 and the outlines that students made from their talk with the food service supervisor. Be sure to emphasize their ideas for improving the lunch program in your school. If possible, allow and encourage students to present their best ideas to the food service supervisor for adoption.

3. Proceed with the "Advanced Activity" if you wish, or else use the quiz mentioned in step 4.

4. **Evaluation:** Distribute Quiz Sheet 13-1 and have students complete it independently. Discuss the answers as a class.

ADVANCED ACTIVITY

Time Needed: Two class periods

Materials Needed: Resource materials (described in step 1)
                              Writing materials
                              Quiz Sheet 13-1

Class Period 1

1. Have students, individually or in pairs, investigate the National School Lunch Program by using at least three *different* resources from the following:

- *Library Research*—Textbooks, magazines, journals, government documents.

- *Interviews*—School food service supervisor or other personnel, administrators, school board members, PTA members, school nutritionist or dietitian.

- *Surveys*—Students, parents, teachers.

- *Record-keeping and Evaluation*—Record foods served in the school lunch and evaluate them according to established guidelines (School Lunch Pattern, Daily Food Guide, Nutrient Analysis) or other quality guidelines.

- *Comparisons*—Observe other institutional food settings (hospitals, restaurants, fast-food businesses, other cafeterias) and compare to the school lunch program.

- *Letter-writing*—Write to government agencies and others who control or investigate guidelines for school food service programs.

2. Students should elicit the aid of the librarian in doing their research.

Class Period 2

1. Have students prepare and present oral reports on their findings.

2. Conduct a large-group discussion on the pros and cons of the school lunch program.

3. Have students issue a statement to their principal, school board director, and/or school food service supervisor that describes ways in which the school lunch program could be improved.

4. **Evaluation:** Distribute Quiz Sheet 13-1 and have students complete it independently. Discuss the answers as a class.

FOLLOW-UP ACTIVITIES

1. Have students report the results of their investigations of the school lunch program at a parent/ teacher meeting. You may want to invite a nutritionist/dietitian to address the issue of nutrition education in the schools. Invite other interested health professionals, such as physicians, nurses, dentists, or health educators. Publicize the meeting in advance to encourage attendance. Afterward, report the outcome of the meeting in the local newspaper.

2. Encourage the school food service personnel to participate in a Nutrition Day, Nutrition Week, or Nutrition Month. Ask them to prepare an especially nutritious meal that the students have planned. Publicize the event through parent/teacher announcements that describe interesting nutrition facts and that are related to the particular theme they have chosen. Send information home to the parents as well.

3. If possible, arrange to have students help plan, prepare, and/or serve meals in the cafeteria. Some schools are not willing or able to allow this kind of participation, but it is worth the asking.

4. Have students write letters to the editors of local newspapers that describe their concerns about the school lunch program.

5. Discuss the school breakfast program, its purpose, value, guidelines, and the possibilities for introducing a school breakfast program in your school.

7. In the school cafeteria, have weekly bulletin boards or displays on nutrition, that use the school lunch menu for a starting point. Also use the daily bulletin or school intercom for such messages. For example, each week could be reserved for presenting a different nutrient. Be sure to include a little information about its background and to identify which foods being served that week contain the nutrient.

7. Make signs that give nutrient values for each food on the cafeteria menu. You could use bar graphs similar to the ones presented in Unit 9.

8. Invite the school food service supervisor to speak on the problems encountered in preparing foods in large quantities and on how these problems are solved.

YOUR SCHOOL LUNCH

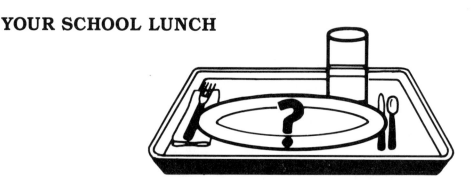

How much do you know about your school lunch? You probably know what foods were served today in the cafeteria. You probably also know which foods are your favorites and which ones you do not like at all. But did you know that students have been eating lunch in school cafeterias since the 1940s? The menus and foods have changed over time, but the basic plan is much the same as it was back then.

The basic school lunch must include certain types and amounts of foods. The government calls this a School Lunch Pattern. Schools that serve lunches following the School Lunch Pattern receive help from the government in the form of food, supplies, money, and technical advice. The following is a chart of the School Lunch Pattern for students ages nine and older.

SCHOOL LUNCH PATTERN
(for ages nine and above)

		Recommended Portion	Minimum Portion
Milk	Unflavored, fluid lowfat, skim, or buttermilk must be offered Whole or flavored milk may be offered	½ pint	½ pint
Meat or Meat Alternate	Lean meat, poultry, or fish Cheese Large egg Cooked dry beans or peas Peanut butter (Or an equivalent quantity of any combination of any of the above)	3 ounces 3 ounces 3 1½ cups 6 tablespoons	2 ounces 2 ounces 2 1 cup 4 tablespoons
Vegetable or Fruit	Two or more servings of vegetable or fruit or both	¾ cup	¾ cup
Bread or Bread Alternate	Must be enriched or whole-grain Bread alternates include rice, macaroni, noodles, other pasta products, other cereal products, such as bulgur or corn grits, and products such as biscuits, rolls, or muffins	10 servings/week	8 servings/week

In addition to the regular lunch, schools may offer other food choices, such as salads or salad bars, sandwiches, soups, and similar a la carte items.

Some schools have Youth Advisory Councils (YACS) to help decide what foods will be served. YACS are groups of students who work together with the school food service supervisor in planning the menus. The students give suggestions about the kinds of foods they would like to eat. If you get involved in the YACS, the food served in the cafeteria *really* becomes your school lunch!

Now that you have studied a little bit about nutrition and know a little more about your school lunch, think about the lunch program at *your* school. Answer the following questions as honestly as you can.

Directions: Using your school's lunch menus from last week, check the lunches to see if they meet the requirements of the School Lunch Pattern described on Sheet 13-1. Check off each of the four requirements on each day's menu.

1. Do the menus at your school follow the School Lunch Pattern? _____ Yes _____ No

2. Does your school offer foods other than the regular lunch? _____ Yes _____ No

   If yes, what other foods does it offer? _____

   _____

   If no, what other foods would you like to have offered? _____

   _____

3. What do you like best about your school lunch program? _____

   _____

   _____

4. What is your major complaint about your school lunch program? _____

   _____

   _____

5. Name several *specific* ways in which your school lunch program could be improved:

   _____

   _____

   _____

6. Do any students in your school help plan, prepare, or serve the school lunch?

   _____ Yes _____ No

7. What do you think is the purpose of having a school lunch program? _____

   _____

   _____

8. How would you feel if there were no school lunch program? _____

   _____

   _____

9. What did (or will) you eat today for lunch? _____

_____

10. Did you eat a lunch that was provided by your school? _____ Yes _____ No

Did you eat a lunch that was carried from home?   _____ Yes _____ No

Did you eat lunch in a restaurant?   _____ Yes _____ No

11. Did your lunch meet the requirements of the School Lunch Pattern? _____ Yes _____ No

12. What could you add to, or subtract from, this lunch to make it fit the School Lunch Pattern?

Add	Subtract

13. Do you think that your lunch was good for you (nutritious)? _____ Yes _____ No

14. Why or why not? _____

_____

_____

_____

QUIZ
YOUR SCHOOL LUNCH

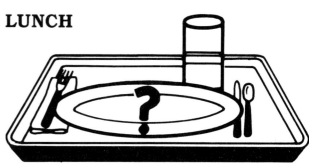

1. Name the four requirements of the School Lunch Pattern:

    1. _____   2. _____

    3. _____   4. _____

2. What did you eat for lunch today?_____

    _____

    What did you eat for lunch yesterday?_____

    _____

3. Evaluate your lunch today and your lunch yesterday according to the School Lunch Pattern requirements:

    a. Are any requirements missing? _____ Yes _____ No

        If yes, what requirements are missing? _____

        _____

    b. If you missed some requirements, what could you have added to make each lunch complete?_____

        _____

4. Place a check mark in front of each menu below if it follows the School Lunch Pattern. If it does not meet the requirements, change the menu so that it does.

    _____ a. hamburger on a bun
              tomato slices
              tossed salad greens   _____ d. macaroni and cheese
              peach cobbler   stewed tomatoes
              milk   whole-wheat bread
                                                            sliced pears and cookies
                                                            milk

    _____ b. beef vegetable soup
              peanut butter sandwich
              carrot and celery sticks   _____ e. cheese pizza
              apple   tossed salad
              milk   orange or banana

    _____ c. spaghetti and meat sauce
              Italian bread
              yellow cake
              milk

Unit 14: The Good Goodies

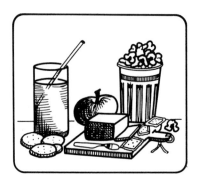

CONCEPTS

–Snacks can contribute valuable nutrients to the total diet.

–Snacks can be relatively easy to plan and prepare.

–A nutritious snack contains foods in which nutrients are dense in relation to calories.

OBJECTIVES

–Students will be able to identify nutritious snacks.

–Students will be able to plan and prepare a nutritious snack.

TEACHER'S UNIT INTRODUCTION

Ever since you were a kid, you've probably heard that snacks are bad for you. Are they? Well, yes ...and no. Yes, if you gobble up foods that are loaded with sugar, salt, and fat but that are low in protein, vitamins, and minerals. But, if you eat snacks in order to supply your body with nutritious foods that your regular meals are lacking, then snacking is a great idea.

Everyone knows you need certain foods for a balanced diet. You can use the Daily Food Guide to select nutritious meals. It makes sense to add snacks from these food groups to your daily diet, particularly if these snacks include foods that you've been missing at mealtimes. A glass of juice after school or before bedtime, for example, contributes to the Fruit-Vegetable group. Peanut butter crackers or an orange, at any time, makes good nutritional sense.

Snacking isn't just milk and cookies after school. It's also munching on an apple while waiting for the bus, nibbling popcorn while watching TV, or eating cheese and crackers at a party. Some of us snack a little; some of us snack around the clock. But whatever your snacking frequency may be, it is *what* you eat that counts. And keeping your eye on your main goal—a balanced daily diet—is most important of all.

In this activity, students will evaluate the nutritional value of snack foods by using the U.S. RDAs. Students will need to know how to use tables, how to calculate percentages, and how to construct bar graphs. You may need to review some of these basic tasks as you describe the activity. The U.S. RDA percentages for nutrients in foods can be found directly on many food labels or in Chart D, "Food Composition Table for Selected Nutrients." To calculate the U.S. RDA percentages for any nutrient in a snack food, use the format described in Unit 7. It may be helpful to have students work in pairs or in small groups.

BASIC ACTIVITY

Time Needed: Two class periods

Materials Needed: Sheet 14-1: "Sample U.S. RDA Bar Graphs"
Sheet 9-1: "U.S. RDA Bar Graph"
Chart D: "Food Composition Table for Selected Nutrients"
Calculators *(optional)*
Quiz Sheet 14-1

Class Period 1

1. First elicit from students a definition of a nutritious snack. Then, provide this definition: A *nutritious snack* is one that contributes nutrients, as well as calories, to the diet. But how many nutrients, and how much of each, should be provided? One widely used rule of thumb for defining a nutritious snack identifies it as one in which the nutrients are dense in relation to the calories.
Complete definitions of a nutritious snack food include:

a. A food is nutritious if the U.S. RDA percentages for at least *four* nutrients in a portion of the food are equal to or greater than the percentage of calories for the same amount of food.

b. A food is nutritious if the U.S. RDA percentages of at least *two* nutrients in a portion of the food are equal to or greater than *twice* the percentage of calories for the same amount of food.

2. Review and define any terms in this definition or in Chart D, "Food Composition Table for Selected Nutrients," that are unfamiliar to the students.

3. Demonstrate how to determine if several different snack foods are nutritious. Examples are shown on Sheet 14-1, "Sample U.S. RDA Bar Graphs." The calories and percentages of the U.S. RDAs are given in Chart D.

a. *Peanuts in shells—10:* 70 calories = 3 percent (of an average total daily calorie intake of 2,500 calories). According to Sheet 14-1, two nutrients—protein and niacin—have percentages that are more than twice the calorie percentage. Therefore, peanuts in shells are a nutritious snack (according to definition 1b. above).

b. *Yogurt, whole milk—1 cup:* 140 calories = 6 percent (of an average total daily calorie intake of 2,500 calories). According to Sheet 14-1, four nutrients—protein, Vitamin A, riboflavin, and calcium—are equal to, or exceed, the calorie percentage. Therefore, yogurt is a nutritious snack (according to definition 1a. above).

c. *Devil's food cake with chocolate icing—1 piece:* 350 calories = 14 percent (of an average total daily calorie intake of 2,500 calories). According to Sheet 14-1, none of the nutrients reach 14 percent of the U.S. RDAs. Therefore, this cake is not a nutritious snack.

4. Distribute a few copies of Sheet 9-1 to each individual, or to each pair of students, or to each small group. Have students select various snack foods to analyze using the method described.

5. On the chalkboard, place the headings "Nutritious," "Nonnutritious," and "Other." Place each of the foods analyzed under one of the headings according to definitions 1a. and 1b. above. If you have determined that a food is nonnutritious, but you believe it has good nutritional qualities that make it an exception to the definitions, place it under the "Other" heading. For example, according to the two definitions, an apple is not a nutritious food because, while it provides 3 percent of the U.S. RDA for calories, it contains only *three* nutrients (Vitamin A, Vitamin C, thiamin) that equal or exceed that level. However an apple *is* a nutritious food, according to most nutritionists, because it is low in calories

and because it contains small amounts of many nutrients, trace minerals, and fiber. Also, an apple is a *whole* food, which means it is minimally processed and not fabricated. Other foods in the "Other" category would include certain desserts, such as ice cream and pudding, which are better snack choices than cakes, cookies, and pastries, because desserts such as ice cream and pudding contribute quite a bit of calcium. However, they do contain added sugar which adds calories.

6. Discuss the foods in the "Other" category, which are often considered "nutritious" but which are labeled "nonnutritious" by the two definitions. There are a variety of reasons why this definition of "nutritious" versus "nonnutritious" does not always work. Encourage students to discuss these reasons and also possible solutions to the problem.

7. Have students plan a nutritious snack for Class Period 2. Use the resources from the References/Resources section at the end of this book for recipe ideas.

Class Period 2

1. Have students prepare and eat the snack.

2. Have the students who prepared the snack explain to the class why the snack is nutritious. In their explanation, students should cite the percentage of nutrients and calories.

3. Proceed with the "Advanced Activity," if you wish, or else use Quiz Sheet 14-1.

4. **Evaluation:** Distribute Quiz Sheet 14-1 and have students complete it independently. Discuss the answers as a class.

ADVANCED ACTIVITY

Time Needed: One class period

Materials Needed: Sheet 14-1: "Sample U.S. RDA Bar Graphs"
Sheet 9-1: "U.S. RDA Bar Graph"
Food composition tables (see References/Resources)
Calculators *(optional)*
Quiz Sheet 14-1

1. Have students work in pairs or in small groups to brainstorm a new definition of *nutritious*. Instruct them to use resources such as food composition tables and introductory nutrition texts (see the References/Resources section at the end of this book).

2. Have each pair or group record their new definition and have them cite examples that fit it. Have them also cite exceptions to their new defintion—that is, foods that are generally considered to be nutritious but that may be labeled "nonnutritious" by their new definition, and foods that may be labeled "nutritious" by the new definition but that have questionable qualities.

3. Begin a large-group discussion so that students may share their definitions with the class.

4. With your assistance, have students decide on the best definition.

5. As an optional activity, have students publicize nutritious versus nonnutritious foods in the school cafeteria, in the school store, or near the vending machines. Students might make posters, banners, or taped announcements for this activity.

6. **Evaluation:** Distribute Quiz Sheet 14-1 and have the students complete it independently. Discuss the answers as a class.

FOLLOW-UP ACTIVITIES

1. Stage a debate surrounding a "questionable" snack food. One team will support the idea that the food is nutritious; the other team will support the idea that it is not nutritious. Give students time to prepare their arguments. Keep score as each side makes a valid point about its view. Foods to consider for the debate might be: apples, bacon, potato chips, ice cream, milkshakes, apple pie, crackers, fruit cocktail, and grape juice.

2. Conduct a *Good Goodies* recipe contest. Each student or student pair, finds or creates a snack recipe. You may choose to have a panel of judges rate either the recipe or the actual prepared snack. Snacks may be made at home or in school. The winning recipe may be published in the school or local newspaper, along with an article about the contest.

3. Have students compile a booklet of *Good Goodie* recipes and sell or freely distribute it within the school or community.

4. Set up a game show called "Nutrition Password." Divide the class into two teams. Prepare lists of snack foods ahead of time (students can do this, but must eliminate themselves from the competition). Each list should include three or four snack foods around a single theme. For example, under the theme of "cold snacks" might be yogurt, ice cream, and orange juice. Pass out the first list to one team. That team's members must use single-word clues to describe each food in succession to the other team, which guesses each food in turn. When all of the foods have been guessed, the theme must be guessed. Score keeping is optional.

SAMPLE U.S. RDA BAR GRAPHS

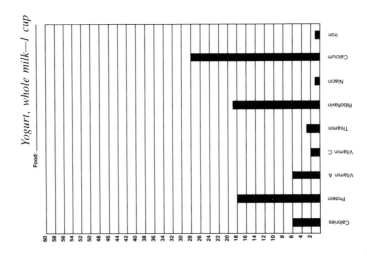

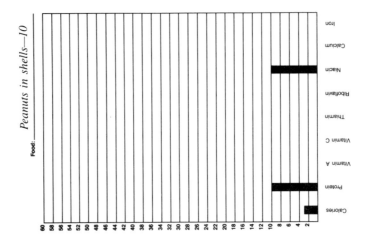

QUIZ
THE GOOD GOODIES

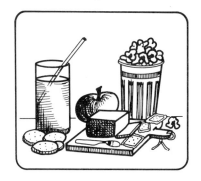

1. Using the table below and the definitions learned in class, state whether each of the following snack foods is nutritious (N), or nonnutritious (NN). Remember, there are *two* definitions that may be used. Show your work on the back of this sheet.

FOOD COMPOSITION TABLE FOR SELECTED NUTRIENTS

FOOD	CALORIES	%†	PROTEIN	VITAMIN A	VITAMIN C	THIAMIN	RIBO-FLAVIN	NIACIN	CALCIUM	IRON
				Percentages U.S. RDA						
apple, 1	80	3	*	3	9	3	2	1	1	1
apple pie, 1 piece	400	16	5	4	5	10	5	6	1	6
bagel, 1	165	7	9	*	*	9	6	6	*	7
bread, cracked wheat, 1 slice	65	3	3	*	*	2	1	4	2	2
cake, plain, 1 slice	320	13	8	9	*	8	7	4	6	5
carrot, raw, 1 medium	35	1	1	178	11	3	2	2	3	3
celery, raw, 1 stalk	5	*	1	2	6	1	1	1	2	1
chocolate chip cookie, 1	60	2	1	*	*	1	1	1	*	1
gelatin (Jell-O), ½ cup	70	3	3	*	*	*	*	*	*	*
grape juice, 4 ounce	85	3	*	*	*	3	2	1	1	2
peanut butter, 1 tablespoon	90	4	6	*	*	1	1	12	1	2

†percentage of 2,500 calories in average daily intake

*none, or less than 1%

Example: __apple__ 80 calories = 3%. According to the table, only 3 nutrients—Vitamin A, Vitamin C, and thiamin—are equal to, or greater than, the calorie value. Therefore, *according to the definition,* an apple is not nutritious.

_____ a. apple pie   _____ e. carrot   _____ h. gelatin (Jell-O)

_____ b. bagel   _____ f. celery   _____ i. grape juice

_____ c. bread, cracked wheat _____ g. chocolate chip cookie   _____ j. peanut butter

_____ d. cake, plain

2. Draw a circle around each food above that is labeled nonnutritious by definition, but which you think is actually nutritious. Then write one sentence telling why you think this definition of nutritious does not always work.

Unit 15: Designing a Personal Diet Plan

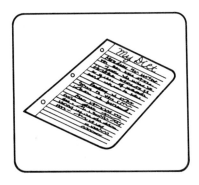

CONCEPTS

–An individual's selection of food is influenced by social, psychological, and biological needs.

–A wide variety of individual food preferences can be used when designing a nutritious diet.

–A nutritious diet can be designed by using the Daily Food Guide.

–A nutritious diet can also be designed by evaluating the diet according to a Nutrient Analysis Method.

OBJECTIVES

–Students will be able to describe the biological, psychological, and social needs a particular food fulfills.

–Students will be able to identify which foods belong to each of the food groups in the Daily Food Guide.

–Students will be able to compare their dietary intake for a specific twenty-four-hour period against an accepted guideline for a nutritious diet and will be able to evaluate the adequacy of their diet.

–Students will be able to plan a day's menu that conforms to an accepted guideline (Daily Food Guide or Nutrient Analysis Method) for a balanced diet.

TEACHER'S UNIT INTRODUCTION

Foodways is a term used to describe the traditional ways in which a society conducts activities connected with food. Foodways describe the reasons why people choose the foods they choose.

The many needs of individuals influence the foodways of a society. These needs can be divided into three main categories: biological, psychological, and social. Short descriptions and examples of each type of need will help to clarify the idea of foodways.

Biological needs are necessary to satisfy the body of an individual. You might think of biological needs as serving the cells, tissues, body organs, and physiological systems of an individual. Hunger is the craving or urgent need for food. Appetite refers either to an instinctive desire to eat, or to a certain taste, or preference, for a particular food. Both hunger and appetite can be satisfied by a variety of individual food choices. The nutritional needs of individuals are only a part of their biological needs.

Psychological needs may also be satisifed by food. Individuals may use food in response to a variety of emotions. Psychological needs differ from individual to individual.

1. *Conditioned response to foods.* Children are especially prone to conditioning by adults. Children may be coaxed or bribed to eat. They may be allowed to refuse food or may be forced to clean their plates. They may be made to feel guilty when they eat or when they do not eat. They may be taught to eat as much as they can, or they may be taught self-control. They may be exposed either to a wide or to a narrow variety of foods. Any of these experiences early in life may lead to conditioned responses to food later on. If children are taught to finish everything on their plates, without regard for hunger, they may, as adults, be conditioned to eat in response to many signals other than hunger.

2. *Emotional weapon or crutch.* Food is often used for emotional purposes, whether in the serving or in the partaking. For example, parents may withhold or lavish food on a child, or on other adults, in response to emotional needs for power or for love. People also use food as release from boredom, tension, sorrow, or from personal inadequacies.

3. *Food and memories.* Individuals can have pleasant or unpleasant memories associated with past experiences with foods. These memories will influence whether or not they will continue to eat those foods. Eating chicken soup when faced with a cold may have been associated with recovery, and so the soup becomes a much-enjoyed food. Likewise, being forced to eat cold, pasty oatmeal as a child may turn an individual against oatmeal forever.

4. *Food taboos and superstitions.* Most cultures have certain foods that are forbidden, or disregarded, for consumption. Food taboos usually exist for irrational or illogical reasons. Hindus are prohibited from eating beef. Zulu women will not drink milk while pregnant. Americans will not eat dog, cat, or horse meat. Superstitions about foods usually reflect the religious, cultural, or economic characteristics of a society, but they may also be linked strongly with an individual's psychological response to foods.

5. *Food and religion.* Food customs and habits are a part of nearly every religion. The communion service of the Christians and the Passover Seder of the Jews are two examples of the role that food plays as a part of religious custom.

Social needs of individuals are as important as biological and psychological needs in determining food choices. Individuals use food as a social status symbol. Foods that cost more, that are exotic, and that are difficult to acquire or prepare may be associated with higher status. Different groups of people regard different foods as having, or not having, status.

Food is also used as a source of communication with others. A parent communicates love for his or her children by serving favorite foods. Employees communicate respect for their bosses by serving expensive, high-quality foods when entertaining them. A teenager communicates rebelliousness, or individuality, by refusing to eat the foods that the rest of the family is consuming.

Food may also be associated with traditional sex roles. For example, males who feel a need to conform to such traditional roles may eat steak and potatoes; females may eat lighter, more feminine-oriented foods, such as salads and fruits.

Meals and foods can also be used to mark occasions or events. Turkey means Thanksgiving, cake with candles a birthday, champagne means a celebration, and coffee means a midmorning break.

Whatever the reason for food choices, an individual's habits are influenced by biological, psychological, and social needs. Many of these needs overlap. It is often difficult to say which need is being filled by the choice of a particular food. Learning about the various reasons or needs behind food choices does, however, allow a person to make more fully conscious and knowledgeable choices. If you are overweight and you know that you are eating because of boredom, you may be able to replace eating with other activities. If you know you are serving a food not because you want to but because it is socially expected, you may choose to serve a different—possibly less expensive and more nutritious—food.

Once you have become familiar with the reasons for eating the foods you do, it is important to analyze and evaluate your diet from a nutritional standpoint. If some of your choices are damaging to your nutritional health, you may decide to make some changes.

There are many different ways to assess individual diets. In this unit, students will learn how to evaluate twenty-four-hour dietary intakes using the Daily Food Guide and/or the Nutrient Analysis Method.

In Unit 11, students learned to use a food frequency form. The diet history is another assessment method that incorporates several nutrition evaluation tools. Diet histories are usually taken by a trained nutritionist or interviewer for the purpose of diagnosing any potential areas of nutritional deficiencies. The diet history gives information not only about food consumed during a specific twenty-four-hour period, but also explores typical food patterns over time (as on the food frequency form). In addition, the diet history usually explores unusual or irregular dietary intakes.

In this unit, students are given a diet history that is designed to be self-administered. It is a less comprehensive (and therefore shorter) record than most professionally administered diet histories. The brevity is necessary to conserve time and to sustain student interest. If students complete their own diet histories, they will be able to make a fairly accurate evaluation of their dietary intake. To help students evaluate their diet histories, instructions have been given within the activities themselves. Because there are no hard-and-fast rules for evaluating the diet history, it would be helpful (but not absolutely necessary) to have a nutritionist or dietitian consult with students, individually or as a group, regarding these dietary evaluations.

Much of the material in this unit should be a review of materials previously learned. By the time most students reach fifth or sixth grade, they have heard of the Daily Food Guide. Unfortunately, most students do not use this tool when choosing their daily diet. The key point of this unit is to impress upon them the ease of using the Daily Food Guide. The alternative approach for planning a menu, the Nutrient Analysis Method, may be new to students. This tool is more difficult to use. The purpose of learning to use such a tool is to enable students to periodically evaluate their diets with a high degree of accuracy. Thus, the Daily Food Guide is useful on a day-to-day basis, whereas the Nutrient Analysis Method is worthwhile for periodic use.

Both the Daily Food Guide and the Nutrient Analysis Method have drawbacks to their use. The Daily Food guide is a simplified tool that does not allow for items such as mixed dishes or new food products. The Daily Food Guide also overemphasizes protein-rich foods by having two separate protein-rich food groups and underemphasizes fruits and vegetables by lumping them into one group. It also underemphasizes the importance of selecting mineral-rich foods, such as whole grains and legumes. However, if a wide variety of foods from all of the groups is selected, chances are a nutritious diet will be achieved.

The Nutrient Analysis Method tends to be lengthy and cumbersome. The accuracy of such an evaluation is worthwhile only for spot-checks of an individual's diet.

BASIC ACTIVITY

Time Needed: Two class periods

Materials Needed: Sheet 15-1: "Foods I Prefer"
Food models or magazine pictures of foods
Chart B: "Daily Food Guide"
Sheets 15-2 through 15-6: "Diet History"
Quiz Sheet 15-1

Class Period 1

1. Have students participate in a brainstorming session on the subject of why they eat what they do. Divide the class into small groups and have a contest to see who can think of the most reasons. Have one group member record the ideas. If students are having difficulty thinking of ideas, give them several examples of situations, such as the following and have them decide whether a biological, psychological, or social need is being met:

   a. I am so happy, I will go buy myself a double-dipper! *(psychological)*

   b. I want the same thing she ordered! *(social)*

   c. I have to drink my milk because Mom tells me I should. *(social)*

   d. I am so hungry after playing ball. *(biological)*

   e. We do not have anything to do tonight. I am so bored—let us go out and have a sundae. *(psychological)*

Limit the number of examples. Encourage students to list at least ten other examples of situations that demonstrate why they eat what they do.

2. Initiate a group discussion about the reasons behind food habits. Stress the variety and individuality of reasons behind food choices. Point out that these reasons sometimes overlap: You eat because you are hungry (biological); you choose a candy bar because you believe it will give you quick energy (psychological).

3. Present the idea of the three categories of needs: biological, psychological, and social. Label them physical, emotional, and social. List the reasons for eating that students identified during their brainstorming session, and classify the reasons under these three categories. Remember that biological needs refer to any needs that are phsyical; psychological needs pertain to the emotional aspects of the individual; and social needs refer to the traditions of the society or group to which the individual belongs.

4. Distribute Sheet 15-1, "Foods I Prefer."

5. Under the column labeled "Foods," instruct students to list all the foods that they prefer. The foods can be single foods, such as raw apples, steak, or whole-wheat bread, or combination foods, such as macaroni and cheese or a tuna salad sandwich. Have students be specific in their description of the foods. Students should list at least twelve foods.

6. Along the top of the page, instruct students to label the columns as you describe them. The following list offers suggestions for headings, but you may choose others that you feel are more appropriate. Use the extra column spaces for your own headings or for those suggested by the class.

   T–Foods that *taste* good to you
   N–Foods you think are *nutritious* or "good" for you
   Y–Foods you ate when you were *young*
   F–Foods your *family* likes
   B–Foods your *buddies* like
   E–Foods you eat when you are *emotional* (bored, lonely, sad, fidgety)
   H–Foods you eat when you are *hungry*

7. Have students check the appropriate categories for each food.

8. Discuss the worksheet results. What patterns do students see in their eating habits? Why do they eat what they do?

Class Period 2

1. Distribute Chart B, "Daily Food Guide." Because this tool is often overused, find out how much students already know. Review the guide only as much as is necessary.

2. Display magazine pictures of foods or food models of a variety of foods.

3. Ask the students to place each food in its food group in the "Daily Food Guide." This activity can be done as a large group, with the teacher displaying the foods and the students orally indicating to which food group each belongs.

4. Distribute Sheets 15-2 through 15-6, the "Diet History" sheets, and have students complete them individually.

5. Have students evaluate their Diet Histories individually by answering the following questions:

a. Do the data on Sheet 15-2 agree or conflict with the data on the twenty-four-hour intake record on Sheets 15-4 through 15-5? For example, if you recorded on sheet 15-2 that you "Hardly Ever" consumed "Milk, Pudding, Custard, Yogurt, Cheese," but your twenty-four-hour intake record showed that you drank three glasses of milk, you have a discrepancy.

b. Do your answers to questions 4, 5, 6, 7, and 8 on Sheet 15-3 correspond with your twenty-four-hour intake record (Sheets 15-4 and 15-5)? For example, if you have checked that you maintain a vegetarian diet, there should be no record of meat, poultry, or fish intake. If there is, you should supply an explanation.

c. Are the descriptions in questions 9, 10, and 11 on Sheet 15-3 accurate? How do they affect your nutrition?

d. Do your answers to questions 12 and 13 on Sheet 15-3 make you think that you should make changes in your dietary habits?

6. After the students have completed step 5, begin a large-group discussion of their findings. Discuss not only their individual diet evaluations, but also the problems with using the "Diet History" as an evaluation tool.

7. Proceed with the "Advanced Activity" if you wish; otherwise use the quiz mentioned in step 8.

8. **Evaluation:** Distribute Quiz Sheet 15-1 and have students complete it independently. Discuss the answers as a class.

ADVANCED ACTIVITY

Time Needed: One or two class periods

Materials Needed: Sheet 15-7: "My Ideal Menu"
Chart A: "Recommended Dietary Allowances"
Chart D: "Food Composition Table for Selected Nutrients"
Chart E: "Dietary Calculation Chart"
Food composition tables *(optional)* (see References/Resources)
Calculators *(optional)*
Quiz Sheet 15-1

Class Period 1

1. Distribute Sheet 15-7, "My Ideal Menu." In introducing this activity, emphasize that for the purposes of this activity there are no restrictions on the cost of the foods, on their availability, on the time or skills needed for preparation, or on other people's needs. Encourage students to use their imaginations. This activity can be introduced the day before the class and used as a homework assignment.

2. Have each student transfer the foods and serving sizes from Sheet 15-7 to Chart E, "Dietary Calculation Chart," in the appropriate food categories. Then, using a food composition table (see the References/Resources section at the end of this book) or Chart D, "Food Composition Table for

Selected Nutrients," students should find the amount of nutrients in each food. They should then subtotal each column and find the grand total for each nutrient. Finally, each student should compare the amount of each nutrient to its RDA, and should note the difference between his or her RDA for energy and the number of calories in food on the menu (+ or −).

3. Students should make evaluations of their ideal menu and decide what specific improvements should be made in their diets.

Class Period 2

1. Many students will not be able to complete the calculations in this activity in one class period. The remaining work can be assigned as homework or can be completed during the next class period.

2. **Evaluation:** Distribute Quiz Sheet 15-1 and have students complete it independently. Discuss the answers as a class.

FOLLOW-UP ACTIVITIES

1. Present students with the names of unusual foods. First, ask them if they would eat the foods without knowing what they were, and why or why not. Then, have them research the foods, and ask them again if they would eat the foods and why or why not.

2. Have students compile a one- to three-day food record composed of everything they eat or drink during the time period chosen. Then, have them analyze food patterns and habits, in chart form, as shown in this example:

FOOD	AMOUNT	WHEN EATEN	WHERE EATEN	WITH WHOM	WHY
orange juice, reconstituted	6 ounces	7 A.M.	kitchen	alone	hunger habit
egg, soft-boiled	1 medium	7 A.M.	kitchen	alone	hunger think it is good for me my father eats them
toast, dry	1 slice	7 A.M.	kitchen	alone	hunger it goes with eggs
potato chips	4 ounce bag	10 A.M.	my locker	friends	everyone else was snacking anxious about test coming up

3. Have students interview other students, parents, siblings, teachers, administrators, and other school personnel to determine their diet histories. Have students use Sheets 15-2 through 15-3 as a pattern for the interviews.

4. Invite a nutritionist, dietitian, or other qualified health professional to speak to the class about dietary assessments. Have the speaker address the class on the variety of methods used to assess diets, including twenty-four-hour recall, three-day diet records, 7-day diet records, dietary histories, weighed food records, and dietary scores.

5. Have students write a few paragraphs describing why they will, or will not, use the dietary tools presented in this unit to help them select a balanced diet.

6. Have students make comments (verbal or written) on the changes they would like to see in their own diets.

FOODS I PREFER

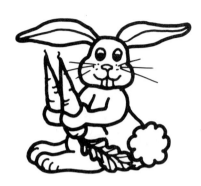

Directions: In the left column, list the names of all of the foods that you like more than others. Then label the tops of the columns as directed by your teacher.

KEY:										
FOODS:										

DIET HISTORY

Directions: Answer each question on Sheets 15-2 through 15-5 as honestly as you can.

1. My eating habits are: _____ excellent _____ good _____ fair _____ poor

2. My appetite is: _____ excellent _____ good _____ fair _____ poor

3. Place a check in the box in each row that indicates how often you eat foods from each food group. Example: If you eat two eggs a week, a hamburger every day, and either chicken or fish for each evening meal, you would check the last box labeled "Three or More Times Per Day."

FOOD GROUPS	Hardly Ever	Several Times Per Week	Once Daily	Two Times Per Day	Three or More Times Per Day
Milk, Pudding, Custard, Yogurt, Cheese					
Animal Proteins (beef, chicken, pork, fish, eggs)					
Vegetable Proteins (beans, nuts, peas)					
Fruit or Juice of: orange, grapefruit, tangerine, strawberries, tomato, green pepper					
Broccoli, Lima Beans, Spinach, Lettuce, Other Greens					
Any other Fruit or Vegetable					
Any type of Cereal, Bread, Roll, Rice, Cracker, Noodles, Macaroni, Spaghetti					
Cakes, Cookies, Pastries, Pies					
Candy					
Soda Pop, Soft Drinks					
Salty Snacks (potato chips, corn chips, etc.)					

4. What food(s) do you eat most often? _____

_____

_____

5. What food(s) do you eat least often? _____

_____

_____

6. Are you on any special diet? _____ yes _____ no   If yes, check which one:

_____ weight control   _____ diabetic   _____ low cholesterol

_____ vegetarian   _____ low salt   _____ other: _____

7. Are you taking any dietary supplements (examples: vitamins, minerals, protein)?

_____ yes _____ no   If yes, please describe: _____

_____

8. Do you have any food allergies or bad reactions to certain foods (indigestion, abdominal pain, diarrhea)? _____ yes
_____ no   If yes, please indicate to which food(s) and how they affect you: _____

_____

9. Do you eat most of your meals: _____ alone _____ with family _____ with friends?

10. Where do you usually eat? (Check one or more.)

_____ home   _____ school dorm or cafeteria   _____ snack bar/coffee shop

_____ own apartment   _____ street vendor   _____ restaurant

_____ youth residence   _____ delicatessen   _____ other: _____

11. Do you ever prepare your own meals? _____ yes _____ no   If yes, which meals and how often? _____

_____

12. What changes would you like to make in your eating habits? _____

_____

13. What problems might you encounter in making these changes? _____

_____

_____

DIET HISTORY:
24-HOUR INTAKE

Directions: Keep a strict record of all foods and beverages you consume in a twenty-four-hour period. Be sure to include soft drinks, gum, snacks, and condiments (ketchup mustard, mayonnaise). For each item, write down the time you eat it, whether it is a meal (M) or a snack (S), a complete description of the food, and the amount you consume.

Time of Day	Meal (M) or Snack (S)	Food Description	Amount

1. Is your twenty-four-hour intake record typical of what you usually eat and drink in one day?

_____ Yes _____ No   If no, revise the twenty-four-hour intake on the chart below to make it more accurate, or make changes on the original chart in another color.

Time of Day	Meal (M) or Snack (S)	Food Description	Amount

2. Is your twenty-four-hour intake record similar to what you usually eat and drink on the weekends? _____ yes _____ no   If no, explain how your weekend diet differs:_____

_____

_____

3. Is your twenty-four-hour intake record similar to what you usually eat and drink during the entire year? _____ yes _____ no   If no, explain how you eat differently during some parts of the year: _____

_____

_____

DIET HISTORY EVALUATION

Directions: Use Chart B, "Daily Food Guide," to evaluate the twenty-four-hour intake record that you recorded on Sheet 15-4 and revised in step 1 of Sheet 15-5. Compile your evaluation on the chart below.

FOOD DESCRIPTION	Amount Eaten	Servings Per Food Group						
		Milk-Cheese	Meat-Fish-Poultry-Beans	Fruit-Vegetable			Bread-Cereal	Fats-Sweets-Alcohol
				Vitamin C-rich	Vitamin A-rich	Other		
Total Number of Servings:								
Recommended Number of Servings:								

MY IDEAL MENU

Directions: Write your ideal menu for one day on this sheet using any pattern of meals you wish. In this activity, there are no restrictions on the cost of the foods, on their availability, on the time or skills needed for preparation, or on other people's needs. Be sure to note the serving sizes for the foods you select.

BREAKFAST:

SNACK:

LUNCH:

SNACK:

DINNER:

SNACK:

QUIZ
DESIGNING A PERSONAL DIET PLAN

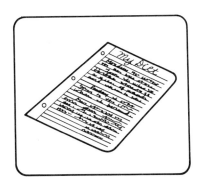

1. List the three categories of needs that are met by food and give an example of each:

   a. _____ need Example: _____

   b. _____ need Example: _____

   c. _____ need Example: _____

2. Place the correct food group number from the key on the right beside each of the foods listed below:

1	Fruit-Vegetable group
2	Bread-Cereal group
3	Milk-Cheese group
4	Meat-Poultry-Fish-Beans group
5	Fats-Sweets-Alcohol group

   a. _____ skim milk

   b. _____ French-style salad dressing

   c. _____ hamburger

   d. _____ whole-wheat muffin

   e. _____ baked potato

   f. _____ chocolate ice cream

   g. _____ butter

   h. _____ applesauce

   i. _____ tuna fish

   j. _____ crackers

   k. _____ pretzels

   l. _____ tomato juice

   m. _____ nonfat dry milk

   n. _____ soybean casserole

   o. _____ soft drink

   p. _____ pancakes

   q. _____ scrambled egg

   r. _____ vanilla pudding

   s. _____ watermelon

   t. _____ peanut butter

3. The following people are having problems with their diets. They are missing foods primarily from a single food group. Name the missing food group for each one.

   a. Mary has been skipping breakfast lately because her bus leaves earlier than usual. For lunch, she usually has an orange, or other piece of fruit, along with a glass of milk. A late-afternoon snack usually consists of cheese and another piece of fruit. For supper, she sits down with her family to a meal of chicken or fish, tossed salad, and a glass of milk. Often she is so hungry after finishing her homework that she eats a tuna salad. Which food group is lacking in Mary's diet?

   _____ To improve her diet, what foods could she eat and when?

   _____

   b. Joey plays basketball after school every day. He is starving when he gets home, and wolfs down two hearty sandwiches of meat and cheese or peanut butter. He usually goes out for a while or he does his homework. Later he grabs another couple of sandwiches and pours down several glasses of milk. In the morning he eats several eggs, bacon, and toast, and at lunch he usually eats pizza and cola. Which food group is lacking in Joey's diet?

   _____ To improve his diet, what foods could he eat and when?

   _____

Unit 16: Discovering Foods with Your Senses

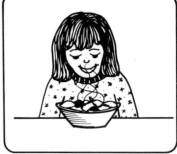

CONCEPTS

–Food can be enjoyed through many senses including taste, smell, sight, sound, and touch.

–Eating a wide variety of foods can be an enjoyable experience if the senses are involved.

OBJECTIVES

–Given an opportunity to taste a variety of foods, students will sample at least three out of five foods.

–Students will be able to name the five senses through which food can be enjoyed.

–Students will be able to give an example of a sensory experience with one food. A sensory experience is a description of one food through the use of the five senses.

TEACHER'S UNIT INTRODUCTION

Discovering food through the senses can be a pleasurable learning experience. Just think of the enjoyment you receive when eating one of your favorite foods! Take a juicy, fresh orange—savor its sweet, zesty taste; relish its refreshing, cool, and wholesome fragrance; notice its bright color; feel its pebbly surface as you peel it; feel the softness and juiciness in your mouth as you eat it; and listen to the muffled, barely audible sound it makes in your mouth.

The purpose of this activity is to alert students to their senses in relation to the enjoyment of food. By paying attention to the senses as they eat, they will not only enjoy their food more, but will avoid overeating because they will eat more slowly.

BASIC ACTIVITY

Time Needed: One class period

Materials Needed: Sheet 16-1: "Tasting Party"
Food for the Tasting Party (see recipe "White on White with Vegetables")
Food preparation equipment (small bowl and mixing spoon *or* blender,
measuring spoons, measuring cups, paring knife, cutting board, plastic wrap,
platters, small paper plates, napkins)
Quiz Sheet 16-1

1. Have the students prepare the recipe "White on White with Vegetables" according to the following recipe.

Ingredients:

1 cup cottage cheese	raw mushrooms	rutabaga sticks
½ cup plain yogurt	celery sticks	green beans
1 small onion, minced	carrot sticks	scallions
1 tsp. lemon juice	zucchini spears	summer squash spears
	turnip chunks	cherry tomatoes

Directions:

a. Mix the first four ingredients in a small bowl or blender until smooth.

b. Cover the dip with plastic wrap and chill.

c. Clean and cut the vegetables. Arrange them on separate platters numbered from 1 to 10.

2. Encourage each student to sample a little of each food. Have the students, working in pairs, complete Sheet 16-1, "Tasting Party." Each food will be fully described when the sheet is completed.

3. Proceed with the "Advanced Activity," if you wish; otherwise use the quiz mentioned in step 4.

4. **Evaluation:** Distribute Quiz Sheet 16-1 and have students complete it independently. Discuss the students' answers while the class enjoys the vegetables and dip.

ADVANCED ACTIVITY

Time Needed: Two class periods

Materials Needed: Sheet 16-2: "Sensory Food Evaluation Lab"
Fluid whole milk
Reconstituted nonfat dry milk
Diluted evaporated milk
Plain crackers (saltines)
Butter
Margarine
Name-brand canned peaches
Store or generic brand peaches

Whole-wheat bread
White bread
Rye bread
Small paper cups
Small paper plates
Napkins
Felt-tip marker
Water
Blindfolds *(optional)*

Class Period 1

1. Introduce this activity as a sensory evaluation lab. The tests that students will be performing are similar to the tests that new food products undergo before they are marketed.

2. Divide the class into four groups.

3. Before conducting sensory evaluations, review the following rules:

a. The samples to be tested should be of the same size, shape, and temperature.

b. The background environment should be quiet.

c. Everyone should be seated.

d. Everyone should have water to drink after each sample.

e. No one should eat (or smoke) thrity minutes prior to the testing.

f. Food samples should be coded randomly by the lab leader, who should remain at the station. This random coding is important because some participants may judge a food by its name and not by its taste, thus reducing the possibility of an objective evaluation.

4. Instruct each group to set up one of the following sensory evaluation labs to serve the whole class. If the students are unfamiliar with the kitchen, or if time is limited, the labs may be set up ahead of time. Make sure there are enough food samples at each lab to allow testing by each student in the class. Students should rotate in groups from one lab station to the next.

Lab #1—Food Ranking

a. Have three types of milk available for tasting: whole milk, reconstituted nonfat dry milk, and diluted evaporated milk. Make sure the milk has been thoroughly chilled.

b. The lab leader should secretly code the cups with either a number or a letter that corresponds to the different kinds of milk.

c. The lab leader should pour approximately one-eighth of a cup of each type of milk into the cups just prior to the arrival of the group at the station.

d. Students should drink a serving of each type of milk.

e. On Sheet 16-2, students should use the codes to rank the samples according to sweetness.

Lab #2—Forced Choice

a. Students should prepare samples of plain crackers (such as saltines); some should be spread with butter and some with margarine.

b. The lab leader should secretly label each plate of crackers with a code number or letter.

c. Students should sample each type of cracker.

d. Students should make a choice of which they prefer. Even if they liked or disliked both, they must still make a choice and indicate it on Sheet 16-2.

Lab #3—Triangle Test

a. Have on hand two brands of a canned fruit (such as peaches). One sample should be a store or generic brand and the other should be a name brand.

b. Students should prepare three samples (per student) of the canned fruit. Two of the samples should be of the same brand, and the third should be of the other brand.

c. The lab leader should secretly label each plate of samples with a code number or letter.

d. The students should taste each grouping of three samples and use all of their senses to detect the differences.

e. On Sheet 16-2, students should mark which two samples are alike and which one is different.

Lab #4—Rating Scale

a. Students should prepare samples of whole-wheat bread, white bread, and rye bread, cutting a quarter of a slice per sample.

b. The lab leader should secretly label each plate of samples with a code number or letter.

c. Students should taste each type of bread and, on Sheet 16-2, they should rate how much they liked each sample. (This lab exercise may be done blindfolded to eliminate biases based on the bread's appearance.)

Class Period 2

1. Following the completion of all labs, begin a large-group discussion of the sensory evaluations. Discuss each lab separately. Be sure to point out the variety of senses that are used to evaluate the foods. End the discussion by having one or more students describe one food using all five senses.

2. **Evaluation:** Distribute Quiz Sheet 16-1 and have students complete it independently. Have student volunteers read aloud their descriptions of foods using the five senses.

FOLLOW-UP ACTIVITIES

1. Conduct experiments to demonstrate the importance of the senses:

a. Blindfold some students and have them taste either mashed potatoes that have been colored with red food coloring or milk that has been colored blue. How does the food color affect the perception of taste?

b. Have some students pinch their noses closed and taste raw potatoes and raw apples. How do these compare?

2. Have students write and illustrate advertisements for nutritious foods. This may be done as either an individual or as a small-group project. Food producers and their advertisers try to appeal to all five senses in developing and marketing their products. Students should use sensory appeal in their ads. Students may also develop a score card to judge the student-developed ads; the highest score should be given to the ad that appeals to the most senses.

3. Students may also participate in a cookbook scavenger hunt to select foods that appeal to all five senses. Have students describe the food or recipe in relation to their five senses.

4. Divide the class into five groups and, by drawing lots, have each group represent one of the five senses. Have each group design and construct a poster that depicts its sense and that illustrates the way in which its sense relates to a variety of foods.

5. Have students plan and prepare a meal. Evaluate it according to the five senses.

TASTING PARTY

Directions: After tasting each food, fill in the questionnaire below with either an answer or a check mark.

FOODS:	#1	#2	#3	#4	#5	#6	#7	#8	#9	#10
What does it *look* like?										
What is the *color*?										
What is the *shape*?										
What does it *sound* like?										
Is the food *crunchy*?										
Is the food *quiet*?										
What does it *taste* like?										
Is it *sweet*?										
Is it *sour*?										
Is it *bitter*?										
Is it *salty*?										
Is it *bland*?										
Is it *spicy*?										
What does it *smell* like?										
Does it have a *strong* aroma?										
Does it have a *weak* aroma?										
What does it *feel* like?										
Is the food *soft*?										
Is the food *hard*?										
Is the food *hot*?										
Is the food *cold*?										

SENSORY FOOD EVALUATION LAB

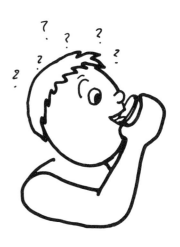

Directions: After you taste the foods at each lab station, fill in the appropriate parts of the questionnaire below.

LAB 1—FOOD RANKING Sweetest milk: _____ In-between milk: _____ Least sweet milk: _____	**LAB 2—FORCED CHOICE** Preferred sample: _____ I liked this sample best because: (Explain using at least one sense.) _____ _____ _____ _____ _____ _____ _____ _____ _____ _____

LAB 3—TRIANGLE TEST

Same samples: _____

_____

Different sample: _____

The samples are different because: (Explain using all five senses):

_____

_____

_____

_____

_____

LAB 4—RATING SCALE

Sample _____: Sample _____: Sample _____:

Like a lot	🙂	🙂	🙂
Like somewhat	🙂	🙂	🙂
Don't care	😐	😐	😐
Dislike somewhat	😠	😠	😠
Dislike a lot	😖	😖	😖

QUIZ
DISCOVERING FOODS WITH YOUR SENSES

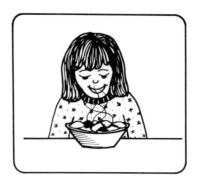

1. Name the five senses you use to enjoy food:

_____

_____

_____

_____

_____

2. Write a short paragraph describing one food you enjoy. Include in your description how each of the five senses contributes to your enjoyment.

_____

_____

_____

_____

_____

_____

_____

_____

_____

_____

_____

_____

_____

_____

_____

_____

_____

_____

_____

_____

SECTION III

SPECIAL DIETS

Unit 17: Energy Balance and Fad Diets

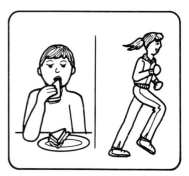

CONCEPTS

–The balance of calories affects body weight in three ways:

  a. To *lose* weight, individuals must consume *fewer* calories than they expend.

  b. To *maintain* weight, individuals must consume *the same number* of calories as they expend

  c. To *gain* weight, individuals must consume *more* calories than they expend.

–Fad diets result in weight loss only when they also follow the principle of caloric balance.

–Nutrition misinformation, especially regarding weight control, is prevalent among teenagers.

–There are many diets available; some are safe and some are hazardous.

–Anorexia nervosa and bulimia are two eating disorders that are accompanied by extreme weight losses and by distorted body images.

OBJECTIVES

–Given a hypothetical situation involving calorie input versus calorie output, students will be asked to identify which situations lead to weight loss, which lead to weight maintenance, and which lead to weight gain.

–Students will be able to plan an individualized and nutritious weight-control diet that specifies the foods to be eaten and the activities to be pursued.

–Students will be able to distinguish between factual and fictitious statements about weight-control diets.

–Students will be able to determine whether or not a diet is safe and well-balanced.

–Students will be able to describe anorexia nervosa and bulimia.

TEACHER'S UNIT INTRODUCTION

Weight control is a popular topic of discussion. Millions of dollars and hours are spent each year by people trying to control their weight. In the United States, this effort looks like a losing battle. More than 10 percent of our school-aged children, nearly 15 percent of our teenagers and young adults, and up to 30 percent of our adults are considered to be obese. That is a *lot* of fat people!

There are several definitions of "fatness." Generally, people who are 20 percent or more above their ideal body weight are considered obese. People 10 percent to 19 percent above their ideal weight are considered overweight. In terms of an individual, consider this simple case of determining obesity.

Mary weighs 153 pounds. Her ideal weight is about 125 pounds. (We will talk about how to determine ideal body weight later.) Twenty percent of 125 pounds is 25 pounds. Adding her ideal weight to this 20 percent margin yields 150 pounds. Weighing in at 153 pounds means that Mary is obese. This method of determining obesity is a simple rule-of-thumb. Depending upon body composition, another girl weighing the same percentage above ideal body weight might not be considered obese if a major proportion of her weight is composed of muscle. Obesity is not always an easy condition to diagnose.

There are several methods of determining ideal body weight, some of which are more complicated than others. Generally, the more complicated methods lead to more accurate measurements. If you want to know if your current weight is ideal, often a simple procedure (such as the "mirror" test) will do.

Here are some of the methods used for determining ideal body weight:

1. *Body Density*—To determine body density, that is, the ratio of body fat to lean body mass (muscle and bone), an "index of specific gravity" can be calculated. Measuring the specific gravity of people involves comparing their body weight under water to their body weight in the air. As the proportion of fat in the body increases, the specific gravity decreases since fat is lighter than lean body mass. Normally, 12 to 18 percent of a man's body weight is fat, whereas 18 to 24 percent of a woman's body weight is composed of fat. This method for determining ideal body weight requires special equipment that may not always be available.

2. *Whole Body Counter*—Using potassium 40, a naturally occurring radioactive isotope of potassium, the amount of lean body mass can be calculated. Subtracting lean body mass from total body weight yields weight of body fat. This method for determining ideal body weight also requires special equipment that may not be available.

3. *Skinfold Measurements*—Using constant-pressure skinfold calipers, the amount of fat in particular places on the body can be measured and compared to a standard. Common places of measurement include triceps (back side of upper arm), subscapular (upper back), and suprailiac (above the pelvic bones).

4. *Ideal Height-Weight Tables*—Weight tables are computed primarily by insurance companies in determining health risks, and they may be used to determine ideal body height-weight. Many, but not all, of the height-weight tables include a provision for body frame size. Frame size may be determined by placing your thumb and middle finger of your left hand around the wrist of your right hand at the widest part. If your thumb and finger overlap beyond the first knuckle, you have a small frame; if they overlap only slightly or if they just meet, you have a medium frame; if they do not meet at all you have a large frame. Of course, these guidelines are not extremely precise. To compensate for imprecision, there are usually a range of ideal body weights that have been computed from average body weights in the United States. Height-weight tables for teenagers are less accurate than those for adults because of the differences in growth rates. (See the "Average Height-Weight Table" on Sheet Sheet 17-1, "Personal Energy Budget.")

5. *Mirror Test*—By looking at yourself naked in a full-length mirror, you will probably be able to judge whether or not you are maintaining ideal body weight. This test may not reveal everything about your weight, but it will give you a good picture of your weight status.

By applying one or more of these methods to yourself, you will be able to determine if you need to lose, maintain, or gain weight. Then, once you have determined this, you need to know how to achieve your goal. There is one major principle behind weight control that is more important than all others, and this is the principle of caloric balance. *Caloric balance means that the number of calories consumed must be balanced with the number of calories expended.*

There are three ways in which this principle affects weight:

1. If fewer calories are consumed than are expended, weight loss occurs.

2. If the same number of calories are consumed as expended, weight is maintained.

3. If more calories are consumed than are expended, weight is gained.

In terms of food, weight control depends on the number of calories in the food you eat. The number of calories equal to one pound of body fat is 3,500. This means that eating an additional 500 calories every day for one week (7 days) will add one pound of body weight. The principle also works in reverse, fortunately. To lose one pound of body weight, you need to eat 3,500 calories less than you use.

Knowing the principle of caloric balance is only the first step in weight control. You must be able to plan a daily diet and exercise program that works for you. Many people look for easy and painless ways of weight control. Fad diets, water pills, hormone shots, or even surgery may seem more desirable than cutting down on calories or increasing exercise. However, the safest and most long-lasting methods are ones that allow for an individualized, nutritious approach to dieting and exercise.

Weight-control diets can be classified into six general categories as follows:

1. High Protein/High Fat/Low Carbohydrate Diets

These diets promote high-protein foods and restrict sources of carbohydrates including fruits, vegetables, breads, cereals, and sometimes milk and milk products. Some of the more recent ones include Dr. Atkin's Diet Revolution, Dr. Stillman's Diet, the Drinking Man's Diet, the Air Force Diet, and the Scarsdale Diet (similar to the others except that it is low in fat).

These diets are nutritionally unbalanced because they eliminate foods from two or three of the food groups in the Daily Food Guide. These diets tend to be low in Vitamin A, the B vitamins, Vitamin C, iron, and calcium.

2. One-Food Diets

These diets prescribe eating "all you can eat" of one or several foods while restricting many others. Examples include the Rice Diet, the Grapefruit Diet, the Banana Diet, and the Yogurt Diet.

These diets are nutritionally unbalanced because they emphasize one food or food group and ignore the others. Usually weight loss occurs because of low calorie intake. These diets are hard to adhere to because they are monotonous.

3. Bizarre Diets

Any odd or unusual diet belongs to this group. The proponents of these diets make unsupported claims concerning the rationale behind the weight loss which might occur. Examples include the HCG Diet (hormone), the Anti-Cellulite Diet, the Fructose Diet, the Last Chance Diet (Protein-Sparing Modified Fast), and the Kelp-B_6-Cider Vinegar-Lecithin Diet.

While these diets may be relatively nutritious, they may also use devices or techniques (such as drugs or formulas) that may be dangerous. Some of the diets may be low in one or more nutrients. The Fructose Diet, for example, limits sources of carbohydrates.

4. Diet Pills, Diuretics, and Laxatives

These drugs, with or without dieting, are purported to stimulate weight loss. Diet pills generally contain mild stimulants to suppress the appetite. Diuretics cause water loss which reduces body weight but not body fat. These methods are generally unsafe in the short run and unsuccessful in the long run.

5. Gimmick Diets

For the most part, these diets are nutritionally sound but incorporate gimmicks or invalid claims regarding weight loss. Examples include the Bread and Butter Diet, the Lazy Woman's Diet, the Easy No-Flab Diet, and the Beautiful Skin Diet.

6. Balanced, Nutritious Diets

These diets encourage use of a variety of foods from the Daily Food Guide. An attempt is made to limit calories and increase activity. Examples include the Weight Watcher's Diet and the Prudent Man's Diet. A nutritious weight reduction diet should lead to a weight loss of one to two pounds per week.

Behavior modification techniques also fall under this category. The behavior modification approach to weight reduction appears to be enjoying recent success. Most behavior modification plans encourage nutritious weight-control diets in addition to increasing exercise. The key to behavior modification is the observance of your own habits and the step-by-step alteration of undesirable patterns of eating and exercising.

These six categories may be helpful in evaluating other diets as they appear on the newsstands. Generally, a sensible weight-control diet includes a wide variety of foods from the Daily Food Guide, limits calories, and encourages additional exercise. The basic rule of weight control—to balance the calories coming in with the calories going out—should be the primary emphasis of any safe weight-control diet. If a gimmick or aid is used to "sell" the diet, be sure to analyze the gimmick as to its safety.

No discussion of weight control is complete without a discussion of the eating disorders that have become prevalent in this country, particularly among teenaged girls. Anorexia nervosa and bulimia appear to afflict 15 percent to 20 percent of young girls in this country. Anorexia nervosa is a disease of self-starvation characterized by a continuous pursuit of extreme, life-threatening thinness, an exaggerated interest in food and in the body, and a general withdrawal from family and friends. Bulimia is a chaotic pattern of eating which includes periods of gorging on large quantities of food (from 3,000 to 20,000 calories) in a short period of time (1 to 2 hours). Gorging is often followed by purging (with self-induced vomiting or laxative abuse) or by severe dieting or fasting. Bulimics generally maintain a normal weight and appearance. Side effects of bulimia are serious and include digestive problems, liver damage, rectal bleeding (with excessive laxative use), dental cavities and erosion of tooth enamel (with vomiting), and electrolyte (mineral) and water balance disturbances.

Teenagers often have trouble recognizing their true body status. Teenage girls, especially, believe that a small amount of fat on their bodies means that they are overweight. It is important to begin teaching teenagers to accept their bodies within a realistic framework. Distorted body images and extreme self-consciousness about physique are common among teenagers. Discussion of this topic may arise within this unit when each student assesses his or her body weight. If you suspect that any of your students is suffering from anorexia nervosa or bulimia, the student should be referred to a counselor or nutritionist specializing in eating disorders.

The activities in this unit give ideas for sensible weight control. Although student materials emphasize weight control through improving dietary habits, it is just as important to keep exercise habits in mind. Follow-up activities that point to the relationship between caloric expenditure and weight control are important to the full understanding of weight control.

BASIC ACTIVITY

Time Needed: Three class periods

Materials Needed: Sheets 17-1 through 17-4: "Personal Energy Budget"
Food composition tables (see References/Resources) *or* calorie counters
Yardstick and scale *(optional)*
Calculators *(optional)*
Sheet 17-5: "Dieting? Dieting!"
Sample diets from popular magazines, newspapers, or books, including two weight-control diets, two athlete's diets, nutritious diets, and fad diets
Sheet 17-6: "Diet Rating"
Quiz Sheet 17-1

Class Period 1

1. Introduce this unit with a short discussion of weight control. Describe the principle of caloric balance.

2. Distribute Sheets 17-1 through 17-4, "Personal Energy Budget," and have students complete them as a large-group activity. Divide them into small groups when they weigh and measure themselves, if you choose to do this in class.

3. As homework, have students record everything they eat and drink for twenty-four hours on the chart called "Today's Diet" on Sheet 17-2.

Class Period 2

1. Have food composition tables or calorie counters available for the calculation of the day's calorie intake on the chart entitled "Todays Diet" on Sheet 17-2.

2. Have students balance their energy budget following the directions on Sheet 17-3.

3. Complete the activity by discussing whether or not the students are in energy balance. Discuss students' answers to the question at the top of Sheet 17-4 (*Answer:* Increase daily activity). Any activity that uses the big muscles of the body at a fairly constant rate for ½ hour or more is good exercise. Elicit ways to increase physical activity from the students (*Answers:* run, swim, bicycle, dance, gymnastics, walking and so forth). Students will propose their individualized exercise plans as the last activity on Sheet 17-4.

Class Period 3

1. Distribute Sheet 17-5, "Dieting? Dieting!" This worksheet should be used as an initiator of discussion. Students should be told that this is not going to be used for a grade.

2. When they have completed all of the items, tell them how to score the quiz: There are *no* true answers; all of the statements are false. The answer key gives explanations of the statements.

3. Discuss the points made in the quiz along with other popular ideas about weight-control diets. Be prepared to send students to additional resources if you are not equipped to answer their questions.

4. Distribute copies of the sample diets you gathered from popular magazines, newspapers, or books, or have the students view the diets on an overhead projector.

5. Using a copy of Sheet 17-6, "Diet Rating" for each sample diet, have the students rate the diets.

6. Discuss the "Diet Rating" sheets as a class, or have individuals or small groups present their evaluations to the class.

7. Proceed with the "Advanced Activity" if you wish; otherwise use the quiz mentioned in step 8.

8. **Evaluation:** Distribute Quiz Sheet 17-1 and have students complete it independently. Discuss the answers as a class.

ADVANCED ACTIVITY

Time Needed: Two class periods

Materials Needed: Sheet 17-6: "Diet Rating"

Class Period 1

1. Begin this lesson with a brief introduction to sources of nutrition information.

2. As a group, have students prepare a list of places in the community that distribute information about weight-control diets. The list could include any or all of the following places:

    a. Physicians' offices

    b. Nutritionists' or dietitians' offices

    c. In magazines and at newsstands

    d. Health food stores

    e. Bookstores

    f. Health clinics

    g. Libraries

3. Individually, or in pairs, have students select one such source and investigate the diet information offered there.

Class Period 2

1. Have the students evaluate the diets using a copy of Sheet 17-6, "Diet Rating," for each diet.

2. After their investigatons, have students report their findings to the class. Encourage discussion of nutritious versus fad diets and how to differentiate between them.

3. **Evaluation:** Distribute Quiz Sheet 17-1 and have students complete it independently. Discuss the answers as a class.

FOLLOW-UP ACTIVITIES

1. Invite a nutritionist or dietitian to speak to the class about fad diets.

2. Have a contest in which students try to create the most bizarre fad diet they can imagine. The students should describe the diets to the other class members. The winner of the contest (the one with the most bizarre diet) should receive the "Rotten Apple" award. Then have students determine ways to make their fad diets nutritious ones.

3. Have students calculate their energy needs by recording their activity for one day and have them compute their energy expenditure using Sheet 17-7, "Energy Expenditure Log."

4. Using Chart G, "Calorie Expenditure by Activity" and a food composition table, have students calculate the number of minutes needed to "burn off" the following foods: an apple, celery stalks, crackers and cheese, french fries, a chocolate bar, apple pie, and any other popular snack food. To do so, find the caloric value of each food in a food composition table. Have students multiply their weight (or an average weight) by the amount of calories expended per minute (given on Chart G). Then divide the number of calories expended by the caloric value of the food. This final number is the number of minutes needed to "burn-off" the calories from each food.

5. Obtain a set of constant-pressure skinfold calipers and a standard skin-fold chart from the school nurse, a local dietitian, or physician (Ross Labs has a plastic model—see References/Resources). Have them demonstrate to you, or to the class, how to properly use them. Measure students' skinfold thicknesses and use the chart to determine if the students are overweight, overfat, of normal weight, or underweight.

6. If there are several students in the class (or in several classes) who have weight-control problems, encourage them to meet after school in a weight-control support group. Consult a manual such as *Taking Charge of Your Weight and Well-Being* (see References/Resources) for ideas about beginning such a group. The students may or may not need a teacher to lead the group.

PERSONAL ENERGY BUDGET

Directions: Sheet 17-1 through 17-4 will help you calculate your "energy budget." First you will determine your ideal body weight. Then you will decide if you weigh too much, too little, or just about the right amount. Next, you will record one full day's calorie intake. Finally, you will balance your energy budget by comparing your calorie intake to your RDA (Recommended Dietary Allowance) for calories.

1. Determining Your Ideal Body Weight

How tall are you? _____ feet _____ inches. How much do you weigh? _____ pounds.
Do you think you are too tall? _____ too short? _____ just right? _____
Do you think you weigh too much? _____ too little? _____ just the right amount? _____

To determine the average weight of a person your age, look at the tables below. There is one table for boys and one for girls. On the correct table, find your age and the average weight of people your age.
The average weight of people my age is: _____ pounds

Next, check the average weight for a person your age. If you are below the average height, your ideal body weight will be on the low side of the weight range. If you are above the average height, your ideal body weight will be on the high side of the range.

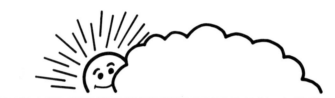

AVERAGE HEIGHT-WEIGHT TABLE FOR AGES 7–17*

| AGE years | Boys | | | | Girls | | | |
	AVERAGE WEIGHT pounds	RANGE IN WEIGHT pounds	AVERAGE HEIGHT inches	RANGE IN HEIGHT inches	AVERAGE WEIGHT pounds	RANGE IN WEIGHT pounds	AVERAGE HEIGHT inches	RANGE IN HEIGHT inches
7	52.5	45.4– 59.6	48.2	46.0–50.4	51.2	43.7– 58.7	47.9	45.7–50.1
8	58.2	49.5– 66.9	50.4	48.1–52.7	56.9	47.5– 66.3	50.0	47.7–52.3
9	64.4	54.6– 74.2	52.4	50.0–54.8	63.0	51.9– 74.1	52.0	49.6–54.4
10	70.7	59.2– 82.2	54.3	51.8–56.8	70.3	57.1– 83.5	54.2	51.6–56.8
11	77.6	64.5– 90.7	56.2	53.6–58.8	79.0	63.5– 94.5	56.5	53.7–59.3
12	85.6	69.8–101.4	58.2	55.3–61.1	89.7	71.9–107.5	59.0	56.1–61.9
13	95.6	77.4–113.8	60.5	57.3–63.7	100.3	82.3–118.3	60.6	58.0–63.2
14	107.9	87.8–128.0	63.0	59.6–66.4	108.5	91.3–125.7	62.3	59.9–64.7
15	121.7	101.1–142.3	65.6	62.5–68.7	115.0	98.8–131.2	63.2	60.9–65.5
16	131.9	113.0–150.8	67.3	64.5–70.1	117.6	101.7–133.5	63.5	61.3–65.7
17	138.3	119.5–157.1	68.2	65.6–70.8	119.0	103.5–134.5	63.6	61.4–65.8

*From *Basic Body Measurements of School Age Children*, Office of Education, U.S. Department of Health, Education, and Welfare.
The ranges given include the cases which fell within the middle two-thirds of those in the sample.

2. Do I Weigh Too Much, Too Little, Or Am I Just Right?

Compare the average weight of people your age to how much you weigh right now.

- If your current weight falls *within* the ideal range, you probably weigh just the right amount.
- If your current weight falls *above* the ideal range, you may weigh too much.
- If your current weight falls *below* the ideal range, you may weigh too little.

3. Record One Full Day's Calorie Intake

Record everything you eat for the next twenty-four hours on the chart below. Be sure to include soft drinks, candy, chewing gum, and other snacks. Also, remember to write down all of the "extras," such as butter on bread or sugar on cereal. Find the number of calories in each food on a food composition table or calorie counter and record it in the column labeled "Calories." Total the calories for the twenty-four-hour period.

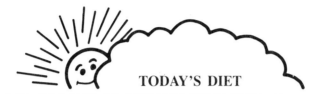

TODAY'S DIET

FOOD	AMOUNT	CALORIES	FOOD	AMOUNT	CALORIES
			COLUMN 2 TOTAL		
			+ COLUMN 1 TOTAL		
COLUMN 1 TOTAL			= GRAND TOTAL		

Look at your completed chart of Today's Diet. Ask yourself, "Do I usually eat about this amount of food, or do I usually eat quite a bit more or less?" If you do usually eat quite a bit more or less, use another color pen to change Today's Diet to make it more typical of how you usually eat. Be sure to change your total calorie count, too.

4. Balance Your "Energy Budget"

A. *Calories in:* The Recommended Dietary Allowances (RDA) for calories are given in the chart below. Find your age and sex on the chart, then look across the table to the two columns labeled CALORIES (Average Intake and Range of Intakes).

The recommended intake of calories for people of my age and sex is _____.

Most healthy people of my age and sex should eat within a range of _____ and _____ calories each day.

AGE & SEX GROUP	WEIGHT (kg.)	WEIGHT (lb.)	HEIGHT (cm.)	HEIGHT (in.)	CALORIES (Average Intake)	CALORIES (Range of Intakes)
1980 RECOMMENDED DIETARY ALLOWANCES						
Males						
7–10	28	62	132	52	2,400	1,650–3,300
11–14	45	99	157	62	2,700	2,000–3,700
15–18	66	145	176	69	2,800	2,100–3,900
19–22	70	154	177	70	2,900	2,500–3,300
Females						
7-10	28	62	132	52	2,400	1,650–3,300
11–14	46	101	157	62	2,200	1,500–3,000
15–18	55	120	163	64	2,100	1,200–3,000
19–22	55	120	163	64	2,100	1,700–2,500

Compare your calorie total on "Today's Diet" to the recommended intake for people of your age and sex. Is it the same, more, or less? _____.

- If you want to *lose* weight, you should eat *less* than your calorie total.
- If you want to *gain* weight, you should eat *more* than your calorie total.
- If you want to stay the *same* weight, you should eat the *same* number of calories as your calorie total.

A good way to gain or lose weight is to do it *slowly*. By eating just 500 calories *less* each day for seven days, you should *lose* about 1 pound. Loss of more than 1 pound per week may be harmful and is likely to be due to water loss or muscle tissue breakdown. By eating just 500 calories *more* each day for seven days, you will *gain* 1 pound. You will gain or lose at this rate because 1 pound of body fat equals 3,500 calories.

> Your energy budget is balanced if you are eating the amount of calories that will help you to reach or maintain your ideal body weight.

B. *Calories out:* Suppose the amount of food you are eating suits you just fine. You do not really want to change your diet. If this is the case, you can still balance your energy budget if it is out of balance. Can you guess how to do this?

_____

If you guessed that you should "change calorie output" or "change activity/exercise habits," you are right!

- If you want to *lose* weight, you should *increase* your activity/exercise.
- If you want to *gain* weight, you should *decrease* your activity/exercise.
- If you want to stay the *same* weight, you should keep your activity/exercise program the *same* as it is now.

On the chart below, write your present activity/exercise program, and also include your ideas for changing it to balance your energy budget if it is out of balance.

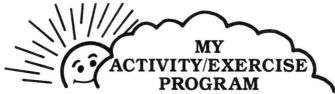

MY PRESENT ACTIVITY/EXERCISE PROGRAM	WHEN I EXERCISE
IDEAS FOR MORE ACTIVITIES	**WHEN I CAN EXERCISE**

IS YOUR ENERGY BUDGET BALANCED TODAY?

DIETING? DIETING!

Directions: Write *true* or *false* for each statement below.

_____ 1. Breads and cereal products are fattening foods and should be eliminated from a weight-control diet.

_____ 2. Using laxatives is one good way to get rid of extra calories.

_____ 3. A baked potato has more calories than a container of fruited yogurt.

_____ 4. You can lose up to five pounds a week safely.

_____ 5. Foods high in protein, such as meat, are also low in calories.

_____ 6. Diet pills help you lose weight because they don't let your calories turn into fat.

_____ 7. Grapefruit and pineapples burn calories.

_____ 8. A girl who weighs 20 percent below her ideal body weight should probably lose five more pounds.

_____ 9. Gelatin is an excellent source of protein.

_____ 10. Since carbohydrates have more calories than either proteins or fats, they should be avoided during a weight-loss program.

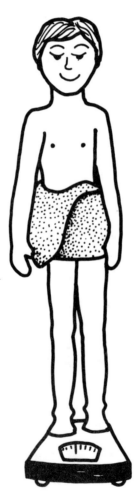

DIET RATING

Directions: Fill out this sheet for each sample diet.

1. Name of the diet: _____

2. Name the source of the diet: _____

3. Place a check mark by each food group below that is included in this diet in *adequate* amounts:

   _____ Fruit-Vegetable Group (four basic servings daily)

   _____ Bread-Cereal Group (four basic servings daily)

   _____ Milk-Cheese Group (four basic servings daily)

   _____ Meat-Poultry-Fish-Beans Group (two basic servings daily)

   _____ Fats-Sweets-Alcohol Group (List items recommended on this diet):

   _____

   _____

4. Does the diet require special products to be purchased? _____ Yes _____ No

5. Does the diet encourage vitamin, mineral, or protein supplements? _____ Yes _____ No

6. Does the diet restrict the amount of water to be consumed _____ Yes _____ No

7. Would the diet be difficult to follow for long periods of time? _____ Yes _____ No

8. Does the diet suggest a great number of pounds to be lost in a short amount of time (more than two pounds per week)? _____ Yes _____ No

9. Does the diet encourage exercise or increased physical activity? _____ Yes _____ No

10. Would you follow this diet? _____ Yes _____ No

OVERALL DIET RATING: _____ EXCELLENT
                        _____ GOOD
                        _____ FAIR
                        _____ POOR

ENERGY EXPENDITURE LOG

Directions: Use the chart below to help you complete the energy expenditure log for a twenty-four-hour period. Then balance your total energy expenditure against your energy intake on Sheet 17-2.

ACTIVITY:	CALORIES*/POUND/MINUTE AT AGES 9–14:
A – SLEEPING (lying still, relaxing)	.008
B – SITTING QUIETLY (reading, writing, taking notes, studying, watching TV, sewing, eating)	.015
C – LIGHT EXERCISE (dressing, personal grooming, light laundry, ironing, light housework such as dusting, dishwashing, cooking, typing, ordinary laboratory work, piano playing, driving)	.020
D – MODERATE EXERCISE (walking at an average pace, active housework, such as making beds, work that requires bending and stretching, babysitting for an active child, volleyball, drum playing)	.032
E – ACTIVE EXERCISE (moderately paced dancing, walking at a brisk pace or uphill, skating, playing Ping Pong, horseback riding, average-paced bicycling, bowling, golfing)	.045
F – VERY ACTIVE EXERCISE (fast paced dancing, running, swimming, basketball, tennis, fast-paced bicycling, football)	.078

*Calculated to include basal metabolic rate and digestion and absorption of food.

Clock Time	Total Minutes	Activity	Energy Level					
			A	B	C	D	E	F
TOTAL	**Hours**							

QUIZ
ENERGY BALANCE AND FAD DIETS

1. Place a check mark in front of each statement you believe is *true*:

_____ a. A weight-control diet should include the following foods: meat, poultry, fish, eggs, beans, nuts, milk, cheese, yogurt, fruits, vegetables, breads, and cereal products.

_____ b. Vitamin and mineral supplements are generally unnecessary for people on a nutritionally balanced weight-loss diet.

_____ c. A person on a weight-control diet should drink plenty of water.

_____ d. A weight-loss goal of eight pounds in four weeks is realistic and safe.

_____ e. A nutritionally sound weight-loss program will lead to a weight loss of one to two pounds per week.

2. Complete these sentences:

a. Anorexia nervosa is _____

_____

b. Bulimia is _____

_____

3. You cannot take off your skin and look in a mirror to see exactly how much body fat you have. You can imagine how much there is, however. When you look in the mirror, you can deduce whether your body fat is decreasing, increasing, or staying the same. For each of the persons below, write whether his or her body fat is staying the same (No Change), increasing (▲), or decreasing (▼).

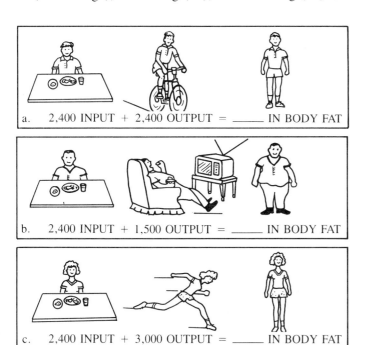

a.   2,400 INPUT + 2,400 OUTPUT = _____ IN BODY FAT

b.   2,400 INPUT + 1,500 OUTPUT = _____ IN BODY FAT

c.   2,400 INPUT + 3,000 OUTPUT = _____ IN BODY FAT

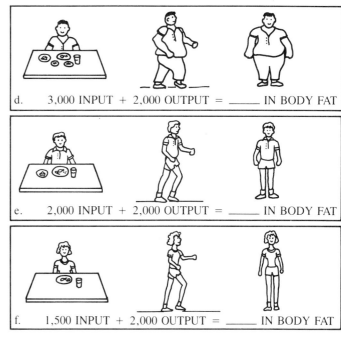

d.   3,000 INPUT + 2,000 OUTPUT = _____ IN BODY FAT

e.   2,000 INPUT + 2,000 OUTPUT = _____ IN BODY FAT

f.   1,500 INPUT + 2,000 OUTPUT = _____ IN BODY FAT

Unit 18: The Athlete's Diet

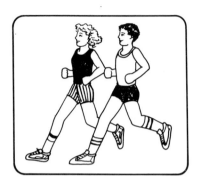

CONCEPTS

–The nutrient needs of athletes are basically the same as those of nonathletes.

–The amount of calories, of water, and, possibly, of sodium needed by athletes may be increased during intensive training and/or performance.

–There is no need for excess protein, vitamins, or minerals in the diets of most athletes. In fact, excessive amounts of these nutrients may be harmful.

OBJECTIVES

–Students will be able to name three substances (calories, water, and sodium) that athletes may have an increased need for during training and performance.

–Students will be able to describe carbohydrate loading and to identify its possible benefits and risks.

–Students will be able to differentiate between facts and fallacies as they apply to the nutritional needs of athletes.

TEACHER'S UNIT INTRODUCTION

The belief that nutrition affects physical performance has been around since well before the days when Popeye ate spinach to gain strength for his fights. It has only been in recent years that systematic research has revealed the biochemical reactions that take place when food produces energy for exercise. This knowledge has enabled nutritionists to support or repudiate specific dietary practices followed by athletes in the hope of improving their performance.

Contrary to popular belief, athletes differ very little from nonathletes when their nutritional needs are compared. Because much confusion and misinformation surrounds this topic, each nutrient will be discussed separately in this unit.

As you are well aware, certain dietary practices or nutrients provide psychological, as well as physical, benefit or harm. Your final evaluation of dietary practices and nutrients will no doubt take their advantages and disadvantages into account.

Vitamins

Daily requirements for vitamins are relatively independent of physical activity; therefore, excessive intakes are not beneficial and could be harmful. Because five or six vitamins of the B complex serve as helpers in energy-yielding reactions during the breakdown of carbohydrate and fat, some coaches have been led to believe that a high intake of B vitamins will result in extra energy for the athlete. There is little evidence to support such a concept. There are dangers in consuming vitamins well above recommended requirements. Furthermore, as energy output increases, energy intake must increase to maintain weight. Taking in more food means getting more vitamins, unless all of the additional food comes from the Fats-Sweets-Alcohol group. Most scientists agree that the vitamin supply provided by a nutritious diet is adequate, and that supplementation is not needed.

Minerals

The body's chemical balance is partly controlled by minerals. We easily consume adequate amounts of these through a nutritious diet. Two minerals in particular are found in the highest concentration in the body fluids—potassium and sodium. Potassium is concentrated inside the cells, and its loss in sweat is small. Thus, loss of potassium is not a serious concern under any but the most extreme conditions, such as very heavy exercise in very hot weather. Even in this case, supplements are not recommended; rather, consumption of extra fruits and vegetables (good sources of potassium) is promoted. Great losses of potassium may occur when athletes use diuretics ("water pills"), a practice sometimes used by wrestlers or gymnasts to qualify for specific weight classes. This practice is dangerous and has no place in the sports scene.

Sodium is concentrated primarily in the fluid outside of the cells. A major function of sodium is to help the body to hold onto water and fluids. Loss of sodium in the form of sodium chloride (salt) occurs through sweating. The amount of sodium lost in sweat increases during exercise in hot, humid weather, and may reach levels as high as 8,000 milligrams daily, although a loss of 4,000 milligrams seems to be more common. It has been found that less sodium is lost in the sweat of well-trained athletes, but no figures exist as to the exact amount. The Estimated Safe and Adequate Daily Dietary Intake of sodium for children seven to ten years of age is between 600 and 1,800 milligrams, and for adolescents eleven years and older, it is between 900 and 2,700 milligrams.

The typical American diet contains quite a bit more sodium than most people need, that is, from 2,300 to 6,900 milligrams a day; this excess salt comes primarily from the addition of table salt to food (table salt, or sodium chloride, is 39 percent sodium). As you can see, an athlete who follows a typical American diet gets adequate sodium, unless his or her sweating is excessive. In these cases, a small increase in sodium intake may be warranted. The best way to do this is simply by adding an extra sprinkle of salt from the salt shaker to food (one teaspoon of salt contains 2,000 milligrams of sodium) or by eating salty items, such as saltines, nuts, snack crackers, or cheese, after practice. A general rule to follow is this: When water loss exceeds five to ten pounds in one contest or practice, consider sodium replacement. Examples of activities that may induce such a water loss include basketball and wrestling of long duration, football practice for long periods in unusually hot weather, and marathon running on hot, humid days.

Salt tablets are *not* the recommended way to replace sodium, because these provide a very high concentration of salt. Excessive salt intake not only impairs an athlete's efficiency during training (due to water retention), but also causes stomach upsets.

Carbohydrates

Carbohydrate loading continues to be surrounded by controversy. Fatigue during long periods of exercise is due to a loss of the stored carbohydrate called glycogen. Changes in diet can alter the body's stores of muscle glycogen, and, in some instances, it is believed to improve performance. The practice of carbohydrate loading benefits only athletes involved in endurance events, such as marathon running or distance swimming. In other types of events, such as wrestling, carbohydrate loading is of no benefit to the athlete, since the body's normal supply of glycogen is more than adequate.

The common procedure of carbohydrate loading begins about one week before a competition. In preparation for the event, the muscles that will be used during it are exercised to exhaustion. This results in a loss of glycogen from the specific muscles used. During the next three days, the athlete follows a relatively low-carbohydrate, high-protein, high-fat diet and continues to exercise using the same muscles. The effect of this part of the regimen is to keep the glycogen content of the exercising muscles low. Three days before the competition, the athlete eats a high-carbohydrate diet (with carbohydrates comprising 60 to 70 percent of the calorie intake), including spaghetti, breads, and beer, along with enough other foods to meet nutritional requirements. This causes the glycogen to increase to a greater than normal level in those muscles (and *only* in those muscles) that were exercised.

Although carbohydrate loading may improve performance in endurance activities, it is not without side effects. During the low-carbohydrate phase of the diet, fatigue, irritability, and nausea have been reported. During the carbohydrate-loading phase, lack of practice may affect the athlete's concept of how he or she will do in the competition. The high glycogen stores may cause a heaviness or stiffness in the muscles, since water is always stored with glycogen. Muscle and kidney damage have also been reported as possible side effects. In athletes aged forty and older, serious side effects involving the heart are definite risks. Finally, fluid and mineral imbalances are also potential risks.

Calories

Physical activity requires calories. Requirements depend on the level of activity and vary with height, weight, and age. Athletes in training require more calories than nonathletes, sometimes as much as or more than 3,000 calories a day. An adjustment in intake is necessary to maintain an appropriate weight.

As you can see, the needs of an athlete differ from those of a nonathlete *only* with respect to calories, water, and sometimes, sodium. Other nutrients in excessive amounts are useless, may possibly be harmful, and are usually expensive.

Athletics have always been an important aspect of school life. Unfortunately, the competitive drive they may encourage often leads students to use unhealthy dietary practices. Dietary restrictions and food fads are frequently followed by students—at times with the encouragement of coaches. Before beginning this unit, it is important to know the dietary suggestions espoused by your school coaches and to understand the validity and/or dangers of these practices. If necessary, discuss these dietary suggestions with a dietitian, or review one of the books in the References/Resources section at the end of this unit.

Students may have additional questions about sports nutrition. Be prepared to offer ideas to them about where to find further information (books, magazines, community resources).

BASIC ACTIVITY

Time Needed: One class period

Materials Needed: Sheet 18-1: "Athlete's Nutrition Facts"
                                        Sheets 18-2 through 18-3: "Build-a-Team Fact or Fallacy Card Game"
                                        Quiz Sheet 18-1

1. Distribute Sheet 18-1, "Athlete's Nutrition Facts," and begin a large-group discussion of the facts and of students' misconceptions about how nutrition relates to exercise.
2. Divide the class into groups of four students apiece.

3. For each group, make one set of "Build-a-Team Fact or Fallacy Card Game" using Sheets 18-2 through 18-3.

4. Describe the following rules of the game to all of the groups:

a. Each student pretends to be a coach for an all-American team.

b. Unfortunately, each coach has only seven members on his or her team and desperately needs three more.

c. Each coach must try to get the team members he or she needs from the other coaches.

d. Coach #1 asks either coach #2, #3, or #4 in his group for one athlete to add to his or her team. The coach who was asked must take a card from the face-down card deck, read the statement to coach #1, and coach #1 must respond with "fact" or "fallacy." If he or she answers correctly, coach #1 gets the athlete and keeps the card. If incorrect, coach #1 gets no one and returns the card to the bottom of the deck.

e. After coach #1's turn, the game continues in a clockwise direction with coach #2 following the same procedure. Coach #2 may even ask coach #1 for his or her newly acquired athlete!

f. The game continues until one coach has completed his or her team.

5. After the game, conduct a short discussion that involves the whole class and that uses the following questions:

• What new information did you discover?

• What facts surprised you?

• What fallacies surprised you?

• How do the needs of athletes differ from the needs of nonathletes?

• What is sodium? Why do we need it? From where do we get most of our sodium?

• What is carbohydrate loading? Who benefits from it? Are there any problems associated with carbohydrate loading?

6. Proceed with the "Advanced Acitivty" if you wish; otherwise use the quiz mentioned in step 7.

7. **Evaluation:** Distribute Quiz Sheet 18-1 and have students complete it independently. Discuss the answers as a class.

ADVANCED ACTIVITY

Time Needed: One class period

Materials Needed: Sheets 18-4 through 18-5: "A Winning Diet"
Props for the play "A Winning Diet": a sign with "Track Practice Starts
Today;" two coach's caps; two whistles; sweatshirts and sneakers for four team
members
Quiz Sheet 18-1

1. Prior to the day of the play, select seven student volunteers to act in and produce the play "A Winning Diet." This play is a vehicle for reinforcing the concept that nutrition can affect athletic performance. A few simple props and a little time invested in rehearsal can transform this activity into a lively play that students may wish to perform for other classes. Have the students collect props and rehearse the play a few times as homework.

2. After the play has been performed for the class, have students individually write a list of nutritional rules that they would expect the track team in the play to follow. The list should come from the play itself. Have students suggest rules in addition to those presented in the play.

3. Conduct a large-group discussion of the rules the students wrote in step 2. Make sure they understand that these rules apply not only to athletes, but to anyone who is active. It is important for students to understand *why* each rule exists. Take another look at the rules on Sheet 18-1 and add the following to them:

- Persons who exercise less should eat less because they need fewer calories. However, they still need the same balance of nutrients.

- Eat a good breakfast. Why? Your body needs to replace the calories and nutrients it used during the night, and it shouldn't have to wait until lunch!

4. **Evaluation:** Distribute Quiz Sheet 18-1 and have students complete it independently. Discuss the answers as a class.

FOLLOW-UP ACTIVITIES

1. Have the students interview an athlete in training and ask the athlete to record everything he or she eats and drinks during a twenty-four-hour period, using Sheet 18-6, "Athlete's Twenty-Four-Hour Intake." Using food composition tables and Table 18-1, the students should then analyze the food recall sheet for calories, protein, sodium, and water. You may need to help students find sodium and water contents in foods not listed on Table 18-1; for these consult food composition tables in the sources listed in the References/Resources section at the end of this book. Some values for water content may be estimated by comparing similar foods. For example, a cookie would be closest to a piece of bread, and tomato sauce would be closest to a vegetable. Have students compare the totals for calories and protein from Sheet 18-6 to: (a) the athlete's RDA for calories and protein, (b) the Estimated Safe and Adequate Daily Dietary Intake of sodium (900–2,700 milligrams depending on age), and (c) the average daily requirement for water (1 milliter per calorie). Ask the students which, if any, values differ and how they differ. Discuss the athlete's needs for extra calories and water. Ask when extra sodium would be needed and how an athlete should obtain the amount needed.

2. Have students list sports in order of priority according to the amount of calories expended using Chart G, "Calorie Expenditure by Activity."

3. Have a panel of athletes discuss their eating habits with the class. Allow the class to support or refute the dietary practices of the athletes based on their knowledge.

ATHLETE'S NUTRITION FACTS

1. The energy and nutrients needed for athletic competition come from digested food that was eaten anywhere from a half day to several weeks prior to their use by the body. A pregame meal requires several hours before the nutrients are able to help the cells.

2. A diet containing excessively oily and fatty foods takes longer to be digested and, therefore, should be avoided before a competition.

3. A normal diet will supply an individual with all of the necessary salt the body needs. The practice of taking salt tablets can lead to a water imbalance in the body and to an upset stomach.

4. There is no evidence that additional amounts of vitamins and minerals, over and above an individual's U.S. RDAs will be of any benefit. An athlete should take care, however, to consume a balanced diet.

5. Dangerous levels of vitamins A and D can accumulate in the body if they are frequently taken in large doses as nutrient supplements.

6. Peak physical performance depends on the replacement of water through moderate fluid intake. Restricting an athlete's water intake before, during, or after exercise can be dangerous to health.

7. The addition of protein to a normally balanced diet will *not* accelerate the growth of muscles.

8. Iron deficiency can be a problem for female athletes with low calorie intakes. A normal American diet supplies about 6 milligrams of iron per 1,000 calories.

9. Additional calories needed for increased activity in exercise should be obtained by an overall increase in the individual's diet, *not* by high-calorie snacks containing few nutrients.

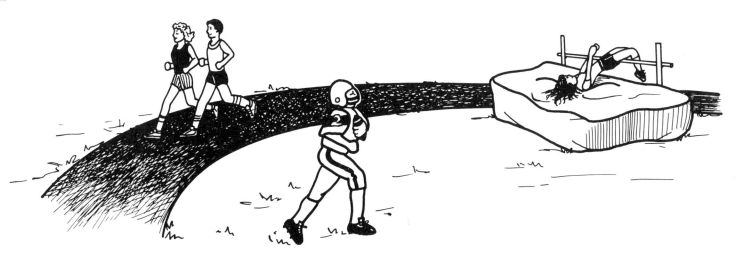

BUILD-A-TEAM FACT OR FALLACY CARD GAME

An athlete needs a lot more protein than a nonathlete of the same age. FALLACY	Because sodium is lost in sweating, an athlete may need extra sodium when he or she practices in very hot weather. FACT	The extra sodium an athlete needs when he or she sweats heavily should always be taken in the form of salt tablets. FALLACY
When an athlete needs extra sodium because he or she has practiced in very hot weather, he or she can get more by adding some salt from the salt shaker to his or her food or by eating something salty. FACT	Water helps to maintain body temperature. FACT	An athlete needs water during practice only when he or she is thirsty. FALLACY
Nutritionists recommend that a pregame meal include a large steak. FALLACY	An athlete can get all of the vitamins he or she needs by following the Daily Food Guide recommendations. FACT	Carbohydrate loading may be useful for people like marathon runners who exercise steadily for a prolonged time. FACT
A weight lifter will perform better if he or she practices carbohydrate loading. FALLACY	Taking extra B vitamins will give an athlete more energy. FALLACY	If an athlete does not get enough water during an event, he or she may develop heat stroke. FACT

BUILD-A-TEAM FACT OR FALLACY CARD GAME

For the athlete, most water is lost through the skin. FACT	Athletes should never drink water before or during a competition. FALLACY	To allow for proper digestion, athletes should eat about three hours before the competition. FACT
Carbohydrate loading has no side effects. FALLACY	Carbohydrate loading may cause heaviness or stiffness in the muscles. FACT	An athlete needs more calories, water, and possibly more sodium, than a nonathlete. FACT
Taking in too much sodium in the form of salt tablets can cause poor performance or stomach upsets. FACT	After a heavy practice, thirst may be satisfied long before the water lost by the body is replaced. FACT	Excess protein (an amount over what is needed) is changed to fat by the body and stored. FACT
An athlete in heavy training should add protein to his or her diet. If the protein is not added, the muscles will not grow properly. FALLACY	Carbohydrate foods, like bread, cereal, and macaroni, leave the stomach faster than protein or high-fat foods. FACT	The stomach should be empty, or nearly empty, before a competition. FACT

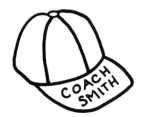

A WINNING DIET

PLACE: The locker room of Central Junior High; the sign on the wall reads "Track Practice
           Starts Today"

TIME: First day of track practice

PLAYERS: Narrator
           Coach Johnston
           Coach Smith
           Player #1
           Player #2
           Player #3
           Player #4

NARRATOR: Coach Smith and Coach Johnston have just finished talking about the track team's performance
                   during the previous year. With a record of five wins and four losses, about all that could be said was
                   that Central *did* have a winning season! What bothered Coach Smith was that members of the team
                   would sometimes perform better in practice than at the track meets. Coach Johnston thought that the
                   team had more ability than past scores had shown.

                   Let's listen in on some of the coaches' ideas for improving the team's record.

COACH   I *know* we have the ability to win, but I don't always see it in the final score.
JOHNSTON:

PLAYER #1:   Coach, what we need is some kind of advantage over the other teams.

PLAYER #2:   Yes, like those pregame steak dinners the football players on TV eat!

PLAYER #1:   I've heard that some of the other students take extra vitamins to give them more energy. Isn't that the
                   kind of advantage we need?

PLAYER #2:   Your're crazy, (*name*)! Extra vitamins don't do you any good, but lots of steak helps you build up
                   your muscles, that is, if you have any. Right, Coach?

COACH SMITH: Whoa folks! Settle down!

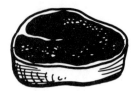

PLAYER #2:   But I'm right...aren't I, Coach?

COACH SMITH: You're right about vitamins. There is no evidence to show that you get any benefit from taking extra
                   vitamins. If you eat a balanced diet, you get all the vitamins your body needs. Improper eating could
                   slow you down, though. That may have been part of our problem last year.

PLAYER #2:   Well, what about all that steak on TV? Steak gives us lots of protein. Don't we need a lot of *extra*
                   protein to perform well?

COACH SMITH: If you eat a balanced diet, you'll get all the protein you need. Extra protein won't help you perform
                   better. Stuffing yourself with a lot of meat just puts on extra *weight* ... and it's expensive!

COACH
JOHNSTON: I agree. When you eat right, you get all of the vitamins and protein you need from your food. I've heard that some team members have a habit of skipping breakfast. (Students look sheepishly around. Several team members look just a little guilty.) That can slow you down . . . in school and on the track. Now, there's something else I'd like us to consider about those pregame meals. I want all of you to think about how long it takes to digest the food you eat.

PLAYER #3:   I get it, Coach. The meal you eat before the game doesn't have enough time to be digested to be of much help.

COACH
JOHNSTON: Right, (name). This is especially true of meals high in fat. I'm afraid this team is not always eating right. It's not enough just to worry about what you eat on the day of the track meet. *Every* meal is important . . . all week long!

PLAYER #4:   Coach, you mean that what I ate *last* week is important for my running *this* week?

COACH SMITH: Yes. Any other questions?

PLAYER #4:   Coach, I read someplace that you need to replace the salt you lose when you sweat. Why don't you give the team salt tablets on really hot days?

COACH SMITH: Is there salt in the food you eat?

PLAYER #4:   Yes . . .

COACH SMITH: By eating food that is salted you get all of the salt your body needs.

PLAYER #1:   I heard that putting large amounts of salt on your food or taking salt tablets can be dangerous to your health.

COACH SMITH: That's right, (name). It can make you retain too much water or give you an upset stomach.

PLAYER #4:   But I get very tired running on hot days. Isn't that because I didn't get enough salt?

COACH
JOHNSTON: Probably not. Maybe you've been forgetting to drink enough water during practice and at the track meets.

PLAYER #3:   I thought drinking water while you exercise might make you sick.

COACH
JOHNSTON: I didn't say to drink the well dry! But you *should* take small amounts of water during practice and at meets, too. Replacing the water you lose from exercising and sweating is just as important as eating right.

COACH SMITH: It could be that poor food habits, such as skipping breakfast, not eating balanced diets, and forgetting to replace lost water, could have held our record down last year.

PLAYER #2:   Let's make up a list of nutrition rules to follow this season!

COACH SMITH: Fine! Any other questions?

PLAYER #2:   Yes! Where are we going to put the trophy? (*The team descends on Player #2.*)

ATHLETE'S 24-HOUR INTAKE

Directions: Record all food and beverages you consume during a full twenty-four-hour period. Be sure to include soft drinks, gum, snacks, and condiments (ketchup, mustard, mayonnaise).

Time Of Day	Meal Or Snack	Food Or Drink	Amount	Calories (Cal.)	Protein (g.)	Sodium (g.)	Water (ml.)
		Totals					
		Recommended Intakes					

Table 18-1

SODIUM AND WATER CONTENTS OF SELECTED FOODS

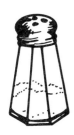 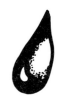

FOOD	AMOUNT	SODIUM	FOOD	AMOUNT	WATER
MILK GROUP: Milk, all types Cheese Cottage cheese	1 cup 1 oz. ½ cup	120 mg. 250 mg. 230 mg.	**MILK GROUP:** Milk, all types	1 cup	160 ml.
MEAT GROUP: Meats: beef, chicken, lamb, pork, turkey (salt added in cooking) Meats: bacon, Canadian bacon, cold cuts, ham, hotdogs Fish, fresh or frozen Egg Beans, dried (cooked)	1 oz. 1 oz. 1 oz. 1 ½ cup	70 mg. 330 mg. 70 mg. 65 mg. 230 mg.	**MEAT GROUP:** Meats, all types Fish, all types Egg Beans, dried (cooked)	1 oz. 1 oz. 1 ½ cup	20 ml. 20 ml. 35 ml. 65 ml.
FRUIT AND VEGETABLE GROUP: Fruits and fruit juices Vegetables, raw Vegetables, cooked (salt added in cooking or canning)	½ cup ½ cup ½ cup	2 mg. 10 mg. 230 mg.	**FRUIT AND VEGETABLE GROUP:** Fruits, all types (canned, without liquid) Vegetables, all types	½ cup ½ cup	85 ml. 70 ml.
BREAD AND CEREAL GROUP: Bread, all types Cereal, all types Spaghetti, macaroni, noodles Rice (instant)	1 slice 1 oz. 1 cup 1 cup 1 cup	120 mg. 230 mg. 2 mg. 7 mg. 606 mg.	**BREAD AND CEREAL GROUP:** Bread, all types Cereal, dry Cereal, cooked	1 slice 1 oz. ½ cup	10 ml. 1 ml. 85 ml.
OTHER: Butter, margarine Oil	1 tsp. 1 tsp.	50 mg. 0 mg.	**OTHER:** Butter, margarine Beverages other than milk	1 tsp. 1 cup	1 ml. 240 ml.
SEASONINGS: Salt	1 tsp.	2,000 mg.			

QUIZ
THE ATHLETE'S DIET

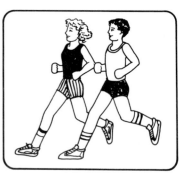

_____ 1. Lack of which of the following nutrients has the quickest effect on a person who is exercising?
   a. Iron   c. Protein
   b. Water   d. Vitamin A

_____ 2. Exercise causes muscles to grow and bones to change shape. Which of the nutrients below are used in both growth and exercise?
   a. Iron CaPAC   c. Water
   b. B vitamins   d. All of the above

_____ 3. Sue has just joined the swim team. She asked her coach if eating large amounts of protein would help her perform better. How should her coach answer this question?
   a. Extra protein is necessary for your muscles to become strong and to perform better.
   b. Salt tablets should be taken with the extra protein.
   c. Extra protein is not necessary if you are already eating a balanced diet.
   d. Only extra protein from meat will help you perform better.

_____ 4. John is scheduled to be the quarterback in the Friday night football game. All week long, he has been eating poorly. Late Friday afternoon, he asks if eating a large, nutritious supper will help him perform well in the game. What should you tell him?
   a. A large, nutritious supper will make up for eating poorly all week long.
   b. Only the protein in the supper will help.
   c. For the most help, he should not drink anything with the supper.
   d. Most of the food will not be digested in time to help.

_____ 5. An athlete needs more _____ than a nonathlete.
   a. Protein   c. Vitamins
   b. Calories   d. Fat

_____ 6. Which most closely describes "carbohydrate loading"?
   a. Eating a lot of honey right before a competition.
   b. Eating a high-fat diet for three days before a competition and having frequent practices.
   c. Eating a pregame meal high in meat and cheese.
   d. Eating a diet high in grain products, fruits, and vegetables during the three days before a competition.

_____ 7. Carbohydrate loading might improve the performance of a:
   a. Marathon runner   c. Weight lifter
   b. Wrestler   d. Football player

SECTION IV

MEAL PLANNING AND PREPARATION

Unit 19   Interpreting Ingredient Labels

Unit 19: Interpreting Ingredient Labels

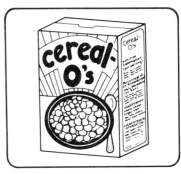

CONCEPTS

–Nutritional labels are required for foods that make nutritional claims, or for foods that have been fortified. Nutritional labels for other food products are optimal.

–If a product has a nutritional label it must meet the specifications set by the Food and Drug Administration (FDA).

–The nutrient content is expressed as a percent of the U.S. RDA for one serving of the food.

–If ingredients are listed on food labels, they must be listed in descending order by weight.

–Food labels may also contain advertisements.

OBJECTIVES

–Students will be able to identify various parts of a food label.

–Students will be able to examine a nutritional label and to determine the amount of vitamins, minerals, calories, and relative ingredient amounts.

TEACHER'S UNIT INTRODUCTION

Food labels can be an invaluable tool for learning about food and nutrition. Labels contain a variety of information ranging from food product descriptions, advertising, recipes, ingredient listings, and nutrition information. The "ingredient listing" and the "nutrition information" parts of the label are the two parts that have strict U.S. government rules specifying how they must appear on the label.

Ingredient Listing

Most processed food products are required to list their ingredients on the food label. The ingredients must be listed by *weight* in *descending* order. For example, the most predominant ingredient (by weight) in the buttermilk pancake mix listed below is "enriched flour." The least predominant ingredient is "artificial color."

Buttermilk Pancake Mix ingredients: enriched flour, sugar, rice flour, baking powder, buttermilk, salt, cornstarch, artificial color.

If flavoring or coloring is used, the specific name of that ingredient need *not* be given. However, the ingredient must be listed as being either *artificial* or *natural.*

Some food products have a "Standard of Identity" and are exempt from the ingredient labeling requirement. A *Standard of Identity* is a recipe that has been established. By law, a food with that name *must* contain the ingredients in the standard recipe. Examples of foods that have a "Standard of Identity" include mayonnaise, ice cream, and catsup.

When nutrition information is included on the label, it must conform to certain standards, including:

1. The nutrition information must be placed to the right of the main display panel.
2. The serving size and number of servings per container must be specified.
3. The number of calories and grams of protein, carbohydrate, and fat per serving must be specified.
4. The percent of the U.S. Recommended Daily Allowances (U.S. RDAs) of eight nutrients (protein, Vitamin A, Vitamin C, thiamin, riboflavin, niacin, calcium, and iron) per serving must be specified.

Here is a sample label with its component parts. (Show this with an opaque projector or make a transparency for use on an overhead projector.)

Average size determined by manufacturer.

Optional: Two types of fat may be listed with the footnote.

Optional: Cholesterol may be listed two ways: total amount and amount/100 grams of food.

Protein is listed twice: above, in its actual amount, and here, as a percentage of the U.S. RDA. This listing is based on a U.S. RDA of 65 grams of low-quality protein or 45 grams of high-quality protein.

Optional: These nutrients (from Vitamin D to pantothenic acid) may be listed. The chosen nutrients must appear in the order presented here.

Optional: Sodium may be listed two ways: total amount and amount/100 grams of food.

U.S. RDA is based on the Recommended Daily Allowances (RDA). They are a single set of recommendations for all active, healthy people. The first eight nutrients (from protein to iron) must appear in the order presented here.

NUTRITION INFORMATION PER SERVING

Serving Size .... ( )
Servings per Container.......................... ( )

Calories .... ( )
Protein...................................... ( ) g.
Carbohydrates .... ( ) g.
Fat .... ( ) g.

  Polyunsaturated** .... ( ) g.

  Saturated** .... ( ) g.
Cholesterol .... ( ) mg.
Sodium..................................... ( ) mg.

PERCENTAGE OF U.S. RECOMMENDED DAILY ALLOWANCES (U.S. RDA)

Protein.............( ) Vitamin B$_6$ ....( )
Vitamin A ....( ) Folacin ....( )
Vitamin C ....( ) Vitamin B$_{12}$...............( )
Thiamin.............( ) Phosphorus ....( )
Riboflavin ....( ) Iodine ....( )
Niacin ....( ) Magnesium ....( )
Calcium.............( ) Zinc ....( )
Iron ....( ) Copper ....( )
Vitamin D...........( ) Biotin ....( )
Vitamin E ....( ) Pantothenic Acid...........( )

**Information on fat content is provided for individuals who, on the advice of a physician, are modifying their total dietary intake of fat.

The ingredient label is useful to the consumer in at least two principal ways:

1. In determining whether one ingredient provides more or less weight than another
2. In identifying whether a food has ingredients that the consumer may want to consume less of or to avoid altogether for health or religious reasons

Nutrition Information

Including nutrition information on the food label is usually voluntary. However, food manufacturers are required by law to include a nutrition label on a food product if

1. Nutrients have been added to the food, that is, the food has been enriched or fortified
2. The manufacturer has made a nutritional claim, for example, "high-protein," "low-cholesterol," "fortified with vitamins", and so forth.

However, manufacturers will often voluntarily put nutrition labeling information on foods that do not meet either of the above two criteria.

Advertisement

Usually food packages have some form of advertisement. It may be a picture or a photograph of the food product or of people enjoying it. Or, the advertisement may use cartoon characters as a trademark. The advertisement is usually designed to catch the eye of consumers and to convince them, as quickly as possible, to buy the product without further examination of the label.

This unit makes use of the information on the U.S. RDAs presented in Unit 7. In Unit 7, it was explained that 100 percent of the U.S. RDAs often exceeds 100 percent of the RDAs for certain age/sex groups. For example, the U.S. RDA for Vitamin A is 5,000 International Units, but the RDA for seven-to-ten-year-old children is only 3,500 IUs and for eleven-to-fourteen-year-old girls it is 4,000 IUs. Thus, seven-to-ten-year-old children need only 70 percent of the U.S. RDA to meet their individual RDA for Vitamin A: eleven-to-fourteen-year-old girls need only 80 percent of the U.S. RDA to meet their individual RDA for Vitamin A. A good rule of thumb about the U.S. RDAs is that if you are *not* a fifteen-to-eighteen-year-old male, you will most likely need substantially *less* than the U.S. RDAs daily. You may wish to have students compare their individual RDAs for selected nutrients to the U.S. RDAs.

On the day prior to implementing this unit, have each student bring to class three food containers or labels that provide nutrition information. Ask them to find at least one label without nutrition information and, if possible, one without an ingredient listing. You might also assign students to bring containers or labels by food groups to ensure a wide variety of labels.

BASIC ACTIVITY

Time Needed: One class period

Materials Needed: Sample food containers or labels *with* nutrition information
Sample food containers or labels *without* nutrition information
Sheets 19-1 through 19-3: "Nutrition Information Labels"
Quiz Sheet 20-1

1. Display or pass around a few of the food containers or labels that do *not* have nutrition labeling information. Ask students if they know why some foods have nutrition labels and some do not.

2. Review the two conditions that make nutrition labeling mandatory (see Teacher's Unit Introduction).

3. Distribute Sheets 19-1 through 19-3, "Nutrition Information Labels." Using the sample food containers and labels, students should complete the worksheets.

4. Following completion of the worksheets, discuss common characteristics, location, and information found on the nutrition label. Make sure the following concepts are understood:

- All labels must have the heading "Nutrition Information."

- The nutrition label must provide a defined set of information including the serving size and number of servings per container. The FDA has translated that a serving size be of an "average, usual, or reasonable size." This is not an iron-clad law, but its flexibility serves a purpose. Let's use a loaf of bread as an example. Since no one is expected to eat the whole loaf, it would serve no purpose to list the total quantities of nutrition in the entire loaf. Either one or two slices is considered to be a proper serving size for a sandwich or buttered toast. Most breads list one slice as the serving size.

- The nutrition label must provide the number of calories and of grams of fat, carbohydrate, and protein, in one serving.

- The nutrition label must provide, per serving, the percent of the U.S. RDAs for the Iron CaPAC nutrients, plus thiamin, riboflavin, and niacin. The use of percentages as a measurement tool makes it easier to plan one's diet. The percentages of the necessary nutrients a food supplies are listed, so there is no need to know what the exact requirements are for each nutrient. The percentage supplied by each food may be used directly.

5. Proceed with the "Advanced Activity," if you wish; otherwise use the quiz mentioned in step 6.

6. **Evaluation:** Distribute Quiz Sheet 19-1 and have students complete it independently. Discuss the answers as a class.

ADVANCED ACTIVITY

Time Needed: One class period

Materials Needed: Food label cut from container (*optional*)
Sheet 19-4: "Hey, What Is In This Food, Anyway?" (three copies per student)
Sheets 19-5 through 19-6: "Mystery Food Labels"
Ten different food containers with nutritional labels
Quiz Sheet 19-11

1. Use the sample food label in the "Teacher's Unit Introduction" (or a real food label cut from its container) under an opaque projector or on a transparency and point out the parts of the label. Include a review of where nutrition information, ingredient listing, and advertisements are located; review also the rules governing their content.

2. Display ten food containers with nutrition labels at stations around the classroom where pairs of students can examine each one. Have each pair evaluate six out of the ten food products using a copy of Sheet 19-4 for each food.

3. Following the activity, conduct a large-group discussion of what students learned about the foods from their labels. Discuss these questions as well:

- Is there enough nutrition information on the labels? Too much?

- Is the nutrition information easy to understand? If needed, how could the label(s) be improved?

4. Distribute Sheets 19-5 through 19-6, "Mystery Food Labels" and have students match the food products with their ingredient labels. You can extend this activity by asking students to bring in "mystery food" containers. Simply make a transparency of each ingredient label (with no identifying food name) and have the class try to guess the mystery food. Or, have the students read their individual ingredient list without showing the food product and have the class guess the product.

5. **Evaluation:** Distribute Quiz Sheet 19-1 and have students complete it independently. Discuss the answers as a class.

FOLLOW-UP ACTIVITIES

1. Have students find and read labels of designated foods that meet the following criteria:

- There are examples from each food group in the Daily Food Guide.

- There are examples of both relatively unprocessed foods (for example, rolled oats) and also of highly processed foods (for example, boxed, sugar-coated cereal).

- There are examples of foods with cholesterol, saturated fat, unsaturated fat, and/or sodium on the label.

2. Have students prepare their own nutritional labels for single foods or dishes listed in food composition tables. Then have a contest where students guess what food the mystery labels describe.

3. Have students look at labels of convenience foods, such as breakfast cereals, breakfast bars, packaged soup, boxed dinners, condiments, cake mixes, and others. You may send students to the grocery store or have them look at foods in either their own kitchen cupboards or in the cupboards in the school's kitchens. Have them list how many times, and in how many products, sugar is listed. Remind them that sugar is also listed as *sucrose, fructose, dextrose, glucose, corn syrup,* and *corn sweetener.* Have them also look for salt or sodium on the label. This activity could also be set up as an investigative game by having students search for foods *without* added sugar or salt.

NUTRITION INFORMATION LABELS

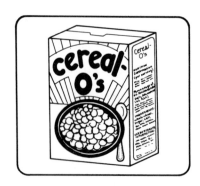

You know that your body needs a variety of nutrients, and that you get those nutrients from the foods you eat. Nutrition information labels, like those you brought to class, help by telling you how *much* of each nutrient is in a serving of the food you eat. Nobody can tell how much Vitamin C is in a glass of orange juice, for example, just by looking at it. That's one of the reasons the Federal Food and Drug Administration (FDA) requires labels on many kinds of foods. Nutrition information labels can help keep track of the nutrients in the foods you eat.

Let's take a look at the labels you brought to class and see what you can learn from them.

1. Do all of your labels have the words "Nutrition Information Per Serving" written at the top?

           Yes   No

Choose one of your labels with nutrition information and answer the following questions:

2. What is the food's name? _____

3. What is the serving size? _____

4. How many calories are in one serving? _____

In addition to the number of calories, the nutrition information lists the grams of fat, carbohydrate, and protein you would get by eating an average portion (one serving) of the food. The information also lists, per serving, the percent of U.S. RDAs for protein and for several vitamins and minerals. If you ate *double* the amount of food in a single serving, you would get *twice* the calories and *twice* the nutrients. You would get only half the calories and nutrients if you ate half a serving.

5. How many calories are in a double serving of your food? _____

Let's look more closely at the information listed under "Percentage of U.S. Recommended Daily Allowances (U.S. RDAs)" on your food label. The amount of protein, vitamins, and minerals are listed as percentages (not grams or milligrams).

For example, an eight-ounce cup of milk provides about 300 milligrams of calcium. The nutrition label tells you that the milk provides 30 percent of the U.S. RDA for calcium. This is because the U.S. RDA for calcium is 1,000 milligrams.

6. $300 \div 1000 =$ _____ . Since percentages express everything in terms of 100, multiply your answer to convert it to percent: _____ %

Percentages are used to make it *easy* for you to find out if the different foods you eat supply all of the necessary nutrients. The recommended daily amount of each nutrient if 100%. Remember: These nutrition labels are used by many different people. Just as the "RDA Doorway to Good Health" in Unit 3 was probably higher than you needed, an amount required to supply 100 percent of a nutrient may be higher than your needs. For many of the Iron CaPAC nutrients and B vitamins, boys and girls aged nine to fourteen years do *not* need 100 percent of the U.S. RDAs. Look at the table on Sheet 19-2 called "Percentages of U.S. RDA for Youth Ages 9–14." What percent of the U.S. RDA is recommended for *you* for each nutrient?

PERCENTAGES OF U.S. RDA FOR YOUTH AGES 9–14

	Protein	Vitamin A	Vitamin C	Thiamin	Riboflavin	Niacin	Calcium	Iron
Girls, ages 9–10	55%	70%	70%	80%	75%	50%	80%	60%
Boys, ages 9–10	55	70	70	80	75	50	80	60
Girls, ages 11–14	70	80	75	80	80	45	120	100
Boys, ages 11–14	70	100	75	90	90	55	120	100

Don't worry if the foods you eat give you more protein, vitamins, and minerals than you need. Your body stores extra amounts of a few nutrients and excretes excesses of the others. Most of the nutrients you need must be replaced each day. You should get a daily supply of protein, Vitamin C, thiamin, riboflavin, niacin, calcium, and iron. A good source of Vitamin A should be supplied in the diet at least every other day.

7. If the label said you get 4 percent of the U.S. RDA of Vitamin C from a glass of milk, how many glasses of milk would you have to drink to get 100 percent of the daily allowance of Vitamin C from milk alone?

_____

8. If you don't want to drink that much milk, name another way to get your Vitamin C:

_____

Milk is a good way to get your protein and calcium, as well as other nutrients, but it is a poor source of Vitamin C. That's why it is important to eat many different types of food. You can get enough of one or two nutrients from one food, and other nutrients from another food, without eating huge amounts of any single food.

Using the three labels you brought to class, we will learn how to count nutrients. Follow the instructions listed below:

Step A: Pick one of your nutrition information labels. Write the food's name and the percentage of each nutrient listed on the chart on Sheet 19-3. Then record the number of calories in one serving.

Step B: Follow Step A for two more of your labels.

9. How would you find out the total percentage of protein supplied by eating one serving of each of the three foods?

_____

_____

Add the percentage supplied by each nutrient when you eat one serving of all three foods and fill in the column marked "Total Calories and % U.S. RDAs from Three Foods."

Step C: Fill in the last column marked "Recommended % of U.S. RDAs for Your Age and Sex" using the information from the chart at the top of this sheet.

	Food #1: _____	Food #2: _____	Food #3: _____	Total Calories and % U.S. RDAs from Three Foods	Recommended % of U.S. RDAs for Your Age and Sex
Calories	_____ cal	_____ cal	_____ cal	_____ cal	_____ cal
Protein	_____ %	_____ %	_____ %	_____ %	_____ %
Vitamin A	_____ %	_____ %	_____ %	_____ %	_____ %
Vitamin C	_____ %	_____ %	_____ %	_____ %	_____ %
Thiamin	_____ %	_____ %	_____ %	_____ %	_____ %
Riboflavin	_____ %	_____ %	_____ %	_____ %	_____ %
Niacin	_____ %	_____ %	_____ %	_____ %	_____ %
Calcium	_____ %	_____ %	_____ %	_____ %	_____ %
Iron	_____ %	_____ %	_____ %	_____ %	_____ %

Did you notice that if you ate only those three foods that were listed, you wouldn't get all of the nutrients you need each day? Also, notice that different foods contain different amounts of each nutrient. That's why it is important to eat *many* kinds of foods. Variety in your diet is very important!

10. On the lines below, write three or four sentences that tell how eating a variety of foods helps you to meet your daily U.S. RDA goals for each student.

_____

_____

_____

_____

_____

_____

_____

_____

_____

_____

_____

_____

_____

_____

Attach your three labels to these sheets.

HEY, WHAT IS IN THIS FOOD, ANYWAY?

NUTRITION INFORMATION PER SERVING:

Serving Size _____

Calories _____

Protein _____ gm./ _____ % U.S. RDA

Carbohydrates _____ gm.

Fat _____ gm.   Sodium _____ mg.
   cholesterol   saturated fat   yes/no
                unsaturated fat yes/no
                  sodium yes/no

<u>% U.S. RDA</u> _____

_____ vitamin A   _____ niacin

_____ vitamin C   _____ calcium

_____ thiamin   _____ iron

_____ riboflavin   yes/no   others

Mmmm Good!!

INGREDIENTS:
Which ingredient is present in the largest

amount? _____
Which ingredient is present in the smallest

amount? _____

MYSTERY FOOD LABELS

Directions: Read each list of ingredients and solve the mystery food! Among the six mystery foods on this sheet and on Sheet 19-6 you will find:

- orange juice
- table mustard
- wheat bread

- thousand island dressing
- yellow cake mix
- breakfast orange drink

1. _____   2. _____

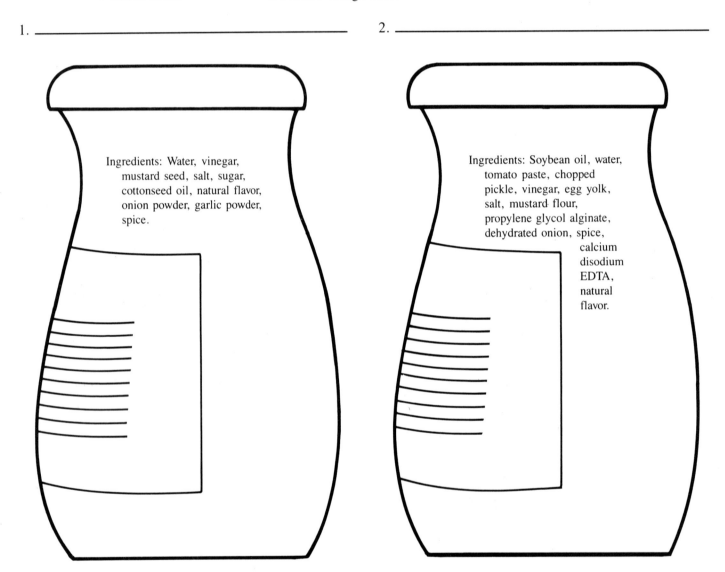

Ingredients: Water, vinegar, mustard seed, salt, sugar, cottonseed oil, natural flavor, onion powder, garlic powder, spice.

Ingredients: Soybean oil, water, tomato paste, chopped pickle, vinegar, egg yolk, salt, mustard flour, propylene glycol alginate, dehydrated onion, spice, calcium disodium EDTA, natural flavor.

3. _____

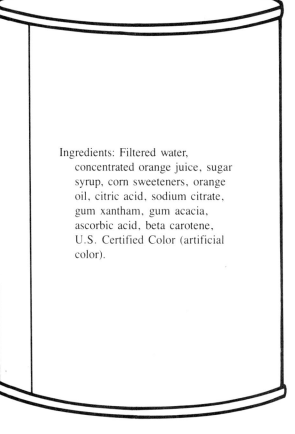

Ingredients: Filtered water, concentrated orange juice, sugar syrup, corn sweeteners, orange oil, citric acid, sodium citrate, gum xantham, gum acacia, ascorbic acid, beta carotene, U.S. Certified Color (artificial color).

4. _____

Ingredients: Filtered water, concentrated orange juice.

5. _____

Ingredients: Wheat flour (bleached flour, malted barley flour) water, whole-wheat flour, nonfat dry milk, brown sugar, yeast, salt, buttermilk, vegetable shortening, wheat gluten, corn syrup, honey, whey, yeast nutrients, mono- and di-glycerides, dough conditioner, corn flour, soy flour, calcium propionate, calcium peroxide.

6. _____

Ingredients: Enriched flour (bleached flour, niacin, iron, thiamin mononitrate, riboflavin), sugar, animal fat and/or partially hydrogenated vegetable oil, shortening, dextrose, modified cornstarch, baking soda, salt, sodium aluminum phosphate, calcium phosphate, propylene glycol, monoesters, mono- and di-glycerides, guar gum, artificial flavor, soy lecithin, artificial color.

QUIZ
INTERPRETING FOOD LABELS

Study the label shown here, then answer the questions below:

1. How many calories are in one serving of this cereal? _____

2. How many calories are added when you eat the cereal with ½ cup whole milk? _____

3. Does a serving of cereal plus milk provide more grams of protein or of carbohydrate? _____

4. If you are nine to fourteen years old, you need 75 percent of the U.S. RDA for Vitamin C. How many servings of this cereal would you have to eat in order to meet your need for Vitamin C? _____

5. If you ate two cups of this cereal, what percent of the U.S. RDA for riboflavin would be supplied by the cereal *alone?* _____

6. How much *more* riboflavin would be supplied by two cups of this cereal *plus* milk? _____

7. Which ingredient is found in the largest amount? _____

8. Which ingredient is found in the smallest amount? _____

9. In what order are the ingredients listed on all food labels?
   a. Alphabetically
   b. Any way the food manufacturer wants to list them
   c. By weight, with the ingredient present in the smallest amount listed first
   d. By weight, with the ingredient present in the largest amount listed first

10. Examine these two cereal ingredient labels:
Brand A: wheat flour, sugar, graham flour, brown sugar, wheat starch, nonfat dry milk, salt, iron, niacin, riboflavin, and thiamin
Brand B: oat flour, defatted soy flour, salt, nonfat dry milk, sugar, wheat starch, wheat germ, iron, niacin, riboflavin, and thiamin
What conclusions can you draw? a. Brand B would probably be lower in sugar than Brand A.
   b. Brand A probably has more salt than Brand B.
   c. Brand B probably has more sugar than Brand A.
   d. Brand B would be a good choice if you were trying to reduce the salt in your diet.

NUTRITION INFORMATION PER SERVING		
SERVING SIZE		1 OZ (⅔ CUP)
SERVINGS PER CONTAINER		14
	1 OZ. CEREAL	1 OZ. CEREAL PLUS ½ CUP VITAMIN D FORTIFIED WHOLE MILK
CALORIES	90	170
PROTEIN	3 g	7 g
CARBOHYDRATE	23 g	29 g
FAT	0 g	4 g
SODIUM	300 mg	370 mg
POTASSIUM	220 mg	395 mg
PERCENTAGE OF U.S. RECOMMENDED DAILY ALLOWANCES (U.S. RDA)		
PROTEIN	4	15
VITAMIN A	*	4
VITAMIN C	25	25
THIAMIN	25	25
RIBOFLAVIN	4	10
NIACIN	25	25
CALCIUM	*	15
IRON	25	25
VITAMIN D	*	10
VITAMIN B₆	25	25
FOLIC ACID	25	25
VITAMIN B₁₂	25	30
PHOSPHORUS	20	30
MAGNESIUM	15	20
ZINC	25	30
COPPER	10	10
PANTOTHENIC ACID	2	6

CONTAINS LESS THAN 2 PERCENT OF THE U.S. RDA OF THESE NUTRIENTS.
INGREDIENTS
WHEAT BRAN, MILLED YELLOW CORN, SUGAR, MALTED CEREAL SYRUP, SALT, SODIUM ASCORBATE (VITAMIN C), NIACINAMIDE, REDUCED IRON, ZINC OXIDE, BHA (A PRESERVATIVE), PYRIDOXINE HYDROCHLORIDE (VITAMIN B₆), THIAMINE MONONITRATE (VITAMIN B₁). FOLIC ACID AND VITAMIN B₁₂. BHT ADDED TO PACKAGING MATERIAL TO HELP PRESERVE FRESHNESS.

SECTION V

Nutrition Issues

Unit 20   A Close Look at Food Advertising

Unit 20: A Close Look at Food Advertising

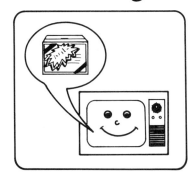

CONCEPTS

- Advertisements are designed to convince the consumer to buy a product.
- Advertisers use a variety of techniques to sell products.
- Highly processed foods are the ones most heavily advertised.
- More than half of the thousands of food commercials watched by children each year are for high-sugar/low-nutrient foods.
- Many food commercials aimed at children convey misleading messages.

OBJECTIVES

- Students will be able to evaluate advertisements (television, radio, magazine, newspaper, or "in-store" ads) according to the criteria described in the unit.
- Students will evaluate food commercials shown during television programs for children on the basis of the techniques used, the level of understanding needed to comprehend the commercial, and the presence and/or accuracy of the nutrition information offered.
- Students will be able to suggest ways to present accurate nutrition information to the television-viewing audience.

TEACHER'S UNIT INTRODUCTION

In a free enterprise system, product promotion makes sense. Therefore, advertising makes sense. In order to survive, companies must sell products, and, in order to sell products, companies must advertise the qualities that make their products special. Deception and misleading information, however, are *not* acceptable means to sell products even if competition is tough. The Federal Trade Commission works to protect you by requiring that advertising be neither deceptive nor unfair. Nevertheless, commercials exist that barely fulfill these requirements. Perhaps this is due to problems in defining exactly what "deceptive" or "unfair" advertising means. Another aspect of this problem is the protection of the media by the First Amendment to the U.S. Constitution, which guarantees freedom of speech and prevents the tightening of governmental control. As a result, it is essential for *you* to become educated about advertising and advertising techniques. With an increased awareness, you will be better equipped to evaluate commercial messages and to make wise decisions in the marketplace.

In most commercials, advertisers appeal to basic psychological needs. The need to feel secure and protected is one such need. Car batteries that are advertised as starting a car immediately in the worst weather and tires that are advertised as holding the car on the road during a storm appeal to our need for safety and security. Another basic psychological need is for love and peer acceptance. A mother who makes terrific cookies for her children earns love; and an office worker who uses the right mouthwash and shampoo is accepted by his or her coworkers.

Advertisers also appeal to the more complex processes of human memory and image association. Slogans that are repeated in an advertisement often establish a familiarity with a product in the consumer's subconscious. Advertisers reason that when the consumer needs to purchase that particular type of product, the chances are good that he or she will choose the most familiar name brand. Associating products with images of popularity, beauty, machismo, happiness, and athletic ability appeals to the human desire to possess such favorable attributes. These intangible qualities are often so much a part of an advertisement that the consumer may come to believe that the *qualities* can be purchased along with the product!

Many of the common advertising strategies are used in all forms of media advertising and for a wide variety of products. Nine of these strategies are:

Strategy 1: <u>Problem/Solution</u>—In this advertising strategy, the person on the screen has a problem. A second person enters the scene with a solution and throws in a sales pitch to the audience. For example, a person in a diner spills a cup of coffee (PROBLEM). The waitress zooms over to clean it up with a special brand of paper towel (SOLUTION), and while she does so, explains the advantages of that particular brand (SALES PITCH).

Strategy 2: <u>Demonstration</u>: This strategy shows the product being used. It is amazing how quickly and perfectly the vegetables are sliced, diced, and chopped by the gadgets on television commercials! This method proved to be particularly effective for one fast-food restaurant. In its commercials, customers were shown tackling big, juicy hamburgers. The campaign, known as "Hot 'n Juicy," played a major role in boosting the company's sales from 2 million to 800 million dollars.

Strategy 3: <u>Personification</u>: This strategy makes the product into a fictitious, living creature. Talking raisins dropping into cereal boxes and hamburgers animated with arms, legs, and faces can promote the product from a novel point of view.

Strategy 4: <u>Testimony</u>: When two or more brands of the same product exist, a convincing strategy is to record the testimony of experts or the opinion of an average, everyday consumer. Do you recognize any of these slogans?

"It really *does* taste like fresh peanuts!"

"I had only one cavity!"

"Four out of five dentists recommend _____ for their patients who chew gum." (Actually, most dentists do not recommend gum chewing at all!)

Strategy 5: <u>Slice of Life</u>: In this strategy, the commercial shows a short story that could happen anywhere. For example, relatives receive a phone call from a son, daughter, or grandchild, and the announcer says, "It's the next best thing to being there." Or, a young boy loses an ice hockey game, and his father gives him a piece of candy to help make him feel better.

Strategy 6: <u>Jingles or Catchy Phrases</u>: These seem to be favorite strategies of advertisers. Most people can identify the products associated with jingles or catchy phrases. Some samples are: "Ring around the collar;" "A piece of the rock;" "Snap, crackle, pop;" and "You deserve a break today!"

Strategy 7: <u>Use of Pleasure Words and Appealing Product Pictures</u>: Strategic words like "happy," "fun," "delicious," "tasty," and "tempting" lead consumers to believe that the product tastes good or that they will feel great if they buy the product. Ask yourself:

"Are Sugar Frosted Flakes really 'GRRREAT!'?"

"Would you describe Campbell's soup as 'Mmmm good!'?"

Words that describe food quality are often accompanied with appealing pictures. Cutting a cake with a feather clearly illustrates tenderness. Close-up photographs of fresh strawberries or peaches can be mouthwatering. Camera angles, special camera lenses, music, sound, and lighting are also often used to enhance a product's best qualities.

Strategy 8: <u>Free Gift</u>: Cereals and some snack items may use the strategy of offering a free toy inside the box or a free toy that can be received by sending in proof-of-purchase seals. This special gift offer increases the desirability of the product. Therefore, if two products of equal quality are available, the fact that one offers something free could become the consumer's basis for deciding to buy that product. (At least, this is what advertisers hope!)

Strategy 9: <u>Endorsement by a Famous Person</u>: A commercial with a well-known personality may capture viewers' attention to a greater extent than if an unknown person appeared with the product. For example, a Jell-O commercial with Bill Cosby may capture children's attention. While the Council of Better Business Bureau's National Advertising Division (NAD) allows all types of endorsers, the National Association of Broadcasters (NAB) tries to minimize this and prohibits the use of celebrities. Commercials that use celebrities continue to exist because only 50 percent of television stations are members of NAB and regulation by the television industry is voluntary.

In the 1950s and 1960s, advertisements for foods were aimed primarily at homemakers. Food commercials were directed toward women concerned with how good the products tasted and with how well they pleased family members. Nutrition as a selling point for foods only became popular in the mid-1970s. The growing interest in health and fitness has caused food product advertisers to include nutritional claims in many of their ads. Nutrition, as well as good taste, now sells food products.

Some techniques used to sell so-called nutrition can be misleading. Although, according to the law, the information presented in the advertisements must be true, the framework that an ad builds around information can be improperly biased. Often, what is *not* said is more important than what *is* said. Some misleading techniques used in presenting nutrition information are:

Technique 1. <u>MORE IS BETTER</u>: Many ads list numbers and percentages of nutrients to illustrate that their food is nutritionally superior. Some commercials stress high numbers such as "100 percent of the U.S. RDAs for 17 nutrients." This implies that more is better or necessary and that their product is superior to another that contains lower amounts, such as 80 percent of the U.S. RDAs for 9 nutrients.

<u>Nutrition Truth</u>: The wide variety of nutrients needed each day(approximately forty different nutrients) can be obtained by choosing a wide variety of foods. Consequently, it is not necessary to purchase highly fortified foods. Generally, we do not receive all of our daily requirement for a nutrient from one food anyway. Rather, the day's nutrient need is contributed from a number of foods in the diet. Implying that a "supernutritious" fortified food is necessary or is better than a nonfortified food is misleading.

Technique 2: <u>NUTRITION BUZZ WORDS</u>: Some ads use currently popular words associated with nutrition to sell food products. It is desirable to associate a food product with terms such as "vitamins," "minerals," "protein," "fiber," "low-calorie," "sugarless," and "natural." To discredit other foods, some ads use negative-appearing words such as "fat," "cholesterol," "sugar," "starchy," "fillers," "additives," and "artificial."

<u>Nutrition Truth</u>: Through the use of desirable nutrition terms, advertisers point out some of the reasons for selecting their food products. For example, Americans can benefit from selecting diets higher in fiber and lower in sugar, salt, and fat. Some terms used in commercials, however, do not have clear-cut definitions and the generalized meanings associated with the terms are not valid. For example, "additives" are popularly associated with health risks and cancer. In fact, not all additives are necessarily harmful. Some are necessary to preserve our food supply and have been thoroughly tested and approved for safety by the Food and Drug Administration.

Each year, children aged two to eleven are exposed to approximately 19,000 to 20,000 commercials on television. The commercials fall into many categories, but the most prevalent one is directed to children and deals with food. Cereals, candy, and other snacks are heavily promoted on television, while a nutritious diet is promoted less than two percent of the time.

There is a heavy emphasis on a limited range of food items. Research indicates that the products advertised are indeed consumed by children. Also, children exert influence on parents to purchase these advertised products. The numerous brands existing among these advertised products create a situation of fierce competition, thus increasing the emphasis placed on advertising.

Food companies advertise heavily so that children will become familiar with their brand name and consequently influence the purchase of their products. Companies vary the flavor, shape, color, or package of their products from that of the competition so that their products will be readily identifiable. One such tool that companies use is to make an association between their product and a particular figure, such as the Trix rabbit or Tony the Tiger. Special slogans or in-pack and mail-order prizes are examples of other methods that promote interest in the brands being advertised.

In order for students to become discriminating consumers, they must become aware of the strategies and techniques used by the product manufacturers. This awareness will allow them to resist the temptation to buy a product simply because the advertisements are appealing. This unit presents teaching strategies designed to encourage students to make self-discoveries regarding commercial advertisements.

BASIC ACTIVITY

Time Needed: Two class periods

Materials Needed: Sheets 20-1 through 20-3: "Who Is Deciding Which Foods I Buy?"
Sheet 20-4: "You Be the Judge!"
Sheet 20-5: "Climb to the Top!"
Quiz Sheet 20-1

Class Period 1

1. Have students complete Sheets 20-1 through 20-3, "Who is Deciding Which Foods I Buy?" If they have difficulty remembering the three particular advertisements, assign these sheets as homework.

In this way, they can watch ads on TV, listen to them on the radio, examine them in magazines and newspapers, and visit a food store to see the displays and signs. If assigned as homework, allow a few days for students to complete the sheets.

2. Conduct a large-group discussion of the students' favorite ads. Explore their reasons for liking the ads they chose. Discuss the influence the ads have on students' decisions to purchase certain food items.

3. Describe and discuss the following list of criteria by which advertisements can be judged:

- The length or size of the advertisement
- The informational content of the advertisement (nutrition information, price, food quality)
- The noninformational content of the advertisement (slogan, jingle, pictures, drawings, recipes, coupon, free gift)
- Motivational factors (how the ad is trying to convince you that you need the food)
- Target audience for the advertisement

4. Distribute Sheet 20-4, "You Be the Judge!" and have students evaluate their three favorite ads on Sheets 20-1 through 20-3 according to the criteria listed in step 3 above. Discuss students' evaluations as a class.

5. Have students discuss how they feel about advertising in general. Is it fair? Should there be more or less control of advertisers? Are people strongly influenced by advertising? Are some people more susceptible than others? Are children more susceptible than teenagers or adults?

Class Period 2

1. List these twelve food groups in the following order on the chalkboard or on a transparency:

Candy and gum	Cereals
Cookies and crackers	Shortenings and oil
Noncarbonated soft drinks	Desserts
Meats and poultry	Carbonated soft drinks
Vegetables	Macaroni and spaghetti
Citrus fruits	Cheese

2. Distribute Sheet 20-5, "Climb to the Top!" Have students fill in the "Nutrient Ladder" by ranking the foods from the list above with the most nutritious food at the top of the ladder and the least nutritious food at the bottom. Students should use only their knowledge of nutrition to order the foods. (There are no right or wrong answers for this activity.)

3. Under "Television Ladder" have students fill in the following foods from top to bottom *in the order given here.* This ranking represents the order of television advertisement concentration, with cereals being the most heavily advertised food product.

Cereals	Carbonated soft drinks
Candy and gum	Meats and poultry
Shortenings and oil	Macaroni and spaghetti
Cookies and crackers	Vegetables
Desserts	Cheese and citrus fruits
Noncarbonated soft drinks	

4. Have students compare and contrast the two lists in a whole-class discussion. Elicit the points that the *least* nutritious foods are the ones most heavily advertised and that the target audience is most likely to be young children.

5. Proceed with the "Advanced Activity" if you wish; otherwise use the quiz mentioned in step 6.

6. **EVALUATION:** Distribute Quiz Sheet 20-1 and have students complete it independently. Discuss the answers as a class.

ADVANCED ACTIVITY

Time Needed: Two class periods

Materials Needed: Sheets 20-6 through 20-7: "What Sells?" (Some students may need a duplicate of Sheet 20-7 to copy their original notes)
Quiz Sheet 20-1

Class Period 1

1. Distribute Sheets 20-6 through 20-7: "What Sells?"

2. Review advertising techniques and strategies (see "Teacher's Unit Introduction").

3. As a homework assignment, have students choose to do one of the following: (1) watch one hour of prime-time television; (2) listen to one hour of radio; (3) review one popular magazine; or (4) review one local daily newspaper. Students should evaluate the ads they observe in the medium chosen and complete Sheets 20-6 through 20-7 for the next class. Some students may need a duplicate of Sheet 20-7 to make a good copy of their notes, which may have been written quickly on the original sheet.

Class Period 2

1. During the next class, reproduce Sheet 20-7 on the chalkboard or make a transparency for use on an overhead projector. Have each student place a check mark under the strategies used by the commercial he or she found to be particularly good. Tally the strategies to find which one was the most frequently used in advertising.

2. Divide the class into groups of four and have the groups compare worksheets to decide which were the best strategies used for each medium. For this activity, you may wish to group students by the medium reviewed. Then begin a whole-class discussion where groups present their findings. Compare and contrast the use of particularly successful strategies by the different media reviewed. Have students decide which strategy was the most successful for each medium.

3. Discuss the pros and cons of each of the most successful strategies in terms of getting the advertiser's message across. Why was one strategy more successful than the others?

4. Calculate the proportion of ads that concerned foods or beverages. Elicit from the students how many of the ads gave nutrition information, what the information was, and if it was accurate. For ads that did not present nutrition information, elicit from students how the advertiser could present this information and what strategies could be used.

5. Discuss the following questions:

• Did you feel skeptical about any of the products advertised? Why?

• Did any ads entice you to buy the product? What "features" sold you?

6. Discuss how commercials appeal to the three basic human needs to feel important, loved, and protected. How were these needs appealed to in the strategies used by the advertisers?

7. **Evaluation:** Distribute Quiz Sheet 20-1 and have students complete it independently. Discuss the answers as a class.

FOLLOW-UP ACTIVITIES

1. Have small student groups create TV or radio commercials for any products they choose (either real or made up by the group), using the strategies they feel are most successful. The commercials should appeal to the basic human needs outlined. Have the groups perform their commercials and follow up each performance with a class critique of the strategies used.

2. Display on a transparency or write on the chalkboard one of the following opinions concerning food advertisements:

"The problem with food advertising is that it uses a lot of clever techniques to make us change our eating habits, but provides very little accurate or useful nutrition information. Food advertising should be limited to the giving of nutrition information."

"One of the major reasons why nutrition is taught in schools is so that people will have accurate and useful nutrition information. They will then be able to make wise food choices. Food advertisements are in direct competition with school nutrition education. Food advertisements should be banned or at least strongly regulated."

Have students read the opinion and discuss any questions they have about it. Then, have them decide which side of the debate they will support. One side is industry-based: They should disagree with the statement and believe that industry is helping nutrition education efforts. The other side is consumer-oriented: They will agree with the statement and believe more control should be exerted on food advertising. Allow students time to prepare their arguments as homework. Have one or two students act as secretaries on the day the debate is conducted to record both sides of the argument. If possible, have students prepare the information in a report to the local newspaper or send information home to parents via the school newsletter.

3. Have students view television for several hours at various times and log the types of food commercials shown. Include a weekday evening, weekday daytime, and Saturday morning. Have them compare and contrast the kinds of food advertisements shown during the different time slots, and have them do the same with the different target audiences that these advertisements are aimed at. Discuss the nutritional impact of these messages.

4. Have a round-table discussion of the pros and cons of stricter control over food advertising. In 1977, Robert Choate of the Control of Children, Media and Merchandising proposed the following:

a. Devices that would separate advertising from regular TV broadcasting: both an announcement and a framelike device to audibly and visually separate commercials

b. Graphic symbols to indicate the relative nutritional worth of a food product

c. Mandatory advertiser-funded messages on nutrition in each broadcast half-hour in which four or more food product commercials appear

Have students discuss how they feel about these regulations.

5. Discuss Public Service Announcements (PSAs) with the students. PSAs are short spots that are aired free-of-charge on television and radio. They must contain useful and nonprofit type of information. Contact a local radio or television station about the possibility of designing and producing a PSA about good nutrition. Some nutrition PSAs are already available, so you could use these and try to convince radio and television stations to air them.

6. Have students design a magazine or newspaper ad for vegetables (or fruits or milk).

7. Study the advertisements for several different brands of the same product. For example, look at ads for several types of ready-to-eat cereals. How are they similar? How are they different?

8. Have a "jingle" contest. Name popular and obscure jingles that advertise food products. Do not say the food product name. Have students recall the products' names. Then ask if they ever buy the product. Does advertising affect what they buy? Why or why not?

Examples of jingles: "Mmmm Good!" (Campbell's Soup)
"Good to the Last Drop" (Maxwell House Coffee)
"It's the Real Thing" (Coca-Cola)
"Have It Your Way" (Burger King)

9. Have students visit a grocery store and report on the percentage of presweetened cereals (compared to all cereals) on the shelves. Have them answer the following questions:

• Have many presweetened cereals used fictional characters to promote the product?

• How many cereals offered premiums for buying a particular brand?

• What companies were represented?

• Which companies had the most shelf space?

• Were there any cereals that did not contain added sugar? Which ones? How are these cereals advertised compared to presweetened cereals?

Conduct a discussion during which students can share their findings.
10. Invite a representative from a food company to speak on the subject of advertising.

WHO IS DECIDING WHICH FOODS I BUY?

Directions: On Sheets 20-1 through 20-3, evaluate your three favorite advertisements—one on TV or radio, one from a magazine or newspaper, and one from an in-store display or sign. Answer the questions below to evaluate each ad.

1. TV OR RADIO COMMERCIAL:

a. Name and describe your favorite TV or radio commercial about food:

_____

_____

_____

_____

b. Why do you like this ad? _____

_____

c. What nutrition information, if any, did you learn about this food from this commercial?

_____

_____

d. Have you ever tried this food?   Yes   No

e. Do you believe this food is as good as the commercial makes it look? Why or why not?

_____

_____

UHF   VHF   ON   OFF

Name ______________________________ Sheet 20-2

2. MAGAZINE OR NEWSPAPER AD:

a. Name and describe your favorite magazine or newspaper ad about food:

____

____

____

____

b. Why do you like this ad? ______________________________

____

____

c. What nutrition information, if any, did you learn about this food from this ad? __________

____

____

d. Have you ever tried this food? Yes No

e. Do you believe this food is as good as the commercial makes it look? Why or why not?

____

____

3. IN-STORE DISPLAY OR SIGN:

a. Name and describe your favorite display or sign in a food store:

_____

_____

_____

_____

b. Why do you like this display or sign? _____

_____

_____

c. What nutrition information, if any, did you learn about food from this display or sign ? __

_____

_____

d. Have you ever tried this food?   Yes   No

e. Do you believe this food is as good as the display or sign makes it look? Why or why not?

_____

_____

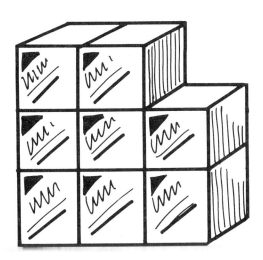
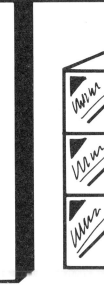
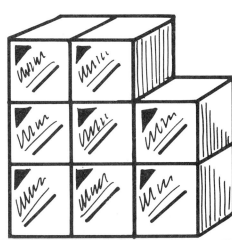

YOU BE THE JUDGE!

Describe the ad	How long or what size is the ad?	What information does the ad tell you about the food?	What else is shown or told in the ad?	How is the ad trying to motivate you to buy the food?	Who is the target audience?
EXAMPLE: This TV ad for "Sunshine Soda" shows children singing and dancing along a stream on a beautiful day. They are all drinking the soda, laughing, and talking.	26 seconds	It tastes good and refreshing. It comes in: 12 oz. or 16 oz. bottles.	catchy song cute children beautiful scenery	The ad makes it look like I will have fun if I drink their product.	children
TV OR RADIO COMMERCIAL:					
MAGAZINE OR NEWSPAPER AD:					
IN-STORE DISPLAY OR SIGN:					

CLIMB TO THE TOP!

**NUTRIENT
LADDER**

**TELEVISION
LADDER**

WHAT SELLS?

Directions: Choose one of the following media and review the ads you observe:

TELEVISION–Watch one hour of prime-time TV (7:30 to 11:00 P.M.)

RADIO   –Listen to one hour of radio at any time

MAGAZINE –Review one popular magazine (Write title on Sheet 20-7)

NEWSPAPER–Review one local newspaper (Write name on Sheet 20-7)

List the products advertised in the medium you chose on Sheet 20-7. For each product, identify the strategy(ies) used to create consumer desire to purchase the product from the list below.

ADVERTISING STRATEGIES AND TECHNIQUES

Problem/Solution	Use of Pleasure Words
Demonstration	Free Gift
Personification	Endorsement by a Famous Person
Testimony	More Is Better
Slice of Life	Nutrition Buzz Words
Jingle or Catchy Phrases	Other (Describe on back of sheet)

To answer "This ad appealed to which need?" choose one of the following:

I – Appealed to basic human need to feel *important*.

L – Appealed to the need to be *loved* or have peer acceptance.

P – Appealed to the need to be *protected* and feel secure.

Decide if you would buy the product based on its advertisement. Describe your reason for choosing to buy it or not to buy it on the back of Sheet 20-7.

After completing Sheet 20-7, write a short paragraph below to answer this question: Do you think food commercials should always supply nutrition information? Never? Sometimes? If so, in what situations?

_____

_____

_____

_____

_____

_____

_____

_____

_____

_____

_____

_____

_____

_____

_____

_____

_____

_____

	Would you buy this product?	This ad appealed to which need? (I,L,P)	Other (Describe)	Nutrition Buzz Words	More Is Better	Endorsement by a Famous Person	Free Gift	Use of Pleasure Words	Jingles or Catchy Phrases	Slice of Life	Testimony	Personification	Demonstration	Problem/Solution
Medium: _____ Time of Observation: _____ Total Number of Ads: _____ Total Number of Food Ads: _____ PRODUCT NAMES:														

QUIZ
A CLOSE LOOK AT FOOD ADVERTISING

1. Name three strategies used by television advertisers to help sell products, and briefly describe each one.

   STRATEGY 1: _____

   _____

   STRATEGY 2: _____

   _____

   STRATEGY 3: _____

   _____

2. Identify two human needs advertisers appeal to in commercials:

   NEED 1: _____

   NEED 2: _____

3. Write a short paragraph describing one TV food commercial you felt was particularly effective. First describe the commercial's "story" line and the scenes or pictures used. Then describe the major strategy(ies) used to sell the product and tell why they were successful. If nutrition information was offered, describe it. If nutrition information was omitted, how could the advertiser offer it?

   _____

   _____

   _____

   _____

   _____

   _____

   _____

   _____

   _____

   _____

   _____

   _____

   _____

   _____

   _____

   _____

   _____

   _____

   _____

APPENDICES

Reproducible Student Charts and Tables
References/Resources
Answer Keys for Units 1-20

RECOMMENDED DIETARY ALLOWANCES[a]

	Age (years)	Weight (kg)	(lb)	Height (cm)	(in)	Protein (g)	Fat-Soluble Vitamins			Water-Soluble Vitamins		
							Vitamin A (μg RE)[b]	Vitamin D (μg)[c]	Vitamin E (mg α-TE)[d]	Vitamin C (mg)	Thiamin (mg)	Riboflavin (mg)
Infants	0.0–0.5	6	13	60	24	kg × 2.2	420	10	3	35	0.3	0.4
	0.5–1.0	9	20	71	28	kg × 2.0	400	10	4	35	0.5	0.6
Children	1–3	13	29	90	35	23	400	10	5	45	0.7	0.8
	4–6	20	44	112	44	30	500	10	6	45	0.9	1.0
	7–10	28	62	132	52	34	700	10	7	45	1.2	1.4
Males	11–14	45	99	157	62	45	1,000	10	8	50	1.4	1.6
	15–18	66	145	176	69	56	1,000	10	10	60	1.4	1.7
	19–22	70	154	177	70	56	1,000	7.5	10	60	1.5	1.7
	23–50	70	154	178	70	56	1,000	5	10	60	1.4	1.6
	51+	70	154	178	70	56	1,000	5	10	60	1.2	1.4
Females	11–14	46	101	157	62	46	800	10	8	50	1.1	1.3
	15–18	55	120	163	64	46	800	10	8	60	1.1	1.3
	19–22	55	120	163	64	44	800	7.5	8	60	1.1	1.3
	23–50	55	120	163	64	44	800	5	8	60	1.0	1.2
	51+	55	120	163	64	44	800	5	8	60	1.0	1.2
Pregnant						+30	+200	+5	+2	+20	+0.4	+0.3
Lactating						+20	+400	+5	+3	+40	+0.5	+0.5

	Niacin (mg NE)[e]	Vitamin B$_6$ (mg)	Folacin (µg)[c]	Vitamin B$_{12}$ (µg)[g]	Minerals Calcium (mg)	Phosphorus (mg)	Magnesium (mg)	Iron (mg)[h]	Zinc (mg)	Iodine (µg)
Infants	6	0.3	30	0.5	360	240	50	10	3	40
	8	0.6	45	1.5	540	360	70	15	5	50
Children	9	0.9	100	2.0	800	800	150	15	10	70
	11	1.3	200	2.5	800	800	200	10	10	90
	16	1.6	300	3.0	800	800	250	10	10	120
Males	18	1.8	400	3.0	1,200	1,200	350	18	15	150
	18	2.0	400	3.0	1,200	1,200	400	18	15	150
	19	2.2	400	3.0	800	800	350	10	15	150
	18	2.2	400	3.0	800	800	350	10	15	150
	16	2.2	400	3.0	800	800	350	10	15	150
Females	15	1.8	400	3.0	1,200	1,200	300	18	15	150
	14	2.0	400	3.0	1,200	1,200	300	18	15	150
	14	2.0	400	3.0	800	800	300	18	15	150
	13	2.0	400	3.0	800	800	300	18	15	150
	13	2.0	400	3.0	800	800	300	10	15	150
Pregnant	+2	+0.6	+400	+1.0	+400	+400	+150	h	+5	+25
Lactating	+5	+0.5	+100	+1.0	+400	+400	+150	h	+10	+50

[a]Adapted from *Recommended Dietary Allowances*, 1980. Washington, D.C.: National Academy Press, with permission. The allowances are intended to provide for individual variations among most normal persons as they live in the United States under usual environmental stresses. Diets should be based on a variety of common foods in order to provide other nutrients for which human requirements have been less well defined.

[b]Retinol equivalents. 1 retinol equivalent = 1 µg retinol or 6 µg beta-carotene.

[c]As cholecalciferol. 10 µg cholecalciferol = 400 IUs of Vitamin D.

[d]α-tocopherol equivalents. 1 mg d-αtocopherol = 1 α-TE.

[e]1 NE (niacin equivalent) is equal to 1 mg of niacin or 60 mg. of dietary tryptophan.

[f]The folacin allowances refer to dietary sources as determined by Lactobacillus casei assay after treatment with enzymes (conjugases) to make polyglutamyl forms of the vitamin available to the test organism.

[g]The recommended dietary allowances for Vitamin B$_{12}$ in infants in based on average concentration (as recommended by the American Academy of Pediatrics) and consideration of other factors, such as intestinal absorption.

[h]The increased requirement during pregnancy cannot be met by the iron content of habitual American diets nor by the existing iron stores of many women; therefore the use of 30–60 mg of supplemental iron is recommended. Iron needs during lactation are not substantially different from those of nonpregnant women, but continued supplementation of the mother for 2–3 months after parturition is advisable in order to replenish stores depleted by pregnancy.

DAILY FOOD GUIDE*

FRUIT-VEGETABLE	BREAD-CEREAL	MILK-CHEESE	MEAT-POULTRY-FISH-BEANS	FATS-SWEETS-ALCOHOL
HOW MANY SERVINGS?				
Four Basic Servings Daily	Four Basic Servings Daily	Basic Servings Daily: *child under 9 2–3 servings *child 9–12 3 servings *teen 4 servings *adult 2 servings *pregnant women 3 servings *nursing women 4 servings	Two Basic Servings Daily	In general, the number of calories you need determines the amount of these "extra" foods you can eat. It's a good idea to concentrate first on the calorie-plus-nutrients foods provided in the other groups.
WHICH FOODS?				
All fruits and vegetables. Include one good Vitamin C source each day. Also frequently use deep-yellow or dark-green vegetables (for Vitamin A) and unpeeled fruits and vegetables and those with edible seeds, such as berries (for fiber).	Select only whole-grain and enriched products. (But include *some* whole-grain bread or cereal, for sure!) Include breads, biscuits, muffins, waffles, pancakes, cereals, pasta, rice, barley, rolled oats, and bulgur.	All types of milk and milk products, including whole, skim, low fat, evaporated, and nonfat dried milks, buttermilk, yogurt, cheese, ice cream, and foods prepared with milk such as puddings or cream soups.	Includes beef, veal, lamb, pork, poultry, fish, shellfish, organ meats, dried peas, soybeans, lentils, eggs, sesame seeds, sunflower seeds, nuts, peanuts, and peanut butter.	Includes butter, margarine, mayonnaise, salad dressings and other fats and oils; candy, sugar, jams, jellies, and syrups; soft drinks and other highly-sugared drinks; alcoholic beverages such as wine, beer, and liquor. Also included are refined but unenriched breads, pastries, and other grain products.
WHAT'S A SERVING?				
Count ½ cup as a serving or a typical portion such as one orange, half a grapefruit or cantaloupe, juice of one lemon, a wedge of lettuce, a bowl of salad, or one medium potato.	Count as one serving 1 slice of bread, ½ to ¾ cup of cooked cereal, cornmeal, grits, pasta, or rice; or 1 oz. of ready-to-eat cereal.	Count an 8 oz. cup of milk as a serving. Equivalent amounts of calcium (but different amounts of calories) are found in the following: 1 cup yogurt, 1½ oz. hard cheese, 1½ cups ice milk or ice cream, or 2 cups of cottage cheese.	Count 2–3 oz. of lean, cooked meat, poultry, or fish without bones as a serving. One egg, ½ to ¾ cup cooked dried beans, dried peas, soybeans, or lentils, 2 Tbsp. peanut butter, or ¼ to ½ cup nuts or seeds count as 1 oz. of meat, poultry, or fish.	No serving sizes have been defined because a basic number of servings is not suggested for this group. Use these foods in moderation.
WHAT'S IN IT FOR YOU?				
Carbohydrates, fiber, Vitamins A and C. Dark-green vegetables are valued for riboflavin, folacin (B vitamins), iron, and magnesium. Certain greens provide calcium. Nearly all fruits and vegetables are low in fat and none contain cholesterol.	Carbohydrates, proteins, B vitamins, iron. Whole-grain products also provide magnesium, folacin (B vitamin), and fiber.	Calcium, riboflavin, protein, vitamins A, B_6, and B_{12}. Milk products also provide Vitamin D when fortified with this vitamin. Fortified lowfat or skim milk products have the same nutrients as whole-milk products but fewer calories.	Protein, B vitamins, iron, phosphorous. Some of these foods also provide zinc, Vitamin A, and magnesium. Foods of animal origin (except fish) are relatively high in cholesterol and saturated fats. Seeds and fish are relatively high in unsaturated fats.	These foods, with the exception of vegetable oils, provide mainly calories. Vegetable oils generally provide Vitamin E and essential fatty acids. Sweets and alcohol provide mainly calories without other essential nutrients.

*Adapted from *Food*, Home and Garden Bulletin Number 228, 1979. Washington, D.C.: U.S. Department of Agriculture.

Chart C

KEY NUTRIENTS IN FOOD*

FAT-SOLUBLE VITAMINS	IMPORTANT FUNCTIONS	IMPORTANT SOURCES
Vitamin A	Helps keep skin clear and smooth Helps keep mucous membranes firm and resistant to infection Promotes normal vision in dim light Helps promote bone growth	Liver, egg yolk Dark-green and orange vegetables Yellowish-pink fruits such as cantaloupe or peaches Butter, margarine, milk, cream, hard cheese, ice cream
Vitamin D (The Sunshine Vitamin)	Assists the body's utilization of calcium and phosphorus in building bones and teeth	Vitamin D-fortified milk Fish liver oils (Sunshine on skin)
Vitamin E	Protects cell membranes from damage Prevents oxidation (destruction) of fats in the body and in food	Meat (especially liver), eggs, vegetable oils Green leafy vegetables Whole-grain cereals, wheat germ
Vitamin K	Maintains normal clotting of the blood	Pork, liver, egg yolk Green leafy vegetables, cauliflower (Synthesized by bacteria in the intestines)

ENERGY NUTRIENTS	IMPORTANT FUNCTIONS	IMPORTANT SOURCES
Proteins	Builds and repairs all tissues such as muscle, blood, and bone Helps form antibodies to fight infection Helps produce enzymes and hormones Supplies energy	Lean meat, fish, seafood, poultry, eggs Milk, cheese, yogurt Dried beans and peas, other legumes Peanut butter, peanuts, other nuts, seeds Breads and cereals
Carbohydrates (Sugar, Starch, and Fiber)	Supplies energy Carries other nutrients present in foods Provides fiber which assists in the elimination of body wastes	Breads and cereals Potatoes, lima beans, corn Dried beans and peas Dried fruits, sweetened fruits Sugar, syrup, jelly, jam, honey
Fats	Supplies large amounts of energy in a small amount of food Supplies essential fatty acids Carries fat-soluble vitamins A, D, E, K	Butter, margarine, shortenings Salad oils and dressings Fatty meats like bacon Marbling in meats Butterfat in milk and cream Nuts and seeds

Adapted from *The Great Vitamin Mystery,* Martin, M. National Dairy Council, Rosemont, IL, 1968.

237

Chart C

WATER-SOLUBLE VITAMINS	IMPORTANT FUNCTIONS	IMPORTANT SOURCES
Thiamin (Vitamin B₁)	Helps promote normal appetite and digestion Helps keep nervous system healthy and prevents irritability Helps body release energy from carbohydrates and fats in food	Meat (especially pork), fish, poultry Eggs Enriched or whole-grain breads and cereals Dried beans and peas Potatoes, broccoli, green leafy vegetables
Riboflavin (Vitamin B₂)	Helps cells use oxygen Helps keep skin, tongue, and lips normal Helps prevent scaly, greasy skin around mouth and nose Helps body release energy from carbohydrates and fats in food	Milk and milk products Meat (especially liver and kidney), fish, poultry, and eggs Green leafy vegetables, broccoli
Niacin	Helps keep nervous system healthy Helps keep skin, mouth, tongue, and digestive tract in healthy condition Helps cells use other nutrients Helps body release energy from carbohydrates and fats in food	Peanut butter Meat (especially liver), fish, poultry Milk and eggs (high in tryptophan) Enriched or whole-grain breads and cereals Dried beans and peas
Pyridoxine (Vitamin B₆)	Helps nervous system tissues function normally Plays a role in red blood cell regeneration Involved in the metabolism of amino acids, fats, and carbohydrates	Liver, pork, ham, salmon Soybeans and lima beans Bananas Yeast Whole-grain cereals Egg yolks Vegetables
Folacin (Folic Acid)	Helps cure (and prevent) megaloblastic anemia Helps enzyme and other biochemical systems function normally	Green leafy vegetables, lima beans, broccoli Liver, kidney Whole-grain cereals Dried beans and peas
Cobalamin (Vitamin B₁₂)	Protects against the development of pernicious anemia Maintains healthy nerves	Eggs, fish, liver, kidney, other meats Milk and milk products
Ascorbic Acid (Vitamin C)	Helps make cementing materials that hold body cells together Helps make walls of blood vessels firm Helps in healing wounds and broken bones Helps body resist infections Helps tissues such as gums and teeth stay healthy	Citrus fruits (orange, grapefruit, lemon, lime) Strawberries, cantaloupe, melons Tomatoes Green peppers, broccoli Green leafy vegetables, cabbage Potatoes

Chart C

MINERALS	IMPORTANT FUNCTIONS	IMPORTANT SOURCES
Calcium	Helps build bones and teeth Helps blood to clot Helps muscles, nerves, and heart to work Helps regulate the use of other minerals in the body	Milk and milk products (low amounts in cottage cheese) Dark-green leafy vegetables Salmon, sardines, and other fish with edible bones Tofu (soybean curd), soybeans, other legumes
Phosphorus	Helps build bones and teeth Helps regulate many internal activities of the body	Liver, fish, poultry, eggs Milk and milk products Whole-grain cereals Nuts
Iron	Combines with protein to make hemoglobin, the red substance in the blood that carries oxygen to the cells	Lean meat (especially liver, kidney), poultry, oysters Dried beans and peas, other legumes Dark-green leafy vegetables Prunes, raisins, dried apricots Fortified, enriched, or whole-grain breads and cereals Molasses
Iodine	Helps the thyroid gland control the rate at which the body uses energy	Seafood, plants grown in soil near salt water, iodized salt
Water	Important in all cells and body fluids Regulates body temperature Transports nutrients to cells and carries wastes away	Water Beverages such as juice or milk Soups Fruits and vegetables

FOOD COMPOSITION TABLE FOR SELECTED NUTRIENTS[a]

Food and Amount	Gm	Calories	%[b]	Protein	Vitamin A	Vitamin C	Thiamin	Riboflavin	Niacin	Calcium	Iron
						Percentages of U.S. RDA					
Almonds, in shell—½ cup	39	120	5	6	*	*	3	11	5	5	5
Apple, fresh—1	138	80	3	*	3	9	3	2	1	1	1
Apple pie—⅐ of 9″ diameter	135	400	16	5	4	5	10	5	6	1	6
Applesauce, sweetened, ½ cup	128	115	5	*	1	2	2	1	*	1	4
Apricots:											
dried—½ cup	65	170	7	5	142	13	*	6	11	4	20
fresh—3	108	55	2	3	57	18	3	3	3	*	3
Asparagus—½ cup	90	20	*	3	16	39	10	10	6	2	3
Avocado—½	114	190	8	4	7	27	9	14	9	1	4
Bacon—2 slices	15	90	4	10	*	*	5	3	4	*	3
Bagel, egg—1	55	165	7	9	*	*	9	6	6	*	7
Baked beans, with pork— ¾ cup	178	220	17	24	5	6	10	3	5	10	18
Banana—1	119	100	4	2	5	20	4	4	4	*	1
Beans, dried, then cooked— ½ cup	128	115	5	11	*	*	4	3	4	4	13
Bean sprouts, cooked— ½ cup	63	20	*	3	*	6	4	4	2	1	3
Beef pot pie—4¼″ diameter	227	560	22	35	37	11	17	16	23	3	23
Beet greens, cooked—½ cup	73	15	*	2	74	18	3	6	1	7	8
Beets, cooked—½ cup	85	30	*	1	*	9	2	2	1	1	2
Biscuit—1, 2½″ diameter	40	155	6	5	1	*	7	5	4	5	4
Blueberries, fresh—½ cup	73	45	2	*	1	17	1	3	2	1	4
Bologna—1 slice, 1 oz.	28	85	3	8	*	*	3	4	4	*	3
Bread, enriched:											
cracked wheat—1 slice	25	65	3	3	*	*	2	1	4	2	2
Italian—1 slice	30	85	3	4	*	*	6	4	4	1	4
rye (light)—1 slice	25	60	2	4	*	*	3	1	4	2	2
white—1 slice	25	70	3	3	*	*	4	3	3	2	4
whole wheat—1 slice	23	55	2	4	*	*	4	2	3	2	3
Broccoli, cooked—½ cup	78	20	*	4	39	116	5	9	3	7	3
Butter—1 Tbsp.	14	100	4	*	9	*	*	*	*	*	*
Cabbage, cooked—½ cup	73	15	*	1	2	40	2	2	1	3	1
Cake:											
devils food, with chocolate icing—1 piece	92	350	14	6	8	*	2	4	1	5	4
yellow, with chocolate icing —1 piece	125	465	19	7	10	*	6	7	4	5	6
yellow, without icing— 1 piece	85	320	13	8	9	*	8	7	4	6	5

Food and Amount	Gm	Calories	%ᵇ	Protein	Vitamin A	Vitamin C	Thiamin	Riboflavin	Niacin	Calcium	Iron
						Percentages of U.S. RDA					
Candy:											
caramels, plain—1 square	10	40	2	1	*	*	*	1	*	2	1
chocolate bar—1 oz.	28	150	6	3	2	1	1	6	*	7	2
gumdrops, starch jelly											
pieces—1 average	2	10	*	*	*	*	*	*	*	*	*
hard—1 average ball	5	20	*	*	*	*	*	*	*	*	1
peanut bar—1 oz.	28	145	6	8	*	*	8	1	13	1	3
peanut brittle—1 oz.	28	120	5	3	*	*	3	1	5	1	4
Cantaloupe—¼, 5″ diameter	133	40	2	1	90	73	4	2	4	2	3
Carrot, raw—1 medium	81	35	1	1	178	11	3	2	2	3	3
Cauliflower, cooked—½ cup	68	15	*	2	1	62	4	3	2	1	3
Celery—1 stalk	40	5	*	1	2	6	1	1	1	2	1
Cereal, ready-to-eat:											
enrichedᶜ—1 oz.	28	110	4	3	*	*	25	25	25	1	13
fortifiedᶜ—1 oz.	28	110	4	5	100	100	100	100	100	4	100
Cheese:											
American—1 slice, 1 oz.	28	95	4	12	5	*	*	7	*	16	*
Parmesan, grated—											
1 Tbsp.	5	25	1	5	1	*	*	1	*	7	*
Chicken, roasted											
breast, ½	98	195	8	65	2	*	5	7	62	1	6
drumstick, 1	52	110	4	31	1	*	2	7	16	1	4
Chicken livers, chopped											
1 cup	140	220	9	76	458	36	14	144	32	2	66
Chicken pie—1 average	302	705	28	61	94	34	23	18	59	5	20
Chili con carne w/beans—											
1 cup	230	305	12	36	3	*	5	16	28	8	33
Chocolate chip cookie—1	12	60	2	1	*	*	1	1	1	*	1
Cocoa, instant powder—											
1 Tbsp.	7	30	1	1	*	*	*	2	*	2	1
Corn, canned—½ cup	83	70	3	3	6	6	2	2	4	*	2
Cornbread—1 piece	42	110	4	4	4	*	3	4	2	4	2
Corn grits, enriched—½ oz.											
dry (½ cup prepared)	123	60	3	2	2	*	3	2	2	*	2
Crackers:											
animal—11 pieces	29	125	5	3	1	*	1	2	*	2	1
butter rounds—9 pieces	30	150	6	3	*	*	8	6	6	4	5
saltines—10 pieces	28	120	5	4	*	*	*	1	1	1	2
Creamed beef on toast—											
⅔ cup/slice	158	280	11	39	8	2	8	19	11	13	16

Food and Amount	Gm	Calories	%[b]	Protein	Vitamin A	Vitamin C	Thiamin	Riboflavin	Niacin	Calcium	Iron
						Percentages of U.S. RDA					
Cupcake:											
yellow, with chocolate icing—											
1 average	46	185	7	3	4	*	2	3	2	2	2
yellow, without icing—											
1 average	33	130	5	3	4	*	3	3	2	2	2
Doughnut, cake, plain—1	42	165	7	3	1	*	5	4	3	2	3
Egg:											
plain—1	51	80	3	14	5	*	3	9	*	3	6
scrambled, with butter—1	64	95	4	13	6	*	3	9	*	5	5
Flounder, fillet, baked, with											
butter—2 oz.	56	115	5	37	*	2	3	3	7	1	4
Fruit Cocktail—½ cup	128	100	4	1	4	4	2	1	3	1	3
Gelatin (Jell-O)—½ cup	120	70	3	3	*	*	*	*	*	*	*
Gingerbread, homemade—											
1 piece	76	275	11	5	1	3	7	6	5	13	23
Graham crackers—4 pieces	28	110	4	3	*	*	1	4	2	1	2
Grapefruit—½	98	40	2	1	2	62	3	1	1	2	2
Grapefruit juice, fresh—4 oz.	123	50	2	1	2	78	3	1	1	1	1
Grape juice—4 oz.	127	85	3	*	*	*	3	2	1	1	2
Grape juice drink,											
enriched–8 oz.	247	110	4	*	*	133	*	*	*	*	*
Grapes, fresh–½ cup	80	55	2	1	2	5	3	1	1	1	2
Green beans, fresh, cooked—											
½ cup	63	15	*	2	7	13	3	3	2	3	2
Hamburger, no roll—1	85	245	10	46	1	*	5	11	23	1	15
Hot dog, no roll—1	44	135	5	12	*	*	4	5	6	*	4
Ice cream, regular—⅔ cup	89	180	7	7	7	*	2	13	*	12	*
Jams and preserves—											
1 Tbsp.	20	55	2	*	*	1	*	*	*	*	1
Ketchup—1 Tbsp.	15	15	*	1	4	4	1	1	1	0	1
Lamb chop—2½ oz.	71	255	10	35	*	*	6	10	18	1	5
Lemonade—8 oz.	248	110	4	1	1	146	4	5	4	1	3
Lettuce, iceberg—½ cup	28	5	*	*	2	3	1	1	*	1	1
Liver, beef—3 oz.	85	195	8	50	908	38	15	210	70	1	42
Macaroni, cooked—½ cup	70	80	3	4	*	*	7	3	4	1	4
Macaroni and cheese,											
prepared from mix—¾ cup	156	290	12	17	11	*	18	12	10	11	*
Maple syrup—1 Tbsp.	19	50	2	*	*	*	*	*	*	*	*
Margarine—1 Tbsp.	14	100	4	*	9	*	*	*	*	*	*
Milk, fluid:											
chocolate, 2% butterfat—											
8 oz.	250	180	7	18	10	4	5	24	2	29	3
evaporated—8 oz.	244	330	13	37	12	8	7	45	2	64	3
nonfat dry, powder—⅓ cup	23	80	3	18	11	2	6	23	1	28	*
skim—8 oz.	245	85	3	19	10	4	5	20	1	30	1
2% butterfat—8 oz.	244	125	5	18	10	4	5	23	1	30	1
whole—8 oz.	244	160	6	18	7	6	5	23	1	29	1

Food and Amount	Gm	Calories	%[b]	Protein	Vitamin A	Vitamin C	Thiamin	Riboflavin	Niacin	Calcium	Iron
							Percentages of U.S. RDA				
Noodles, enriched, cooked—											
½ cup	80	100	4	7	1	*	8	4	5	1	7
Oatmeal, cooked—½ cup	123	67	3	4	*	0	7	1	1	1	4
Ocean perch:											
breaded, fried—2½ oz.	70	160	6	30	*	*	5	5	6	2	5
broiled, 2½ oz.	65	60	2	27	*	*	4	4	6	2	5
Onions, raw—½ cup	85	30	1	2	1	14	2	2	1	2	2
Orange, fresh—1	131	65	3	2	5	109	9	3	3	5	3
Orange juice, fresh—4 oz.	123	55	2	1	5	103	7	2	3	1	1
Oysters, raw—6	90	60	2	18	6	*	6	12	12	6	30
Pancakes—1, 4″ diameter	27	60	2	3	1	*	3	4	1	6	2
Papaya—¼ average	114	50	2	1	40	28	2	1	1	3	3
Peach:											
canned, water packed—											
½ cup	122	40	2	1	11	6	1	2	4	1	2
fresh–1	100	40	2	1	27	12	1	3	5	1	3
Peanut butter—1 Tbsp.	15	90	4	6	*	*	1	1	12	1	2
Peanuts:											
in shell—10	18	70	3	10	*	*	*	*	10	*	*
salted—¼ cup	36	210	8	14	*	*	8	3	31	3	4
Pear, fresh—1	164	100	4	2	1	11	2	4	1	1	3
Peas, fresh, cooked—½ cup	80	60	2	7	9	27	15	5	9	2	8
Pepper, green, raw—1	164	35	1	3	14	350	9	8	4	2	6
Pineapple, water pack—											
1 slice	58	25	1	*	1	7	3	1	1	1	1
Pizza with cheese—⅐ of 10″											
diameter	57	140	6	8	5	6	7	8	5	9	5
Plum, fresh—1	28	20	*	*	2	2	1	1	1	*	1
Popcorn, plain—1 cup	12	45	2	2	*	*	*	1	1	*	2
Pork chop—3 oz.	85	330	13	47	*	*	54	14	25	1	16
Potato:											
baked—1	165	145	6	6	*	52	10	4	13	1	6
chips—14	28	160	6	2	*	8	4	1	7	1	3
french fries—½ cup	55	150	6	4	*	19	5	3	9	1	4
Pretzels, thin sticks—											
47 pieces	28	110	4	4	*	*	*	1	1	1	2
Prune juice—4 oz.	128	100	4	1	*	4	1	1	3	2	29
Prunes–10 medium	96	240	10	*	30	10	10	10	10	10	20
Pudding, chocolate, prepared											
from mix—½ cup	144	155	6	19	3	3	2	12	1	15	*
Pumpkin pie—⅐ of 9″											
diameter	135	290	12	12	49	4	8	13	5	11	7

Food and Amount	Gm	Calories	%[b]	Protein	Vitamin A	Vitamin C	Thiamin	Riboflavin	Niacin	Calcium	Iron
						Percentages of U.S. RDA					
Pumpkin seeds, hulled—¼ cup	35	195	8	16	1	1	6	4	4	2	22
Raisins—¼ cup	42	125	5	2	*	1	4	1	1	2	5
Rice, enriched—½ cup	103	110	4	3	*	*	8	4	5	1	5
Roast beef—3 oz.	85	365	15	37	*	*	3	7	15	1	12
Roll:											
hamburger—1	40	120	5	5	*	*	8	4	7	3	4
hard—1 medium	25	80	3	4	*	*	4	3	3	1	3
Salad oil—1 Tbsp.	14	120	5	*	*	*	*	*	*	*	*
Shrimp, cooked—½ cup	55	65	3	30	1	*	*	1	5	6	10
Sloppy Joe—¾ cup	187	205	8	26	10	26	8	10	15	8	12
Sodas:											
club—12 oz.	356	*	*	*	*	*	*	*	*	*	*
cola type—12 oz.	370	145	6	*	*	*	*	*	*	*	*
cream—12 oz.	371	160	6	*	*	*	*	*	*	*	*
fruit-flavored—12 oz.	372	170	7	*	*	*	*	*	*	*	*
root beer—12 oz.	370	150	6	*	*	*	*	*	*	*	*
Soup, canned:											
chicken noodle—1 cup	241	75	3	6	14	*	3	4	7	2	4
cream of chicken, prepared with water—1 cup	244	120	5	5	11	*	2	4	4	3	3
vegetarian vegetable—1 cup	241	70	3	3	60	2	3	3	5	2	6
Soup, dehydrated:											
beef noodle—1 cup	251	40	2	3	*	2	8	3	4	1	2
chicken noodle—1 cup	252	55	2	5	1	*	5	3	4	3	3
Spaghetti with meatballs and tomato sauce—1 cup	248	330	13	41	32	37	17	18	20	12	21
Spinach, cooked—½ cup	90	20	*	4	146	42	4	7	2	8	11
Steak—3 oz.	85	330	13	43	1	*	3	9	20	1	14
Strawberries, whole—½ cup	75	30	1	1	1	73	2	3	2	2	4
Stuffed pepper, beef—1 average	185	320	13	43	29	277	13	20	18	15	18
Sugar:											
brown—1 Tbsp.	14	50	2	*	*	*	*	*	*	1	3
white, granulated—1 Tbsp.	12	45	2	*	*	*	*	*	*	*	*
Sunflower seeds, hulled—¼ cup	38	215	9	14	5	*	50	5	10	5	15
Sweet potato, baked—1	146	205	8	5	237	54	9	6	5	6	7
Tangerine—1	86	40	2	1	7	44	3	1	0	2	2
Tomato:											
canned, juice—4 oz.	122	25	1	2	20	33	4	2	5	1	6
fresh—1 medium	123	30	1	2	22	47	5	3	4	2	3
Tuna, canned—½ cup	80	160	6	51	1	*	3	6	48	1	8
Turkey:											
dark meat—3 oz.	85	155	6	52	*	*	3	12	14	2	11
white meat—3 oz.	85	140	6	54	*	*	2	7	27	2	8
Turnip greens, cooked—½ cup	73	15	*	3	91	83	7	10	2	13	4
Turnips, cooked—½ cup	78	20	*	1	*	28	2	2	1	3	2
Veal roast—3 oz.	85	200	8	53	*	*	4	13	23	1	15
Watermelon, fresh—1 piece	426	140	6	5	50	70	30	8	4	3	4
Yogurt:											
skim milk—1 cup	227	125	5	29	*	3[c]	6	31	1	45	1
whole milk—1 cup	227	140	6	18	6	2	3	19	1	28	1

[a]*Nutrients in Foods.* Leveille, G. A., Zabik, M. E., and Morgan, K. J. The Nutrition Guild, Cambridge, MA, 1983.

[b]Percent of 2,500 calories.

[c]For more precise information refer to package label of specific cereal.

*None or less than one percent.

DIETARY CALCULATION CHART

Name of Food and Amount Eaten	Calories	Protein (gms)	Vitamin A (IUs)*	Vitamin C (mgs)	Thiamin (mgs)	Riboflavin (mgs)	Niacin (mgs)	Calcium (mgs)	Iron (mgs)
Milk-Cheese Group:									
Subtotal:									
Meat-Poultry-Fish-Beans Group:									
Subtotal:									
Fruit-Vegetable Group:									
Subtotal:									

DIETARY CALCULATION CHART

Name of Food and Amount Eaten	Calories	Protein (gms)	Vitamin A (IUs)*	Vitamin C (mgs)	Thiamin (mgs)	Riboflavin (mgs)	Niacin (mgs)	Calcium (mgs)	Iron (mgs)
Bread-Cereal Group:									
Subtotal:									
Fats-Sweets-Alcohol Group:									
Subtotal:									
Grand Total:									
Recommended Dietary Allowance:									
Difference (+ or − RDA)									

*IUs stand for International Units which are standard units of measurement. A similar measurement, Retinol Equivalents (REs), may replace IUs. To convert IUs to REs divide IUs by 5.

HEIGHT/WEIGHT AND
RECOMMENDED ENERGY INTAKE*

Age and Sex Group	Weight		Height		Energy	
	kg.	lb.	cm.	in.	needs in calories	range in calories
infants						
0.0–0.5 year	6	13	60	24	kg. × 115	95– 145
0.5–1.0 year	9	20	71	28	kg. × 105	80– 135
children						
1–3 years	13	29	90	35	1,300	900–1,800
4–6 years	20	44	112	44	1,700	1,300–2,300
7–10 years	28	62	132	52	2,400	1,650–3,300
males						
11–14 years	45	99	157	62	2,700	2,000–3,700
15–18 years	66	145	176	69	2,800	2,100–3,900
19–22 years	70	154	177	70	2,900	2,500–3,300
23–50 years	70	154	178	70	2,700	2,300–3,100
51–75 years	70	154	178	70	2,400	2,000–2,800
76+ years	70	154	178	70	2,050	1,650–2,450
females						
11–14 years	46	101	157	62	2,200	1,500–3,000
15–18 years	55	120	163	64	2,100	1,200–3,000
19–22 years	55	120	163	64	2,100	1,700–2,500
23–50 years	55	120	163	64	2,000	1,600–2,400
51–75 years	55	120	163	64	1,800	1,400–2,200
76+ years	55	120	163	64	1,600	1,200–2,000
pregnancy					+300	
lactation					+500	

*Adapted from *Recommended Dietary Allowances*, 1980. Washington, D.C.: National Academy Press, with permission.

The data in this table have been assembled from the observed median heights and weights of children, together with desirable weights for adults for mean heights of men (70 inches) and women (64 inches) between the ages of eighteen and thirty-four years as surveyed in the U.S. population data (DHEW/NCHS).

Energy allowances for the young adults are for men and women doing light work. The allowances for the two older groups represent mean energy needs over these age spans, allowing for a 2% decrease in basal (resting) metabolic rate per decade and a reduction in activity of 200 calories per day for men and women between fifty-one and seventy-five years: 500 calories for men over seventy-five years; and 400 calories for women over seventy-five. The customary range of daily energy output is shown for adults in the range column and is based on a variation in energy needs of ±400 calories at any one age, emphasizing the wide range of energy intakes appropriate for any group of people.

Energy allowances for children through age eighteen are based on median energy intakes of children of these ages followed in longitudinal growth studies. Ranges are in the 10th and 90th percentiles of energy intake to indicate range of energy consumption among children of these ages.

CALORIE EXPENDITURE BY ACTIVITY

Directions: This table shows the number of calories burned per pound of body weight. To calculate your energy expenditures, multiply the appropriate figure on the chart by your body weight in pounds. If you spent more or less time in any activity, you will need to adjust your calculations as shown in the example.

EXAMPLE:

You weigh 100 pounds and spend 30 minutes doing class work:

$$(0.3 \text{ calories/pound}) \times 100 \text{ pounds} = 30 \text{ calories}$$

Your friend weighs 100 pounds and spends 15 minutes doing class work:

$$(0.3 \text{ calories/pound} \div 2) \times 100 \text{ pounds} = 15 \text{ calories}$$

Daily Activities	Calories Burned Per Pound* 30 min.	60 min.
Brick Laying	3.4	6.8
Calisthenics	1.0	2.0
Car Repairs	0.8	1.6
Carpentry or Farm Chores	0.8	1.6
Chopping Wood	1.4	2.8
Class Work	0.3	0.6
Conversing	0.4	0.8
Dancing	1.0	2.0
Dressing or Showering	0.6	1.2
Driving	0.6	1.2
Eating	0.3	0.6
Gardening and Weeding	1.2	2.4
House Painting or Metal Working	0.7	1.4
Housework	0.8	1.6
Motorcycling	0.7	1.4
Mountain Climbing	2.0	4.0
Mowing Grass	0.8	1.6
Office Work	0.6	1.2
Personal Care	0.9	1.8
Pick and Shovel Work	1.3	2.6
Resting in Bed	0.2	0.4
Sawing Wood	1.6	3.2
Shoveling Snow	1.5	3.0
Sleeping	0.2	0.4
Standing–no activity	0.3	0.6
Standing–light activity	0.5	1.0
Walking (3 mph)	1.0	2.0
Walking–downstairs	1.3	2.6
Walking–upstairs	3.4	6.8
Watching TV	0.2	0.4
Working in Yard	0.7	1.4
Writing	1.0	2.0

Sports Activities	Calories Burned Per Pound* 30 min.	60 min.
Archery	1.0	2.0
Badminton or Volleyball	1.1	2.2
Baseball	1.0	2.0
Basketball	1.4	2.8
Bicycling on level (10 mph)	1.6	3.2
Bowling	1.3	2.6
Canoeing	1.4	2.8
Fencing	1.0	2.0
Football	1.7	3.4
Golf	1.1	2.2
Handball	1.9	3.8
Horseback Riding	1.4	2.8
Ping Pong	0.8	1.6
Rowing	1.0	2.0
Running (6 mph)	2.5	5.0
Sailing	0.6	1.2
Skating	2.0	4.0
Skiing	1.9	3.8
Soccer	1.8	3.6
Squash	2.1	4.2
Swimming	1.4	2.8
Tennis	1.9	3.8
Water skiing	1.5	3.0
Wrestling, Judo, or Karate	2.6	5.2

*Figures include calories spent for basal metabolism and digestion of food.

References/Resources

FOOD AND NUTRITION INFORMATION AND EDUCATION RESOURCES CENTER

What is FNIC?

FNIC is an information center that serves people who are interested in human nutrition, food service management, and food technology.

What does FNIC do?

The Center acquires and lends books, journal articles, and audiovisual materials that deal with foods and nutrition. The AV collection includes films, filmstrips, slides, audiocassettes, videocassettes, posters, charts, games, and transparencies. The Center's collection ranges from children's materials through professional resources.*

Who uses FNIC?

FNIC serves many kinds of users, including school administrators, food service managers, teachers, and nutritionists.

What is FNIC's lending policy?
* You may borrow an unlimited number of books for a period of one month.
* You may borrow up to three audiovisual items at a time, for a period of two weeks. (Do not order them more than one month ahead of the date on which they will be used.)
* There is no charge for any of the materials.

How do I reach the Center?

Street Address:	10301 Baltimore Boulevard
	Beltsville, MD 20705
Mailing Address:	FNIC
	National Agricultural Library
	Room 304
	Beltsville, MD 20705
Telephone:	(301) 344-3719 (Twenty-four-hour telephone monitor)
Office Hours:	Monday–Friday 8:00 A.M. to 4:30 P.M.

---

*Many of the references and resources in this kit are available through FNIC.

FOOD COMPOSITION TABLES

"Nutritive Value of Foods" *Home and Garden Bulletin #72*. U.S. Department of Agriculture. Superintendent of Documents, U.S. Government Printing Office, Washington, DC, 20402, 1981. $4.50.

Food Values of Portions Commonly Used. Pennington, J. A., and Church, H. N. Harper & Row, New York, 1984. $7.64.

"Nutritive Value of American Foods in Common Units" *Agricultural Handbook #456*. U.S. Department of Agriculture. Superintendent of Documents, U.S. Government Printing Office, Washington, DC, 20402, 1981. $8.50.

Handbook of the Nutritional Content of Foods. Watt, B. K., and Merrill, A. L. Dover Publications, Inc., New York, 1975. $5.50.

RELIABLE SOURCES OF NUTRITION INFORMATION

American College of Nutrition (ACN)
100 Manhattan Ave. #1606
Union City, NJ 07087
(201) 866-3518

The American Dietetic Association (ADA)
430 North Michigan Ave.
Chicago, IL 60611
(312) 280-5000

The American Heart Association (AHA)
7320 Greenville Ave.
Dallas, TX 75231
(214) 750-5300

Center for Science in the Public Interest (CSPI)
1755 S. St., NW
Washington, DC 20009
(202) 332-9110

The Children's Foundation (CF)
1420 New York Ave., NW
Suite 800
Washington, DC 20005
(202) 347-3300

Community Nutrition Institute (CNI)
1146 10th St., NW
Washington, DC 20036
(202) 833-1730

Environmental Nutrition
52 Riverside Dr., 15th Floor
New York, NY 10024

Food and Drug Administration (FDA)
U.S. Dept. of Health and Human Services
5600 Fishers Lane
Rockville, MD 20857

Food and Nutrition Service (FNS)
U.S. Department of Agriculture
Washington, DC 20250

Food Research and Action Center (FRAC)
2011 I St., NW
Washington, DC 20006
(202) 452-8250

National Dairy Council (NDC)
6300 N. River Rd.
Rosemont, IL 60018
(312) 696-1020

National Nutrition Consortium (NNC)
24 Third St., NE, Suite 200
Washington, DC 20002
(202) 547-4819

The Nutrition Foundation
888 17th St., NW
Washington, DC 20006
(202) 872-0778

The Society for Nutrition Education (SHE)
1736 Franklin St.
Oakland, CA 94612
(415) 444-7133

SOFTWARE*

APPLE PIE
- From DDA
- $229.95
- Apple II + , IIe (48K), DOS 3.3, Radio Shack TRS-80 Model III or IV, one disk drive.

This package includes the programs: YOU ARE WHAT YOU EAT!, JUMPING JACK FLASH!, GREASE, SALTY DOG, MUNCHIES, SWEET TOOTH, and FOOD FOR THOUGHT. Programs may be purchased separately. Descriptions and prices of each program follow.

YOU ARE WHAT YOU EAT!
- From DDA
- $79.95
- Apple II + , IIe (48K), DOS 3.3, Radio Shack TRS-80 Model III or IV, one disk drive; printer optional.

This program analyzes a meal or an entire day's diet and will produce a printout of the analysis. The analysis includes ideas for improving the diet or meal; total calorie, sodium, and cholesterol intake; and a bar graph which illustrates how close the diet comes to meeting the RDA for protein and 7 vitamins and minerals.

JUMPING JACK FLASH!
- From DDA
- $34.95, includes instruction booklet.
- Apple II + , IIe (48K), DOS 3.3, Radio Shack TRS-80 Model II/IV one disk drive; printer optional.

This program helps students to examine the number of calories they expend when working, playing, and resting. It can be used with YOU ARE WHAT YOU EAT! to teach energy balance and weight control concepts. Designed for junior and senior high students and the general public.

GREASE
- From DDA
- $27.95, includes instruction booklet, student worksheets.
- Apple II + , IIe (48K), DOS 3.3, Radio Shack TRS-80 Model III/IV, one disk drive.

This is a program about fat, cholesterol, and their association with heart disease. Students can determine the amount of fat in a meal or diet. They can also learn about fat in fast foods by ordering a meal from one of three fast-food restaurant chains. The amount of fat in a food is translated into an equivalent number of teaspoons. Designed for junior and senior high students and the general public.

SALTY DOG
- From DDA
- $27.95.
- Apple II + , IIe (48K), DOS 3.3, Radio Shack TRS-80 Model III/IV, one disk drive.

This program examines the role of sodium in the diet, including sodium's effect on blood pressure. Bar graphs are used to compare the amount of salt found in foods. Students can analyze a meal or a day's diet to determine its sodium content, and can learn to identify food having high levels of sodium by playing the computer game SODIUM SLEUTH.

MUNCHIES
- From DDA
- $34.95, includes instruction card.
- Apple II + , IIe (48K), DOS 3.3, Radio Shack TRS-80 Model III/IV, one disk drive.

This program is designed to help junior and senior high students make wiser snack choices. Students can examine the nutrient profile of a wide array of popular snacks and can compare the nutrient profiles of snacks.

SWEET TOOTH
- From DDA
- $27.95.
- Apple II + , IIe (48K), DOS 3.3, Radio Shack TRS-80 Model III or IV, one disk drive.

This program answers questions frequently asked about sugar. Students learn to recognize "hidden" sources of sugar by playing the computer game CUBE CITY. This game graphically illustrates the amount of sugar in food by comparing it to sugar cubes.

FOOD FOR THOUGHT

- From DDA

- $34.95, includes instruction card.

- Apple II +, IIe (48K), DOS 3.3, Radio Shack TRS-80 Model III/IV, one disk drive.

This program is a "test your I.Q." type game. There are seven categories of questions and two difficulty levels (novice and expert). A series of questions about the selected topic is asked. The computer indicates whether the correct answer was selected and then explains the answer. Designed for junior and senior high students and the general public.

EAT SMART NUTRITION COMPUTER PROGRAM

- 1981. From The Pillsbury Company, M/S 3286, Pillsbury Center, Minneapolis, MN 55402.

- $19.75, includes 5¼" diskette, 25-page teacher's manual, 30 copies of worksheets and pamphlets, 4 activity sheet masters.

- Apple II +, IIe, or III (48K), disk drive; monitor, printer (optional).

An economical, easy-to-use program for junior high and high school students as well as adults, this software analyzes an individual's diet for one day. The program was designed to create awareness of key nutrients in the diet and of ways to improve diets through individual food choices. A concise food worksheet enables users to code and input food items for analysis as percent Recommended Dietary Allowances (RDAs) for eight nutrients in six age/sex categories. Total sodium, cholesterol, and percent calories from fat are also listed in the analysis. The description of calories as percent RDA, both on-line and in the documentation, is somewhat confusing because total calories are listed rather than percentages. The program is easy to follow if the user's guide supplements the on-line instructions.

With a data base of 136 representative foods, the scope of the program is limited. Other foods can be coded by using a substitution list in the kit. Analysis includes three meals (up to 9 items each) and three snack periods. The program provides analysis of individual food items, three meals, and combined snacks, as well as the total intake. Dietary recommendations are generated in response to the levels of nutrients and calories in the analysis. Recommendations are generally accurate and seem appropriate for the intended audience.

Significant features of this kit are the worksheets and follow-up activities. Educationally sound, these activities seem interesting and likely to enhance learning.

Because it is capable of rapidly providing practical, accurate information at health fairs, the program has potential to arouse interest in nutrition. Used with the related activities, it could also involve users in improving their food habits.

Reviewed by Ruth McNabb Dow, Ph.D., R.D., Associate Professor, School of Home Economics, Eastern Illinois University, Charleston, IL 61920.

EATING MACHINE

- Thorne, B. S., 1982. From Muse Software, 347 N. Charles St., Baltimore, MD 21201.

- $49.95, includes 5¼" diskette, 3-page instruction guide, 65-page user's manual.

- Apple II + or IIe (48K), disk drive; monitor, printer (optional).

As you examine the "consequences" of the foods you choose in your diet by comparing a day's food selection with the RDA and U.S. Dietary Goals, you will find this program entertaining, as well as educational.

Viewing the display monitor, users choose a daily menu from 500 foods listed in 11 food categories. Standard serving sizes are offered for easy input. After the user selects the day's menu, the program provides feedback, including extensive graphics. Total calories, protein, vitamins A and C, calcium, iron and sodium intake are compared to the RDA using bar graphs, sound enhancement, and a smiling or frowning face. If the user's nutrient intake is within the RDA range, the computer displays a smile. If the intake is above the range in calories or soidum, a frown appears. A bar graph also illustrates the percentage of calories provided by protein, carbohydrates, fats, and alcohol.

A short instruction guide contains enough information to run the program; the user's manual provides additional instructions for altering the data base, analyzing a recipe, and storing personal files. Program weaknesses, although noted in the manual, relate more to a new user than to the program's design. Because the new user is unfamiliar with the way in which foods are listed in the 11 food categories, initially data entry will be time consuming.

Students and adults will find the program's graphics helpful in understanding the importance of proper food selection.

Reviewed by Pam Boyce, Program Leader, Family Living Education, Michigan State University, Cooperative Extension Service, 103 Human Ecology Building, East Lansing, MI 48824.

EATS

- Byrd-Bredbenner, C., 1981. From Pennsylvania State University, Nutrition Education Center, University Park, PA. 16802.

- $75.00; includes 5½" diskette, 59-page user's guide, 7-page factsheet.

- Apple II + or IIe (48K), disk drive; monitor, printer (optional).

This program is designed to help teens and adults become more aware of the composition and nutritional adequacy of their diets. The program quickly analyzes reported dietary intake for one day. It then prints total calories and sodium; percent of calories from protein, fat, and carbohydrate; and percent of the RDA for selected nutrients. For nutrients in short supply (less than ⅔ RDA), the program reports a few of their functions and sources. However, the printout does not include a listing of the foods entered, so it is not easy to check for errors in data entry.

Once the program is loaded, even the novice should be able to use it and make corrections with ease. The user's manual gives clear directions and conveniently arranges foods both alphabetically and by food group. Estimating portion size to enter may occasionally pose a problem, especially for those weak in the use of decimals. Because about 700 foods are coded and the sodium intake is reported to the nearest hundredth of a milligram, the user might wrongly assume that the results are highly accurate. In fact, the data base includes only 90 different food groups; items similar in nutrient content have been grouped together via the coding system. However, provided the users are told that the results are rough estimates, the output is sufficiently accurate for nutrition education purposes. The information presented in the printout and the fact sheet is basically sound, although not always easily understood by the lay person.

This program is likely to appeal to people who are curious about how their diet stacks up and what they might do to make it better. The program can be used independently, but having a nutritionist available to answer questions is recommended.

Reviewed by Carol West Suitor, M.S., R.D., Assistant Director of Education, Frances Stern Nutrition Center, New England Medical Center, 171 Harrison Ave., Boston, MA 02111.

FAST FOOD MICRO-GUIDE

- Schrank, J., 1983. From The Learning Seed, 21250 N. Andover, Kildeer, IL 60047.
- $36.00, includes 5¼″ diskette, 10-page user's guide.
- Apple II (48K), disk drive; TRS-80 Model III (48K), disk drive, monitor, printer (optional).

This program analyzes the nutrient content of meals eaten in nine fast-food restaurants. The nutritional analysis would interest anyone who eats at these restaurants on a regular basis, such as high school students or people who travel and frequent these establishments. The nutritional analysis is provided for each meal selected at the chosen restaurant and includes: total calories; percentage of calories from fat; grams of protein; percentages of the RDA for vitamins A and C, B vitamins (riboflavin, thiamin, niacin), calcium, and iron; and milligrams of sodium. The program also provides statements regarding the adequacy of the intake. An example of one of the statements is, "Your meal is good in vitamin B but is lacking in vitamin A, C. You can get additional vitamin A, C from carrots, eggs, dairy products and fresh vegetables, citrus fruits, tomatoes, potatoes, dark-green vegetables." Because the program does not specify which foods on the list provide a particular nutrient, individuals with limited nutrition knowledge may be misled.

The program meets its objective of analyzing the nutritional content of a meal consumed at a fast-food restaurant. Overall, the program is easy to use despite the lack of documentation. However, there is no capability to store the data or make corrections during data entry, which can be frustrating for the user. The analysis is rapid and offers the user immediate feedback. The appearance of the printout is monotonous with varying-length one-line statements, some with words hyphenated incorrectly. The analysis provided appears to be valid, and I recommend this program as a supplement to other more complete diet/nutrient analysis software.

Reviewed by Janet H. Gannon, M.S., R.D., Nutritionist/Project Manager, Capital Systems Group, Inc., 11301 Rockville Pike, Kensington, MD 20895.

GRAB A BYTE

- 1983. From the National Dairy Council, 6300 N. River Road, Rosemont, IL 60018.
- $40, includes 5¼″ diskette, 8-page instructor's guide, 8-page user's guide.
- Apple II+ (48K) or IIe (64K), DOS 3.3, disk drive; monitor, printer (optional).

Developed for use with seventh through ninth-grade students, GRAB-A-BYTE uses three programs in an educational game format to review and reinforce previously taught nutrition concepts. GRAB-A-GRAPE, the first program, begins with the student selecting four categories of questions from the following: fast foods, food facts, food and sport, food basics, weight control, and body building. The student picks the desired category and level of difficulty, and is provided an answer for which he or she must choose the correct question. Depending on its difficulty, each question is assigned a score of one to three points. Incorrect responses are fully explained, and correct ones reinforced. Styled after the popular TV quiz show "Jeopardy," this program impressed me as an innovative and effective way of teaching nutrition.

The second program, NUTRITION SLEUTH, invites the student to become "Inspector Good Diet," and try to solve four nutrition mysteries—each a case in which a teenager's diet is low in a certain nutrient. Similar to the game Hangman, the object is to spell the name of the deficient nutrient by guessing one letter at a time. Wrong guesses elicit up to three clues. Depending on how readily the mystery is solved, the program confers ratings of "Flatfoot," "Detective," or "Super Sleuth." I found this game enjoyable, but a bit too short—a few more mysteries would, I am sure, be well-received by teachers and students alike.

HAVE-A-BYTE, the final program allows students to construct a meal of up to eight foods that is analyzed for calories and eight nutrients. The program presents the analysis in terms of "percent of daily needs" for the appropriate age/sex group. If desired, the students can try to improve the meal's nutritional value by adding or deleting foods, or they can select an entirely different meal for comparison. If a printer is available, printouts of the calorie and nutrient profile of each meal further enhance the educational worth of this program. Unfortunately, the program does not provide the percent of calories from fat, protein, and carbohydrate. Additional teacher information to guide interpretation of the table of "percent of daily needs" would also have been valuable. However, neither of these omissions seriously detracts from the overall usefulness of this program.

An instructor's guide lists several "suggestions for success," and provides a helpful chart that identifies activities in *Food . . . Your Choice Level 4,* that teach the content covered in this set of three programs. Other Dairy Council resources are also identified. A user's guide provides detailed descriptions of each program and contains the 90-item food list that is used with HAVE-A-BYTE.

The three programs show how sound nutrition information and effective educational approaches can be brought together with the creative application of microcomputer technology to yield excellent results.

Reviewed by James Krebs-Smith, M.P.H., R.D., Instructor, Nutrition Program, The Pennsylvania State University, University Park, PA 16802.

NUTRITION SIMULATION

- Anderson, C., and M. Johnson, 1983. From EMC Publishing, Changing Times Education Service, 300 York Avenue, St. Paul, MN 55101.
- $55.00, includes 5¼″ diskette, 26-page teacher's guide; $80.00, includes same items with back-up disk.
- Apple II+ or IIe (48K), DOS 3.3, disk drive; monitor.

This simulation provides an opportunity to practice the basic skills of meal management with nutritional and economic concerns in mind. In the first of the three parts of the program, the user goes on the shopping spree with a specific amount of money and a list of 95 foods to choose from. In the second section the user plans menus for three days. The third section provides the user with an evaluation of the food choices in terms of cost, calories, and nutritional quality.

The evaluation compares grocery expenses to a twenty-dollar daily limit. The program also compares the calculated calorie intake to a rough estimate of calorie needs based on values for ideal weight and activity level. The number of servings eaten from each of the Five Food Groups is compared to suggested intakes.

The simulation can be done for any or all seasons, with food prices varying accordingly. To make the program realistic, the developers have included "freebie" food sampling, special holiday needs, unexpected eating opportunities, and unplanned purchases. The price lists can be updated by the teacher.

Although the program does not discuss specific nutrients, it does stress the effects of the method of preparation on the caloric value of a food. Some basic information concerning the Five Food Groups is given at the beginning of the simulation; however, the teacher needs to further clarify the program's use. The accompanying guide should be read carefully and used to orient a user during the first time through the program. The short version takes about an hour for the novice user; the long version may take three or more hours to complete. The program allows the user to save work to continue at a later time. This simulation provides a thorough test of basic food purchasing and meal planning skills.

Reviewed by Joan A. Yuhas, Ph.D., R.D., Assistant Professor, School of Home Economics, Ohio University, Athens, OH 45701.

NUTRITION TUTORIAL

- Anderson, C., 1983. From EMC Publishing, 300 York Ave., St. Paul, MN 55101.
- $55, includes 5¼″ diskette, 12-page user's guide; $80, includes same items with back-up disk.
- Apple II+ or IIe (48K), DOS 3.3, disk drive; monitor (color preferred).

The program objectives are to teach the basic food groups, recommended food group servings, definitions of nutrition terms, functions and sources of selected nutrients, relationship of calories to activity level, nutrition labeling, and menu planning considerations. In an interactive, user-friendly style, the program teaches very basic concepts at a level appropriate for junior high, high school, or adult audiences with limited previous exposure to nutrition. The use of color graphics and sound enhances the user's experience.

The menu-driven program allows the user to focus on specific program units: food groups, serving sizes, nutrients and calories, nutrition labeling, and menu planning. Within each unit, blocks of instructional material are followed by mastery exercises with varied response formats. The use of case studies and sample menus provides practical application of concepts and stimulates decision-making. Program analysis of user's food intake by food groups personalizes the program and may increase user interest. Documentation provides useful ideas for application and follow-up activities.

Units on food groups and serving sizes are the best developed. The program provides minimal information on selected nutrients and calories; and nutrition labeling and menu planning units are limited in scope. Some concepts such as "healthful" versus "not healthful" snacks and "high" versus "low" calorie foods need follow-up explanations to avoid possible misunderstandings. A noticeable inaccuracy is the statement that as people grow older, they need fewer servings from the dairy group.

The program's educational design is sound and stimulating, and the visual design is excellent. However, without content corrections or supplemental information a user might seriously misunderstand some of the program's messages.

Reviewed by Martha S. Brown, Ph.D., R.D., Associate Professor, School of Home Economics, Eastern Illinois University, Charleston, IL 61920.

NUTRITION VOLUME 1

- 1982. From Minnesota Educational Computing Consortium, 3490 Lexington Ave., N., St. Paul, MN 55112.
- $37, includes 5¼″ disk, 53-page user's guide.
- Apple II+ or IIe (48K), disk drive; monitor.

This program provides a nutrient analysis of a one-day food intake. It draws on a data base of 598 foods that are coded before using the software. The analyzed information is compared with the 1980 RDA. Some of the program objectives are: (1) to list foods that are key sources of selected nutrients; (2) to determine whether eating patterns need to be changed; (3) to identify basic nutrients and their functions; (4) to classify foods according to the Four Food Groups; and (5) to develop acceptable criteria for food selection. The target audiences are high school students and adults.

The program analyzes the following nutrients: calories, protein, carbohydrate, fat, Vitamin A, Vitamin C, calcium, and iron. If an individual is low in a nutrient, the amount (in mg or IU) is displayed. The program indicates the additional amount of each nutrient needed to meet the RDA and provides a list of food sources of nutrients.

Users indicate serving size in terms of a reference serving size (e.g., 1.0, .5, 1.25, etc.). The program is easy to use because the food list is arranged alphabetically, and it utilizes a wide variety of common foods. It does not attempt to analyze fast foods, but it does list some snack foods by brand names.

The software package meets its stated objectives, both with the computer program as well as with the student materials included in the user's booklet. This program is designed for beginning nutrition students. Although limited in number, the nutrients analyzed are sufficient for students at this level.

The documentation is complete and includes introductory materials, lesson ideas, data base information, follow-up ideas for students, and instructions for using the Apple computer and printer. The documentation is complete, easy to read, appropriate for the audience, accurate, and well-done.

One of the program's unusual features is a listing of the five foods from the intake that provided the greatest number of calories. This program, by nutrition professionals, is well-done and should help free the beginning nutrition student from the struggle with lengthy computations.

Reviewed by Nancy Dillon, Owner, Strictly Software, 4321 N. 39th St., Phoenix, AZ 85018.

NUTRITION VOLUME 2

- 1982. From Minnestoa Educational Computing Consortium, 3490 Lexington Ave., N., St. Paul, MN 55112.
- $37.00, includes 5¼″ program diskette, 5¼″ back-up diskette (limited usage), 53-page support manual.
- Apple II+ or IIe (48K), disk drive; monitor.

Junior high and high school students as well as adults can use this two-program package as an effective aid for analyzing the composition of food intake in relation to their body processes and activities. "Lean" estimates and evaluates an individual's calorie intake and energy expenditure for 1–3 days. A limited statement of deficiencies is given for other nutrients. The program is designed to help individuals compare their weight with established weight ranges for age, sex, height, and body structure; and to set a weight goal. The program also analyzes the diet and activities to see whether the goals are being met. "Recipe" determines how specific foods meet caloric and nutrient needs of an individual. This program indicates how a food or foods meet the RDA for calories, protein, carbohydrate, fat, iron, calcium, riboflavin, thiamin, niacin, Vitamin A, and Vitamin C for individuals in various age and size groups.

The foods list is workable but somewhat limited (432 foods); it contains no fast-food or packaged items and few combination dishes. Although somewhat difficult for secondary students to understand without an explanation, the graphs of the nutrient totals are usuable once students comprehend what is being illustrated. The printed analysis is complete, but its format requires considerable paper, which can be costly.

A well-written support manual gives excellent background information, goals, sample runs, technical information, and seven useful student handouts. The strengths outweigh the weaknesses, and for the price the program is a good one.

Reviewed by Kathleen S. Willson, B.S., M.A., Instructor, Home and Family Life Education, Cascade Junior High, 610 Riverview Dr., N.E., Auburn, WA 98002.

---

*Reviews from the *Journal of Nutrition Education* 16(2):80–110, 1984.

REFERENCES/RESOURCES FOR UNITS 1–20

UNIT 1–NUTRITION OVERVIEW: PROTEINS, CARBOHYDRATES, AND FATS

Books

Blood and Guts—A Working Guide to Your Own Insides. Allison, L. Little Brown & Company, Boston, 1976. $11.45 (paper $6.70).

Focus on Food. Peck, L. B., Moragne, L., Sickler, M. S., and Washington, E. O. McGraw-Hill, Inc. New York, 1974. $19.60.

Food and Your Future. White, R. B. Prentice-Hall, Inc., Englewood Cliffs, NJ. No date. $21.28.

Food for Today. Kowtaluk, H. and Kopan, A. O. Chas. A. Bennett Company, Inc., Peoria, IL, 1977. Text ed. $19.96; Student guide $3.96.

Food: Where Nutrition, Politics and Culture Meet—An Activities Guide for Teachers. Katz, D. and Goodwin, M. T. Center for Science in the Public Interest, 1755 S Street, NW, Washington, DC 20009, 1976. $5.50.

Good for Me! All About Food in Thirty-Two Bites. Burns, M. Little, Brown & Company, Boston, 1978. $8.95.

Jane Brody's Nutrition Book. Brody, J. Bantam Books, New York, 1981. $7.95.

The No-Nonsense Guide to Food and Nutrition: The Facts for Everybody . . . by The People Who Know. McGill, M. and Pye, O. New Century Publishing, Inc., Piscataway, NJ, 1982. $8.95.

Nutrition Concepts and Controversies. Hamilton, E. M. and Whitney, E. West Publishing Company, St. Paul, MN, 1985. $20.95.

What's to Eat? The U.S. Department of Agriculture Yearbook. Superintendent of Documents, U.S. Government Printing Office, Washington, DC 20402, 1979. $8.50.

You Are What You Eat: A Common Sense Guide to the Modern American Diet. Gilbert, S. Macmillan Inc., New York, 1977. $10.95.

Booklets

"Building a Better Diet." Superintendent of Documents, U.S. Government Printing Office, Washington, DC 20402, 1979. $28.00/100 copies.

"Food" *Home and Garden Bulletin #228.* Superintendent of Documents, U.S. Government Printing Office, Washington, DC 20402, 1980. $6.00.

"Guide to Good Eating." National Dairy Council, 6300 N. River Road, Rosemont, IL 60018, 1974. $0.05

"Guide to Wise Food Choices." National Dairy Council, 6300 N. River Road, Rosemont, IL 60018, 1978. $0.35.

"How Your Body Uses Food." National Dairy Council, 6300 N. River Road, Rosemont, IL 60018, 1972. $0.60.

"Nutrition." Distribution Center, 7 Research Park, Cornell University, Ithaca, NY 14850, 1976. Series of 12 lessons $20.00; flip chart, $6.00; activity book, $5.50.

"Nutrition Source Book." National Dairy Council, 6300 N. River Road, Rosemont, IL 60018, 1978. $2.00.

"Your Food—Chance or Choice." National Dairy Council, 6300 N. River Road, Rosemont, IL, 60018, 1974. $0.45.

Audiovisuals

Eating On the Run. Alfred Higgins Productions, 9100 Sunset Boulevard, Los Angeles, CA 90069, 1975. Film, 16mm, color, 15½ minutes. $305.00 (rental $31.00).

Food, Energy and You. Perennial Education, Inc., 930 Pitner Ave., Evanston, IL 60202, 1978. Film, 16mm, color, 20 minutes. $375.00 (rental $38.00).

Food Models. National Dairy Council, 6300 N. River Road, Rosemont, IL 60018, 1974. $6.50 (small set); $9.00 (large set).

Guide to Good Eating. National Dairy Council, 6300 N. River Road, Rosemont, IL 60018, 1978. Poster. $1.10.

How a Hamburger Turns into You. Perennial Education, Inc., 930 Pitner Ave., Evanston IL 60202, 1978. Film, 16mm, color, 19 minutes. $350.00 (rental $36.00).

Key Nutrients. Professional Health Media Services, Box 922, Loma Linda, CA 92354, 1980. Poster. $4.95.

Soup's On! NASCO, 901 Janesville Avenue, Fort Atkinson, WI 53538. No date. Game. $17.50.

Super Sandwich. Home Economics School Service, P.O. Box 802, Culver City, CA 90230-0802, No date. Game. $15.95.

What's Good to Eat? Perennial Education, Inc., 930 Pitner Ave., Evanston, IL 60202, 1978. Film, 16mm, color, 17 minutes. $320.00 (rental $29.00).

UNIT–2 NUTRITION OVERVIEW: VITAMINS, MINERALS, AND WATER

Books

Jane Brody's Nutrition Book. Brody, J. Bantam Books, New York, 1981. $7.95.

The No-Nonsense Guide to Food and Nutrition: The Facts for Everybody . . . by the People Who Know. McGill, M. and Pye, O. New Century Publishers, Inc., Piscataway, NJ, 1982. $8.95.

Realities of Nutrition. Deutsch, R. M. Bull Publishing Company, Palo Alto, CA, 1976. $12.95.

Booklets

"Food" *Home and Garden Bulletin #228.* Superintendent of Documents, U.S. Government Printing Office, Washington, DC 20402, 1980. $6.00.

"The Great Vitamin Mystery." National Dairy Council, 6300 N. River Road, Rosemont, IL 60018, 1974. $0.60.

"Nutrition Source Book." National Dairy Council, 6300 N. River Road, Rosemont, IL 60018, 1978. $2.00.

Audiovisuals

Soup's On! NASCO, 901 Janesville Avenue, Fort Atkinson, WI 53538, No date. Game. $17.50.

Super Sandwich. Home Economics School Service, P.O. Box 802, Culver City, CA 90230-0802, No date. Game. $15.95.

Vitamins from Food. Perennial Education, Inc., 930 Pitner Ave., Evanston, IL 60202, 1978. Film, 16mm, color, 18 minutes. $340.00 (rental $35.00).

Vitamins: What Do They Do? Alfred Higgins Productions, Inc., 9100 Sunset Boulevard, Los Angeles, CA 90069, 1982. Film, 16mm, color, 21 minutes. $375.00 (rental $38.00).

Wheels. NASCO, 901 Janesville Avenue, Fort Atkinson, WI 53538, No date. Game. $17.50.

"Yardsticks for Nutrition." Distribution Center, 7 Research Park, Cornell University, Ithaca, NY 14850, 1973. Leader's portfolio, $1.50; teaching guide, $0.25.

UNIT–3 RDA DOORWAY TO GOOD HEALTH

Books

Focus on Food. Peck, L.B., Morgane, L., Sickler, M. S. and Washington, E.O. McGraw-Hill Inc., New York, 1974. $19.60.

Introductory Nutrition. Guthrie, H. A. The C. V. Mosby Company, St. Louis, MO, 1983. $23.95.

Recommended Dietary Allowances. Food and Nutrition Board. National Academy of Sciences, Printing and Publishing Office, 2101 Constitution Ave., NW, Washington, DC 20418, 1980. $8.00.

Audiovisual

Super Sandwich. Home Economics School Service. P.O. Box 802, Culver City, CA 90230-0802. No date. Game. $15.95.

UNIT–4 RDA METERSTICK TO GOOD NUTRITION

Books

Introductory Nutrition. Guthrie, H. A. The C. V. Mosby Company, St. Louis, MO, 1983. $23.95.

Recommended Dietary Allowances. Food and Nutrition Board. National Academy of Sciences, Printing and Publishing Office, 2101 Constitution Ave., NW, Washington, DC 20418, 1980. $8.00.

Booklet

"NRC—RDA Sheet." National Dairy Council, 6300 N. River Road, Rosemont, IL 60018, 1980. $0.05.

Audiovisuals

Soup's On! NASCO, 901 Janesville Ave., Fort Atkinson, WI 53538. No date. Game. $17.50.

What's Good to Eat? Perennial Education Inc., 930 Pitner Ave., Evanston, IL 60202, 1978. Film, 16mm, color, 17 minutes. $320.00 (rental $29.00).

UNIT–5 THE THREE Bs: MEETING YOUR RDAs

Books

Metabolics—Putting Your Food Energy to Work. Lamb, L. Harper & Row, Inc., New York, 1974. $12.95.

Principles of Nutrition. Wilson, E. D., Fisher, K. H. and Fuqua, M. E. John Wiley & Sons, Inc., Toronto, Canada, 1979. Text, $31.95; Teacher Manual and Workbook, $8.95.

Realities of Nutrition. Deutsch, R. M. Bull Publishing Company, Palo Alto, CA, 1976. $12.95.

Recommended Dietary Allowances. Food and Nutrition Board. National Academy of Sciences, Printing and Publishing Office, 2101 Constitution Ave., NW, Washington, DC 20418, 1980. $8.00.

Booklet

"The Great Vitamin Mystery." National Dairy Council, 6300 N. River Road. Rosemont, IL 60018, 1974. $0.60.

Audiovisuals

What's Good to Eat? Perennial Education Inc., 930 Pitner Ave., Evanston, IL 60202, 1978. Film, 16mm, color, 17 minutes. $320.00 (rental $29.00).

Wheels. NASCO. 901 Janesville Avenue, Fort Atkinson, WI 53538, No date. Game. $17.50.

UNIT–6 YOUR RDA FOR ENERGY

Books

Introductory Nutrition. Guthrie, H. A. The C. V. Mosby Company, St. Louis, MO, 1983. $23.95.

Nutrition Concepts and Controversies. Hamilton, E. M. N. and Whitney, E. N. West Publishing Co., St. Paul, MN, 1985. $20.95.

One Fat Summer. Lipsyte, R. Bantam Books, New York, 1978. $2.25.

Principles of Nutrition. Wilson, E. D., Fisher, K. H. and Fuqua, M. E. John Wiley & Sons, Inc., Toronto, Canada, 1979. Text, $31.95; Teacher's Manual and Workbook, $8.95.

Recommended Dietary Allowances. Food and Nutrition Board. National Academy of Sciences, Printing and Publishing Office, 2101 Constitution Ave., NW, Washington, DC 20418, 1980. $8.00.

Audiovisual

Good Loser—The Weight Control Game. NASCO, 901 Janesville Avenue, Fort Atkinson, WI 53538, No date. Game. $17.50.

UNIT 7–RDA IN THE U.S.A.

Books

Food and Your Well Being. Labuza, T. P. West Publishing Company, AVI Publishing Company, Inc., Westport, CT, 1977. Text, $17.95; Instructor's Manual and Study Guide, $7.50.

The No-Nonsense Guide to Food and Nutrition: The Facts for Everybody ... by the People Who Know. McGill, M. & Pye, O. New Century Publishing, Inc., Piscataway, NJ, 1982. $8.95.

Realities of Nutrition. Deutsch, R. M. Bull Publishing Company, Palo Alto, CA, 1976. $12.95.

Booklets

"Nutrition Labeling—How It Can Work for You." The National Nutrition Consortium, Inc., Nutrition Labeling, P.O. Box 4110, Kankakee, IL 60901, 1975. $3.00.

"Nutrition Labeling: Tools for Its Use." Superintendent of Documents, U.S. Government Printing Office, Washington, DC 20402, 1983. $4.75.

Audiovisuals

Food Models. National Dairy Council, 6300 N. River Road, Rosemont, IL 60018, 1974. $6.50 (small set); $9.00 (large set).

Read the Label—Set a Better Table. Food and Drug Administration, 5600 Fishers Lane, Rockville, MD 20857, 1976. Film, 16mm, color, 10 minutes. $130.00 (free rental).

UNIT 8–IDENTIFYING NUTRIENT-RICH FOODS

Books

Deliciously Low: The Gourmet Guide to Low-Sodium, Low-Fat, Low-Cholesterol, Low-Sugar Cooking. Roth, H. New American Library, New York, 1983. $17.50.

Introductory Nutrition. Guthrie, H. A. The C. V. Mosby Company, St. Louis, MO, 1983. $23.95.

Realities of Nutrition. Deutsch, R. M. Bull Publishing Company, Palo Alto, CA, 1976. $12.95.

Booklet

"Nutrition Source Book." National Dairy Council, 6300 N. River Road, Rosemont, IL 60018, 1978. $2.00.

Audiovisuals

Food Models. National Dairy Council, 6300 N. River Road, Rosemont, IL 60018, 1974. $6.50 (small set); $9.00 (large set).

U.S. RDA Comparison Cards. National Dairy Council, 6300 N. River Road, Rosemont, IL 60018, 1974. Learning kit, 57 cards. $7.50.

UNIT 9–DETERMINING NUTRIENT DENSITY IN FOOD

Book

Realities of Nutrition. Deutsch, R. M. Bull Publishing Company, Palo Alto, CA, 1976. $12.95.

Booklet

"Nutrition Labeling: Tools for Its Use." Superintendent of Documents, U.S. Government Printing Office, Washington, DC 20402, 1983. $4.75.

Audiovisuals

Food Models. National Dairy Council, 6300 N. River Road, Rosemont, IL 60018, 1974. $6.50 (small set); $9.00 (large set).

Index of Nutritional Quality Food Profiles. Chec Systems, Utah State University Foundation, 47 N. Main Street, Logan, UT 84321, 1983. Food composition cards. $60.00.

Nutrient Density Nutrition Education Curriculum, for Grades K-6. Chec Systems, Utah State University Foundation, 47 N. Main Street, Logan, UT 84321, 1979. Teaching kit, including 3 sets of profile cards. $398.00.

U.S. RDA Comparison Cards. National Dairy Council, 6300 N. River Road, Rosemont, IL 60018, 1974. Learning kit, 57 cards. $7.50.

UNIT 10–EATING RIGHT, FEELING WELL

Books

Food and People. Lowenberg, M.E., Todhunter, E. N., Wilson, E. D., Savage, J. R. and Lubawski, J. L. John Wiley & Sons, Inc., New York, 1979. $30.95.

Looking In: Exploring One's Personal Health Values. Read, D. A. Prentice-Hall, Inc., Englewood Cliffs, NJ, 1977. $13.95.

Nutrition, Behavior and Change. Gifft, H. H., Washban, M. B. and Harrison, G. G. Prentice-Hall, Inc., Englewood Cliffs, NJ. 1972. $24.95.

Audiovisuals

Even a Strong Body Can Be Diseased. Center for Science in the Public Interest, 1755 S Street, NW, Washington, DC 20009, 1979. Poster. $3.00.

Nutrition for Young People: You Are What You Eat. Guidance Associates, Inc., Communications Park, Box 3000, Mount Kisco, NY 10549, 1983. 6 filmstrips, 6 tape cassettes, teacher's guide. $199.50.

UNIT 11– HOW DO YOU STACK UP NUTRITIONALLY?

Books

Food and People. Lowenberg, M. E., Todhunter, E. N., Wilson, E. D., Savage, J. R. and Lubawski, J. L. John Wiley & Sons, Inc., New York, 1979. $30.95.

Food Fight: A Report on Teenagers' Eating Habits and Nutritional Status. Olsen, L. Citizens Policy Center, 1515 Webster Street #401, Oakland, CA 94612, 1984.

Food: Where Nutrition, Politics and Culture Meet: An Activities Guide for Teachers. Katz, D. and Goodwin, M. T. Center for Science in the Public Interest, 1755 S Street, NW, Washington, DC 20009, 1976. $5.50.

Looking In: Exploring One's Personal Health Values. Read, D. A. Prentice-Hall, Inc., Englewood Cliffs, NJ. 1977. $19.95.

Nutritional Assessment in Health Program. Christakis, G. American Public Health Association, Inc., 1015 Eighteenth Street, NW, Washington, DC, 1973. $6.00.

Nutrition Concepts and Controversies. Hamilton, E. M. N. and Whitney, E. N. West Publishing Co., St. Paul, MN, 1985. $20.95.

The No-Nonsense Guide to Food & Nutrition: The Facts for Everybody . . . by the People Who Know. McGill, M. and Pye, O. New Century Publishing, Inc., Piscataway, NJ, 1982. $8.95.

Booklets

"Background and Issues Paper in the School Foodservice and Child Nutrition Programs." The American School Foodservice Association, 4101 E. Ilif Avenue, Denver, CO 80222-9989, 1979. $0.50.

"Nutrition and Your Health." Superintendent of Documents, U.S. Government Printing Office, Washington, DC 20402, 1980. $2.25.

"Your Food—Chance or Choice?" National Dairy Council, 6300 N. River Road, Rosemont, IL 60018, 1974. $0.45.

Audiovisuals

Nutrition: Food and Health. Guidance Associates, Inc., Communications Park, Box 3000, Mount Kisco, NY 10549, 1983. 151 slides, 2 tape cassettes, teacher's guide. $169.50.

Nutrition for Teenagers Only. Pleasantville Media, Box 415, Pleasantville, NY 10570, 1984. 3 filmstrips, 3 cassettes, teacher's guide. $139.00.

UNIT 12–START THE DAY BETTER WITH BREAKFAST

Books

Good Breakfast Book: A Bringing-Back-Breakfast Cookbook. Goldbeck, N. and Goldbeck, D. G. P. Putnam's Sons, New York, 1976. $5.95.

Introductory Nutrition. Guthrie, H. A. The C. V. Mosby Company, St. Louis, MO, 1983. $23.95.

Booklet

"Food in the Morning." Media Services Printing, Room D-10, New York State College of Human Ecology, Cornell University, Ithaca, NY 14853. Four lessons, teaching guides, student handouts. $1.50.

Audiovisual

Eating on the Run. Alfred Higgins Productions, 9100 Sunset Boulevard, Los Angeles, CA 90069, 1975. Film 16mm, color, 15½ minutes. $305.00 (rental $31.00).

UNIT 13–YOUR SCHOOL LUNCH

Book

Eating Better at School: An Organizer's Guide. Center for Science in the Public Interest, 1755 S Street, NW, Washington, DC 20009, 1980. $2.50.

Booklets

"Doing More with Less" Innovative Ideas for Reducing Costs in the School Nutrition Program." Food Research and Action Center, 1319 F Street, NW, Suite 500, Washington, DC 20004, 1983. $10.00.

"Resources for Food Service Personnel." The Nutrition Education Center, The Pennsylvania State University, Benedict House, University Park, PA 16802, 1981. $3.00

Audiovisuals

Eating on the Run. Alfred Higgins Productions, 9100 Sunset Boulevard, Los Angeles, CA 90069, 1975. Film, 16mm, color, 15½ minutes. $305.00 (rental $31.00)

Merchandising School Lunch: A Nutrition Approach. CNETP Publications, Dept. of Nutritional Sciences, University of Connecticut, V-17, Storrs, CT 06268. Box of materials. $50.00.

UNIT 14–THE GOOD GOODIES

Books

The Good Goodies: Recipes for Natural Snacks 'n' Sweets. Dworkin, S. Rodale Press, Emmaus, PA, 1974. $7.95.

The Junk Food Alternative: High-Nutrient Snacks, Desserts and Quick Meals. Burum, L. 101 Productions, San Francisco, CA, 1980. $5.95.

Sweet and Natural: Desserts Without Sugar, Honey, Molasses, or Artificial Sweeteners. Warrington, J. The Crossing Press, Trumansburg, NY, 1982.

Booklet

"Nutrition Labeling: How It Can Work for You." National Nutrition Consortium, Nutrition Labeling, P.O. Box 4110, Kankakee, IL 60901, 1980. $3.00.

Audiovisuals

U.S. RDA Comparison Cards. National Dairy Council, 6300 N. River Road, Rosemont, IL 60018, 1974. Learning kit, 57 cards. $7.50.

Your Snacks—Chance or Choice? National Dairy Council, 6300 N. River Road, Rosemont, IL 60018. Poster. $0.65.

UNIT 15–DESIGNING A PERSONAL DIET PLAN

Books

The Fannie Farmer Cookbook, 12th edition. Cunningham, M. Bantam Books, New York, 1983. $5.95.

Food and People. Lowenberg, M. E., Todhunter, E. N., Wilson, E. D., Savage, J. R. and Lubawski, J. L. John Wiley & Sons, Inc., New York, 1979. $30.95.

Nutritional Assessment in Health Programs. Christakis, G. American Public Health Association, Washington, DC, 1973. $6.00.

Nutrition, Behavior and Change. Gifft, H. H., Washban, M. B. & Harrison, G. G. Prentice-Hall, Inc., Englewood Cliffs, NJ. 1972. $24.95.

Nutritious and Delicious: A Collection of 200 Taste-Tempting Recipes That Are Good and Good for You. Roginski, P., editor. Greater Cincinnati Nutrition Council, 2400 Reading Rd., Cincinnati, OH 45202, 1982. $7.50.

Recommended Dietary Allowances. Food and Nutrition Board. National Academy of Sciences, Printing and Publishing Office, 2101 Constitution Ave., NW, Washington, DC 20418, 1980. $8.00.

Teenage Nutrition and Physique. Huenemann, R. L., Hampton, M. C., Behnke, A. R., Shapiro, L. R. and Mitchell, V. W. Charles C. Thomas Publishers, Springfield, IL, 1974. $13.75.

What's to Eat? U.S. Department of Agriculture Yearbook. Superintendent of Documents, U.S. Government Printing Office, Washington, DC 20402, 1979. $8.50.

You Are What You Eat: A Common Sense Guide to the Modern American Diet. Gilbert, S. Macmillan, Inc., New York, 1977. $10.95.

Booklets

"Food" *Home and Garden Bulletin #228.* Superintendent of Documents, U.S. Government Printing Office, Washington, DC 20402, 1980. $6.00.

"Guide to Wise Food Choices." National Dairy Council, 6300 N. River Road, Rosemont, IL 60018, 1978. $0.35.

Audiovisuals

Guide to Good Eating. National Dairy Council, 6300 N. River Road, Rosemont, IL 60018. 1978. Poster. $1.10.

Nutrition on the Run. Sunburst Communications, 39 Washington Ave., Pleasantville, NY 10570, 1984. 3 filmstrips, 3 cassettes, teacher's guide. $139.00.

UNIT 16–DISCOVERING FOODS WITH YOUR SENSES

Books

Food: Where Nutrition, Politics and Culture Meet—An Activities Guide for Teachers. Katz, D. and Goodwin, M. T. Center for Science in the Public Interest, 1755 S Street, NW, Washington, DC 20009, 1976. $5.50.

Handbook of Food Preparation. American Home Economics Association, 2010 Massachusetts Avenue, NW, Washington, DC, 1980. $8.00.

Realities of Nutrition. Deutsch, R. M. Bull Publishing Company, Palo Alto, CA, 1976, $12.95.

Understanding Nutrition. Whitney, E. N. and Hamilton, E. M. N. West Publishing Company, St. Paul, MN, 1984. $24.95.

Booklet

"Food" *Home and Garden Bulletin #228.* Superintendent of Documents, U.S. Government Printing Office, Washington, DC 20402, 1980. $6.00.

UNIT 17–ENERGY BALANCE AND FAD DIETS

Books

The Art of Starvation: A Story of Anorexia and Survival. Macleod, S. Schocken Books, Inc., New York, 1982. $12.95.

The Family Health Cookbook. White, A. and The Society for Nutrition Education. David McKay Co., Inc., New York, 1980. $9.95.

For Teenagers Only: Change Your Habits to Change Your Shape. Ikeda, J. P. Bull Publishing Co., Palo Alto, CA, 1980. $6.95.

Nutrition, Weight Control and Exercise. Katch, F. I. and McArdle, W. D. Lea & Febiger, Philadelphia, PA, 1983. $18.50.

Rating the Diets. Berland, T. The New American Library, Inc., New York, 1980. $3.95.

Taking Charge of Your Weight and Well-Being. Nash, J. and Ormiston, L. Bull Publishing Co., Palo Alto, CA, 1978. $13.95.

Weight Watchers' Food Plan Diet Cookbook. Nidetch, J. The New American Library, Inc., New York, 1980. $13.95.

Booklets

"Calories & Weight: The U.S.D.A. Pocket Guide." Superintendent of Documents, U.S. Government Printing Office, Washington, DC 20402, 1981. $3.75.

"Cut Down on Calories." The Nutrition Education Center, The Pennsylvania State University, Benedict House, University Park, PA 16802, 1981. Single copy free.

"Exchange Lists for Meal Planning." American Dietetic Association, 430 N. Michigan Avenue, Chicago, IL 60611, 1976. $0.75.

"Fad Diet Frauds." The Nutrition Education Center, The Pennsylvania State University, Benedict House, University Park, PA 16802, 1981. Single copy free.

"Food and Your Weight." Superintendent of Documents, U.S. Government Printing Office, Washington, DC 20402, 1977. $4.50.

"Guidelines for Anthropometric Measurement." Ross Laboratories, Educational Services, 625 Cleveland Ave., Columbus, OH 43216, $1.00.

"Weight Control." The Nutrition Education Center, The Pennsylvania State University, Benedict House, University Park, PA 16802, 1981. Single copy free.

"Weight Control Source Book." National Dairy Council, 6300 N. River Road, Rosemont, IL 60018, 1983. $1.00.

"Your Calorie Catalog." National Dairy Council, 6300 N. River Road, Rosemont, IL 60018, 1983. $0.25.

Audiovisuals

Anorexia-Bulimia. Marshfilm, Box 8082, Shawnee Mission, KS 66208, 1984. Filmstrip, audiocassette, 10 minutes. $3.25.

Calipers. Ross Laboratories Educational Services, 625 Cleveland Ave., Columbus, OH 43216. Plastic skinfold calipers. $3.00.

Calories–Food and Activity. Media Services Printing, Room D-10, New York State College of Human Ecology, Cornell University, Ithaca, NY 14853, 1978. Flip chart. $3.00.

Dangerous Dieting: The Wrong Way to Lose Weight. Pleasantville Media, Box 415, Pleasantville, NY 10570, 1984. 3 filmstrips, 3 cassettes, teacher's guide. $145.00.

Dieting—The Danger Point. McGraw-Hill Films, 110 5th Street, Del Mar, CA 92014, 1981. Film, 16mm, color, 20 minutes. $335.00 (rental $36.00).

Energy—Our Food and Our Needs. AV Resource Center, 8 Research Park, Cornell University, Ithaca, NY 14850, 1984. Set of 65 slides, illustrated script, study guide. $30.00 (rental $12.00).

Fad Diet Circus. Sterling Educational Films, 241 E. 34th Street, New York, 1975. Film, 16mm, color, 15 minutes. $275.00.

Fat Chance! Audiovisual Services, Special Services Building, The Pennsylvania State University, University Park, PA 16802, 1978. Videocassette, color, 29 minutes. $165.00 (rental $16.50).

Food$ense—Reducing Diets. Audiovisual Services, Special Services Building, The Pennsylvania State University, University Park, PA 16802, 1976. Videocassette, color, 8 minutes. $75.00 (rental $10.50).

Nutrition: Foods, Fads, Frauds and Facts. Guidance Associates, Inc., Communications Park, Box 3000, Mount Kisco, New York 10549-0900, 1974. Filmstrip, audiocassette. $129.50.

Wasting Away: Understanding Anorexia Nervosa and Bulimia. Guidance Associates, Inc., Communications Park, Box 3000, Mount Kisco, New York 10549-0900, 1984. 4 filmstrips, 4 cassettes, teacher's guide. $159.50.

UNIT 18—THE ATHLETE'S DIET

Books

The Athlete's Kitchen. Clark, N. Van Nostrand Reinhold, 7625 Empire Dr., Florence, KY 41042, 1981. $10.95.

Bodyworks: The Kid's Guide to Food and Physical Fitness. Bershad, C. and Bernick, D. Random House, New York, 1981. $8.99.

Food for Sport. Smith, N. Bull Publishing Co., Palo Alto, CA, 1976. $6.95.

Food Power: A Coach's Guide to Improving Performance. National Dairy Council, 6300 N. River Rd., Rosemont, IL 60018, 1983. $10.00.

Nutrition and Athletic Performance. Darden, E. The Athletic Press, Pasadena, CA, 1976. $7.95.

Rating the Diets. Berland, T. The New American Library, Inc., New York, 1980. $3.95.

The Sports-Nutrition Kit. Food and Nutrition Division, Arizona Department of Education, 1535 N. Jefferson, Phoenix, AZ 85007, 1982. $10.83.

Booklets

"Athletics and Nutrition: Fact and Fiction." The Nutrition Education Center, The Pennsylvania State University, Benedict House, University Park, PA 16802, 1981. Single copy free.

"Athletics and Nutrition: Fuel for Fitness." The Nutrition Education Center, The Pennsylvania State University, Benedict House, University Park, PA 16802, 1981. Single copy free.

"A Guide to Food, Exercise and Nutrition." National Dairy Council, 6300 N. River Road, Rosemont, IL 60018, 1984. $0.50.

"Nutrition and Your Health." Superintendent of Documents, U.S. Government Printing Office, Washington, DC 20402, 1981. $2.25.

"The Sodium Content of Your Food." Superintendent of Documents, U.S. Government Printing Office, Washington, DC 20402, 1981. $4.25.

Audiovisuals

Fad Diet Circus. Sterling Educational Films, 241 E. 34th St., New York, 1975. Film, 16mm, color, 15 minutes. $275.00.

Food for Fitness. Butterick Publishing Co., 708 Third Ave., New York, NY 10017, 1979. Filmstrip, audiocassette, wall chart, 8 spirit masters, teacher's guide. $39.00.

Nutrition and Exercise. Sunburst Communications, 39 Washington Ave., Pleasantville, NY 10570, 1980. Two filmstrips, audiocassettes, study guide. $99.00.

Nutrition for Sports: Facts and Fallacies. Alfred Higgins Productions, Inc., 9100 Sunset Blvd., Los Angeles, CA 90069, 1982. Film, 16mm, color, 20 minutes. $395.00 (rental $40.00).

UNIT 19–INTERPRETING FOOD LABELS

Books

The No-Nonsense Guide to Food and Nutrition: The Facts for Everybody . . . by the People Who Know. McGill, M. and Pye, O. New Century Publishers, Inc., Piscataway, NJ, 1982. $8.95.

Realities of Nutrition. Deutsch, R. M. Bull Publishing Co., Palo Alto, CA, 1976. $12.95.

Nutrition Source Book. National Dairy Council, 6300 N. River Road, Rosemont, IL 60018, 1978. $2.00.

Booklets

"Nutrition Labeling: Tools for Its Use." Superintendent of Documents, U.S. Government Printing Office, Washington, DC 20402, 1983. $4.75.

"Nutrition Labels and the U.S. RDA." Food and Drug Administration, 5600 Fishers Lane, Rockville, MD 20857, 1981. Single copy free.

Audiovisuals

Label Literacy: How to Read Food Packaging. Sunburst Communications, 39 Washington Ave., Pleasantville, NY 10570, No date. 2 filmstrips, 2 audiocassettes, teacher's guide. $99.00.

Read the Label—Set a Better Table. Food and Drug Administration, 5600 Fishers Lane, Rockville, MD 20857, 1976. Film, 16mm, color, 10 minutes. $130.00.

UNIT 20–A CLOSE LOOK AT FOOD ADVERTISING

Book

The Feeding Web: Issues in Nutritional Ecology. Gussow, J. D. Bull Publishing Co., Palo Alto, CA, 1978. $14.95 (paper $11.95).

Answer Keys

UNIT 1: Nutrition Overview:
      Proteins, Carbohydrates, and Fats

SHEET 1-6:

What Is the Answer?

less; more
more; less
the same; the same

The Balancing Act

increase
increase
no change
decrease

SHEET 1-7

Which three nutrients give you energy?

(1) carbohydrates
(2) proteins
(3) fats

List some activities that require energy:

(Accept any activities that require movement, such as swimming, running, walking, or bicycling. Acceptable answers may also include body functions, such as breathing or digesting food.)

SHEET 1-10

Which food groups provide a lot of carbohydrates?

Fruit-Vegetable group
Bread-Cereal group
Fats-Sweets-Alcohol group

Which food groups provide a lot of proteins?

Milk-Cheese group
Meat-Poultry-Fish-Beans group

Which food groups provide a lot of fats?

Milk-Cheese group
Meat-Poultry-Fish-Bean group
Fats-Sweets-Alcohol group

Carbohydrate Corner

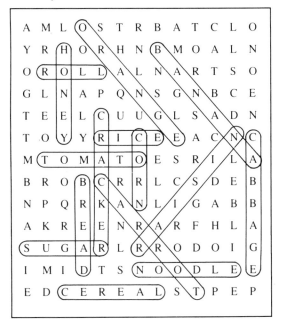

SHEET 1-11:

Protein Pad

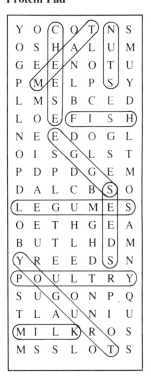

Sheet 1-11

Foods with Fat

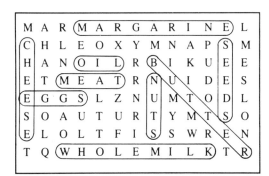

Laying a Good Foundation Summary Chart

NUTRIENTS	FUNCTIONS	FOOD SOURCES
PROTEINS	—To make and repair tissue and blood cells —Can provide energy —Promote growth	Meat, poultry, fish, eggs, legumes, nuts, seeds, milk, cheese, yogurt
CARBOHYDRATES	—To provide energy	Breads, biscuits, muffins, waffles, pancakes, macaroni, noodles, rice, oats, all fruits and vegetables, sugar, honey
FATS	—To provide energy —To carry fat-soluble vitamins A, D, E, K	Oil, butter, margarine; most foods from Meat-Poultry-Fish-Beans group; many foods from Milk-Cheese group
VITAMIN A	—To help with vision especially in dim light —To promote healthy skin and bone growth	Dark-yellow fruits and vegetables; dark-green vegetables
VITAMIN C	—To strengthen blood vessels —To help in wound healing —To contribute to bone and tooth formation	Citrus fruits and juices; many other fruits and vegetables
B VITAMINS Thiamin Riboflavin Niacin	—To promote healthy nerves —To promote the use of fats, carbohydrates, and proteins	Foods in Meat-Poultry-Fish-Beans group; foods in Bread-Cereal group; riboflavin in Milk-Cheese group
CALCIUM	—To make and repair bones and teeth —To help muscles and nerves work	Dark-green, leafy vegetables, sardines, some seafoods; foods in Milk-Cheese group
IRON	—To carry oxygen in the blood	Foods in Meat-Poultry-Fish-Beans group and Bread-Cereal group
WATER	—To transport materials through the body —To help the body eliminate wastes	All foods and beverages

QUIZ SHEETS 1-1 through 1-2:

1. a. decrease
   b. increase
   c. NC
2. d
3. a
4. b
5. c
6. c
7. a, b, c
8. a, c, d
9. b, c, d
10. c
11. d
12. c
13. a. 1. provides energy
       2. builds body tissues
    b. 1. provides energy
       2. carries fat-soluble vitamins
    c. 1. provides energy

UNIT 2: Nutrition Overview: Vitamins, Minerals, and Water

SHEET 2-7:

True or False
false
true
true

List three foods rich in protein:
(Answers may include any meat, fish, poultry, dried beans, bread, or cereal.)

List three foods rich in Vitamin D:
milk, eggs, butter

List three foods rich in Vitamin C:
(Answers may include any citrus fruit or juice, or any of the following fruits and vegetables: strawberries, cantaloupe, tomatoes, spinach, turnip greens, broccoli.)

SHEET 2-8:

List three foods rich in calcium:
(Answers may include any foods from the Milk-Cheese group.)

List three foods rich in Vitamin A:
(Answers may include any dark-yellow or orange fruits or vegetables, or any dark-green vegetable.)

Is it possible that food made Ku Sung grow taller?
Yes

What five nutrients made her bones grow?
Calcium, Vitamin A, Vitamin C, Vitamin D, protein

What foods in Ku Sung's American diet have these nutrients?
Calcium: any food from the Milk-Cheese group
Vitamin A: any dark-yellow or orange fruit or vegetable, or any dark-green vegetable
Vitamin C: any citrus fruit or juice; or any of the following fruits and vegetables: strawberries, cantaloupe, tomatoes, spinach, turnip greens, or broccoli
Vitamin D: milk, eggs, butter
Protein: any meat, fish, poultry, dried beans, bread, or cereal

SHEET 2-9:

Foods for Healthy Skin:

C   Limes
C   Strawberries
A   Apricots
A   Squash
C   Oranges
AC Broccoli

AC Spinach
C   Fresh Lemonade
A   Peaches
C   White grapefruit
A   Carrots
AC Turnip greens

SHEET 2-10:

Name one other role of calcium:
To help bones grow and become strong.

Name two other roles of Vitamin C:
To help bones grow and become strong. To keep skin healthy and to help in wound healing.

Match the foods with the nutrients:
Calcium: Cheese, Pudding, Milk, Yogurt, Ice Cream
Vitamin C: Tomato, Grapefruit, Strawberries, Cantaloupe, Oranges

Where Is the Vitamin A?

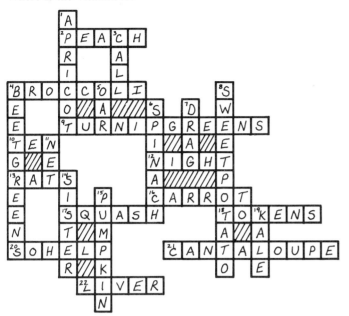

SHEET 2-12:

Place an *X* next to the foods that help you have healthy nerves:

___ Tomatoes	_X_ Cheese	___ Oranges
_X_ Meat	_X_ Eggs	_X_ Milk
_X_ Cereal	___ Apricots	___ Carrots
_X_ Bread	_X_ Dried beans	___ Grapefruit
___ Squash	and peas	_X_ Rice

SHEET 2-13:

Unscramble these words:

Rolls	Tomatoes	Fish	Noodles
Peas	Broccoli	Beans	Beverages
Nuts	Water	Seeds	
Milk	Eggs	Poultry	

SHEET 2-15:

Word Search 1

VITAMIN C

Strawberries
Cantaloupe
Watermelon
Potato
Tangerine
Tomato
Orange

VITAMIN A

Peach
Liver
Squash
Pumpkin
Spinach
Carrots

CALCIUM

Cheese
Milk
Ice Cream
Broccoli
Yogurt
Beans

SHEET 2-16:

Word Search 2

IRON	PROTEIN
Avocado	Cheese
Beans	Chicken
Blueberries	Egg
Chili	Fish
Greens	Hamburger
Hamburger	Legumes
Liver	Milk
Pork	Nuts
Spinach	Peanuts
Veal	Turkey
Whole Wheat	Veal

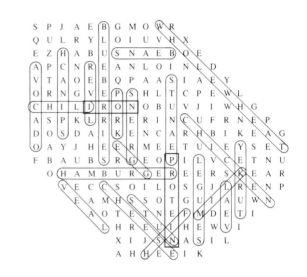

SHEET 2-17:

Iron CaPAC Anagrams

Unscrambled Word	Iron CaPAC Nutrients
food	Iron CaPAC
nutrient	Iron CaPAC
calcium	*
iron	*
nutrition	Iron CaPAC
growth	A, Pro
oxygen	Iron
blood	Iron, Pro
protein	*
tissue	Iron CaPAC
clot	Ca
teeth	Ca, C
bones	Ca, C
ascorbic acid	*
Vitamin A	*
energy	Iron
nerves	Ca
repair	Pro
build	Pro
skin	A
infection	C
gums	C
eyes	A
healing	C

*This is an Iron CaPAC nutrient; no answer required in this space.

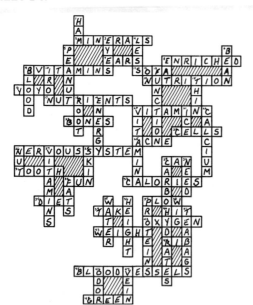

UNIT 3: RDA Doorway to Good Health

QUIZ SHEET 3-1:

1. a
2. c
3. b

UNIT 4: RDA Meterstick to Good Nutrition

SHEET 4-1:

1. Iron CaPAC
2. iron, calcium, protein, Vitamin A, Vitamin C

SHEET 4-2:

3. a. and b.:

Nutritious Food Chart

Nutrient	Food	Nutrient Amount	Stars
Iron	Beef pot pie	4.1 mg.	**
	Chili con carne	4.3 mg.	
	Gingerbread*	4.1 mg.	
	Liver, beef	7.5 mg.	***
	Oysters	4.8 mg.	
	Prunes	4.0 mg.	
Calcium	Cheese, American	163 mg.	
	Milk, chocolate	285 mg.	
	Milk, skim	300 mg.	
	Milk, whole	290 mg.	
	Yogurt, skim milk	452 mg.	
	Yogurt, whole milk	216 mg.	
Protein	Beef pot pie	23 g.	**
	Chicken breast	31 g.	
	Liver, beef	22 g.	***
	Pork chop	26 g.	
	Tuna	23 g.	
	Veal roast	22 g.	
Vitamin A	Beet greens	3,697 I.U.	
	Cantaloupe	4,505 I.U.	**
	Carrot	8,910 I.U.	
	Liver, beef	45,390 I.U.	***
	Sweet potato	11,826 I.U.	
	Turnip greens	4,567 I.U.	**
Vitamin C	Broccoli	70 mg.	
	Cantaloupe	44 mg.	**
	Orange	65 mg.	
	Pepper, green	210 mg.	
	Strawberries	44 mg.	
	Turnip greens	50 mg.	**

*Gingerbread is a good source of iron *only* when it is made with blackstrap molasses.

SHEET 4-3:

5. a. beef pot pie
      liver, beef
      cantaloupe
      turnip greens

   b. These foods contain large amounts of two or more of the Iron CaPAC nutrients. Therefore, you get more of these nutrients for the amount of food you eat. Compared to the other foods, these foods are more nutritious.

6. a. 2.7 mg. iron
   b. 163 mg. calcium
   c. 6 g. protein
   d. 8,910 IU Vitamin A
   e. 28 mg. Vitamin C

7. a. 7–10 yrs.—10 mg. iron
      11–14 yrs.—18 mg. iron
   b. 7–10 yrs.—3.7 hamburgers
      11–14 yrs.—6.7 hamburgers
   c. 7–10 yrs.—10 mg. iron point
      11–14 yrs.—18 mg. iron point

SHEET 4-4:

8. a. 7–10 yrs.—800 mg. calcium
      11–14 yrs.—1200 mg. calcium
   b. 7–10 yrs.—4.9 slices cheese
      11–14 yrs.—7.4 slices cheese
   c. 7–10 yrs.—800 mg. calcium point
      11–14 yrs.—1200 mg. calcium point

9. a. children 7–10 yrs.—34 g. protein
      boys 11–14 yrs.—45 g. protein
      girls 11–14 yrs.—46 g. protein
   b. children 7–10 yrs.—5.7 eggs
      boys 11–14 yrs.—7.5 eggs
      girls 11–14 yrs.—7.7 eggs
   c. children 7–10 yrs.—34 g. protein point
      boys 11–14 yrs.—45 g. protein point
      girls 11–14 yrs.—46 g. protein point

SHEET 4-5:

10. a. children 7–10 yrs.—3500 IU Vitamin A
       boys 11–14 yrs.—5000 IU Vitamin A
       girls 11–14 yrs.—4000 IU Vitamin A
    b. children 7–10 yrs.—.4 carrot
       boys 11–14 yrs.—.6 carrot
       girls 11–14 yrs.—.4 carrot
    c. children 7–10 yrs.—3500 IU Vitamin A point
       boys 11–14 yrs.—5000 IU Vitamin A point
       girls 11–14 yrs.—4000 IU Vitamin A point

11. a. children 7–10 yrs.—45 mg. Vitamin C
       children 11–14 yrs.—50 mg. Vitamin C
    b. children 7–10 yrs.—1.6 tomato
       children 11–14 yrs.—1.8 tomato
    c. children 7–10 yrs.—45 mg. Vitamin C point
       children 11–14 yrs.—50 mg. Vitamin C point

SHEET 4-6:

12. a. Yes
    b. (This question will be difficult to answer since no exact definition has been given for what constitutes a high level of a nutrient in a food. Students can use Chart C, "Key Nutrients in Foods," but answers will vary because, again, no frame of reference has been provided. Accept answers that seem reasonable based on Chart C. Then discuss this dilemma with the students. Appropriate answers would be:

    hamburger—iron and protein
    cheese—calcium, protein, and Vitamin A
    egg—protein, iron, and Vitamin A
    carrot—Vitamin A
    tomato—Vitamin A and Vitamin C

13. *Cheese* is the correct answer because the cheese is higher than the other foods in three of the five Iron CaPAC nutrients. The nutrients in which it is higher are calcium, protein, and Vitamin A.

14. and 15. (These answers will vary, but the foods chosen should be ones that are found to be high in two or more nutrients based on an examination of the nturients listed for the food in either Tables 4-1 through 4-2, "Energy and Iron CaPAC Table" or Chart C, "Key Nutrients in Foods.")

QUIZ SHEET 4-1:

1. d
2. d
3. b
4. b

UNIT 5: The Three Bs: Meeting Your RDAs

SHEET 5-1:

B VITAMINS DEFICIENCY CHART

ILLNESS	BEHAVIOR OF PERSONS WITH ILLNESS	APPEARANCE OF PERSONS WITH ILLNESS	DIET OF PERSONS WITH ILLNESS	MISSING NUTRIENTS	FUNCTIONS OF MISSING NUTRIENTS
pellagra	nerve disturbance insanity death	reddening of skin, especially on body parts indigestion diarrhea soreness and irritation of tongue weight loss	cornmeal corn pone salt pork hominy molasses white flour sweet potatoes greens	niacin tryptophan	helps keep nervous system healthy helps keep skin, mouth, tongue, digestive tract, in healthy condition helps cells use other nutrients helps body release energy from carbohydrates and fats in food
beriberi	paralysis death	withered leg and arm muscles leg swelling enlarged heart	polished rice	thiamin (vitamin B₁₂)	helps promote normal appetite and digestion helps to keep nervous system healthy and to prevent irritability helps body release energy from carbohydrates and fats in food

SHEET 5-6:
Rich sources (20 percent of the RDA) of the B vitamins, for students in the age groups listed below, include any foods whose nutrient content exceeds the following values:

	Children ages 7–10	Boys ages 11–14	Girls ages 11–14
Thiamin	.24 mg.	.28 mg.	.22 mg.
Riboflavin	.28 mg.	.32 mg.	.26 mg.
Niacin	3.2 mg.	3.6 mg.	3.0 mg.

TABLE 5-1:
Circled values should be:

FOODS HAVING 20% RDA FOR ONE B VITAMIN	B VITAMIN VALUES THAT SHOULD BE CIRCLED: Thiamin (mg.)	Riboflavin (mg.)	Niacin (mg.)
beans, navy	.26*		
beef pot pie	.25*	.27*	4.5
chicken breast			12.5
chicken livers	.20*	2.44	6.2
chicken pot pie	.34	.30*	11.8
chili con carne			3.0*
hamburger, no roll			4.6
lamb chop			3.5*
liver, beef	.22*	3.56	14.0
macaroni and cheese	.27*		
milk			
chocolate		.40	
skim		.34	
whole		.39	
peas	.22*		
pork chop	.96	.28*	5.8
stuffed pepper, beef		.33	3.6
tuna in oil			9.5
yogurt, skim milk		.52	
yogurt, whole milk		.32	
*Some students, usually boys aged 11–14 years, will not circle these values because these students' RDAs are higher than the other students' RDAs.			

TABLE 5-1, *(continued)*
Note that, depending on age and sex, certain values will be circled legitimately for some students and not for others. Make sure that students tie this activity to the concept that the RDA is different for different students in the same class.

Alert students to the fact that attaining the RDA for the B vitamins depends upon combining foods. You may find that completion of the three examples provides an opportunity to reinforce the prevailing belief in the desirability of food variety in diets. The values for the three examples should be:

SHEET 5-6:

Example 1	Thiamin (.24, .28 & .22 mg)*	Riboflavin (.28, .32 & .26 mg)*	Niacin (3.2, 3.6 & 3.0 mg)*
Oatmeal	.10	.02	.1
Milk, whole	.07	.39	.2
Total	.17	.41	.3

SHEET 5-7:

Example 2			
Hamburger patty	.08	.18	4.6
2 Slices bread, white	.12	.10	1.2
1 Serving french fries	.07	.04	1.7
2 Packets tomato catsup	.02	.02	.4
Total	.29	.34	7.9

Example 3			
Hamburger patty	.08	.18	4.6
2 Slices bread, white	.12	.10	1.2
2 Packets catsup	.02	.02	.4
1 Cup milk, whole	.07	.39	.2
Total	.29	.69	6.4

*20% RDA, respectively for children 7–10, boys 11–14, and girls 11–14

Yes; Examples 2 and 3 meet twenty percent of the RDAs for all three nutrients.

QUIZ SHEETS 5-1 through 5-2:

1. c   6. d
2. c   7. a
3. b   8. c
4. c   9. a
5. c   10. a

UNIT 6: Your RDA for Energy

1. 1,700   6. No, men need more.
2. 2,800   7. They decline.
3. 2,100   8. a. Age
4. 2,700   b. Sex
5. 2,000   9. 2,400
10. The younger child needs energy for growth. The man is not growing and has a lower basal metabolic rate.
11. No. Sitting is a sedentary activity. The average person also gets activity that could be considered "light" or "moderate" each day.
12. Yes. The average adult male or female does not spend most of his or her day doing the heavy lifting and other activities that are involved in construction work, and which burn up quite a few calories.

QUIZ SHEET 6-1:

1 c   5. a. A large four-year-old boy
2. b   b. An eighteen-year-old boy who plays varsity
3. d   basketball
4. c   c. A girl who takes a walk after school
                     d. A male wrestler

UNIT 7: RDA in the U.S.A.

QUIZ SHEET 7-1:

1. a   4. b
2. d   5. b
3. c   6. c

UNIT 8: Identifying Nutrient-Rich Foods

QUIZ SHEET 8-1:

1. c
2. d
3. c
4. a. beans, dried
   b. pudding
   c. beans, dried *or* chicken
   d. broccoli
   e. asparagus *or* broccoli *or* peas
   f. peas
   g. broccoli *or* pudding
   h. chicken *or* peas

UNIT 9: Determining Nutrient Density in Food

SHEET 9-1:

U.S. RDA Bar Graphs for Nutrient Density

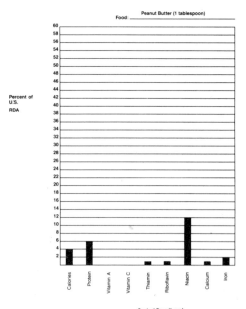

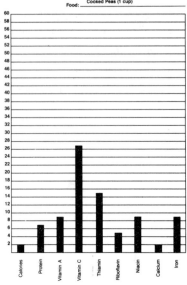

SHEET 9-2:

SHEET 9-2:

1. Yes
2. The second criterion—equal to or greater than 2 for at least two nutrients
3. Both of them
4. Nutrient-dense
5. Protein, Vitamin A, thiamin, riboflavin, calcium, and iron are all greater than 3%
6. Vitamin A = 2   thiamin = 1
   riboflavin = 3   calcium = 1
   iron = 2

SHEET 9-3:

7. Yes
8. Because eggs have a nutrient density equal to or greater than 2 for the *four* nutrients
9. The first criterion
10. Both criteria
11. (Answers depend on choices made by students. Practically all vegetables meet one or both of these criteria.)
12. Neither of these qualifies as a nutrient-dense food.
13. Yes
14. Because each of the foods supplies valuable amounts of one or more nutrients. An apple has a nutrient density of 3 for Vitamin C and supplies fiber to the diet; flounder has a nutrient density of 7 for protein and 1 for niacin.
15. Neither of these foods has a nutrient density of 1 for any nutrients.
16. (Answers will vary, but should include foods that are high in sugar and/or fat and that have low nutrient densities for all nutrients.)

QUIZ SHEET 9-1:

1. a   3. b
2. b   4. b

QUIZ SHEET 9-2:

5. d   7. b
6. b   8. c

UNIT 10: Eating Right, Feeling Well

SHEET 10-1:

(Students' answers will vary. The important criterion to use in judging their responses is to make sure the answers are completely descriptive and honest.)

QUIZ SHEET 10-1:

(Students' paragraphs will vary. In each paragraph, check to make sure the three components of good health are discussed: the physical, mental, and emotional aspects. Examples of each are provided in step 2 of the "Basic Activity.")

UNIT 11: How Do You Stack Up Nutritionally?

SHEET 11-1:

Each block of Sheet 11-1: "Food Frequency Form" identifies the number of points to be assigned for meeting that intake pattern. Post the Score Chart below on the chalkboard, bulletin board, or make a transparency of it for an overhead projector so that students may score their forms independently. The total possible score is 45. Any score below 35 is considered an inadequate diet.

SCORE CHART

Food Groups	Hardly Ever	Several Times Per Week	Once Daily	Two Times Per Day	Three or More Times Per Day
MILK, PUDDING, CUSTARD, YOGURT, CHEESE	0	3	7	10	10
ANIMAL PROTEINS (beef, chicken, pork, fish, eggs)	0	3	7	10	10
VEGETABLE PROTEINS (beans, nuts, peas)	0	3	4	4	4
FRUIT or JUICE OF: orange, grapefruit, tangerine, strawberries, tomato, green pepper	0	2	4	4	4
BROCCOLI, LIMA BEANS, SPINACH, LETTUCE, OTHER GREENS	0	3	4	5	5
any other FRUIT or VEGETABLE	0	0	2	2	2
any type of CEREAL, BREAD, ROLL, RICE, CRACKER, NOODLES, MACARONI, SPAGHETTI	0	0	0	7	10

TOTAL SCORE = ___45___

SHEET 11-2:

1. *False.* Honey, like brown sugar and white sugar, is a source of readily available carbohydrates. The small amounts of other nutrients in honey are not significant.

   Of all the sweeteners, blackstrap molasses and sorghum are the most nutritious choices because they have good amounts of calcium and iron. However, all sources of sweeteners should be kept to a minimum because they contain excess calories.

2. *True.* A medium potato has about 90 calories; a large apple has about 125 calories. Remember, it is the butter and sour cream on your potato that adds calories.

3. *False.* An average kiss burns about 9 calories.

4. *True.* Athletes, like anyone else, need some protein. Protein is found in meat, but also in poultry, fish, eggs, legumes, seeds, milk, cheese, grains, and cereals. You do not have to eat meat to get enough protein. Eating more protein than is needed to rebuild body cells (including muscle cells) does not help to build extra muscle.

5. *True.* Many of the B vitamins function in nerve transmission.

6. *False.* Potatoes lose many of their nutrients in the process of making potato chips. In addition, potato chips have added fat and salt (sodium), which are generally found in excess in the American diet and which should be avoided.

7. *False.* Large doses of Vitamin C can cause the body to adapt to a higher *required* intake, can increase the possibility of kidney stone formation, and, if taken during pregnancy, can result in rebound scurvy (Vitamin C deficiency) in the infant at birth.

8. *False.* Ingredients of food labels are listed in order of decreasing weight. The first ingredient listed has more weight than any other ingredient, the second ingredient has the second highest weight, and so on.

9. *False.* Small amounts of Vitamin A are important for a healthy skin, but there is some evidence that Vitamin A, applied topically or taken orally, will alleviate acne once it has developed. The idea that Vitamin A will cure acne came from findings that Vitamin A deficiency sometimes results in a condition resembling acne.

10. *False.* Like anything else, carbohydrates in moderate amounts, are not fattening. *Excess* protein, fat, and carbohydrate *all* turn to fat.

SHEET 11-3:

(There are no "correct" answers to this activity. This tool is used simply to assess students' attitudes to see how they feel about nutrition. A shift to a more positive attitude is desirable, but there are no right or wrong ways to feel.)

SHEET 11-8:

1. Yes
   a. He is not getting enough high-quality protein.

   b. Combine two kinds of plant foods to form a high-quality protein *or* add milk and cheese to his diet.
2. (A variety of answers is acceptable.)
3. (A variety of answers is acceptable.)

SHEET 11-9:

1. No
2. (A variety of answers is acceptable.)
3. (A variety of answers is acceptable.)

SHEET 11-10:

1. Yes
   a. She does not have a source of vegetables, nor a source of breads or cereals.
   b. Out in space there is little chance of getting additional food.
2. (A variety of answers is acceptable.)
3. (A variety of answers is acceptable.)

QUIZ SHEET 11-1:

(Students' responses will vary. Check for complete and thoughtful answers.)

UNIT 12: Start the Day Better with Breakfast

QUIZ SHEET 12-1:

1. a. Add 1 serving from Fruit-Vegetable group
   b. √
   c. √
   d. √
   e. Add 1 serving from Milk-Cheese group
   f. √
2. (Answers will vary. Menu should contain 1 serving from Milk-Cheese group, 0–1 serving from Meat-Poultry-Fish-Beans group, 1 serving from Fruit-Vegetable group, and 1 serving from Bread-Cereal group.)
3. Breakfast resupplies the body with energy.
   Breakfast resupplies the body with nutrients.
4. c

QUIZ SHEET 12-2:

5. d   7. a
6. d   8. b

UNIT 13: Your School Lunch

QUIZ SHEET 13-1:

1. 1. Milk
   2. Meat or meat alternate
   3. Vegetable or fruit
   4. Bread or bread alternate
2. (Answers will vary.)
3. (Answers will vary.)

4. a. √
   b. √
   c. Add vegetable or fruit
   d. √
   e. Add milk

UNIT 14: The Good Goodies

QUIZ SHEET 14-1:

1. a. NN   e. N   h. NN
   b. NN   f. N   i. NN
   c. NN   g. NN   j. NN
   d. NN

2. Circled foods should include the apple, the bagel, the bread, the grape juice, and the peanut butter. (Short answers will vary.)

UNIT 15: Designing a Personal Diet Plan

QUIZ SHEET 15-1:

1. a. Biological (Example: hunger, appetite)
   b. Psychological (Example: emotions, religion, familiarity)
   c. Social (Example: occasions, events, communications)

2. a. 3   f. 3   k. 2   p. 2
   b. 5   g. 5   l. 1   q. 4
   c. 4   h. 1   m. 3   r. 3
   d. 2   i. 4   n. 4   s. 1
   e. 1   j. 2   o. 5   t. 4

3. a. Bread-Cereal group
      Any foods from the Bread-Cereal group, any time of day
   b. Fruit-Vegetable group
      Any foods from the Fruit-Vegetable group, any time of day

UNIT 16: Discovering Foods with Your Senses

QUIZ SHEET 16-1:

1. Sight, taste, sound, touch, smell
2. (Answers will vary, but check to make sure all of the five senses are mentioned.)

UNIT 17: Energy Balance and Fad Diets

SHEET 17-5:

1. *False.* Many selections of breads and cereal products are lower in calories than other foods. For example, compare the calorie value of a slice of bread to a 1-ounce slice of cheese (70 calories versus 95 calories), and of 1 cup of ready-to-eat cereal to just ¼ cup of peanuts, shelled (110 calories versus 210 calories). In any weight-control diet, it is important to include a variety of foods from the Daily Food Guide.
2. *False.* Laxatives cause foods to pass through the intestines so quickly that some of the calories are not absorbed. Regular use of laxatives can be dangerous. Misuse of laxatives can lead to rectal bleeding, digestive problems, and electrolyte and water balance disturbances.
3. *False.* A large baked potato has about 145 calories compared to fruited yogurt which has 230 calories.
4. *False.* Recommended weight loss is 1 to 2 pounds per week.
5. *False.* High-protein foods generally have more calories than other foods because they often contain considerable amounts of fat.
6. *False.* Diet pills are designed to suppress the appetite. They generally contain milk stimulants.
7. *False.* Grapefruit has no special qualities to help burn calories. One-half of a grapefruit has about 40 calories. It may provide a sense of fullness if eaten before a meal and, thus, may reduce the intake of food.
8. *False.* Anyone who weights 20 percent below ideal body weight is considered underweight. It is important *not* to lose weight if you are already underweight.
9. *False.* Gelatin is a source of protein that lacks several essential amino acids, which makes it an inferior source of protein.
10. *False.* Carbohydrates have the same number of calories as proteins, ounce-for-ounce, and less than half the calories that an equal weight of fat provides.

QUIZ SHEET 17-1:

1. a. ✓   b. ✓   c. ✓   d. ✓   e. ✓
2. a. A disease of self-starvation characterized by a continuous pursuit of extreme, life-threatening thinness, an exaggerated interest in food and body, and a general withdrawal from family and friends.
   b. A chaotic pattern of eating that includes periods of gorging on large quantities of food within a short period of time; gorging is often followed by purging (with self-induced vomiting or laxative abuse) or by severe dieting or fasting.
3. a. NC   b. ♠   c. ♥   d. ♠   e. NC   f. ♥

UNIT 18: The Athlete's Diet

QUIZ SHEET 18-1:

1. b   2. d   3. c   4. d   5. b   6. d   7. a

UNIT 19: Interpreting Food Labels

SHEET 19-1:

1. Some will have nutrition labels and some will not.
2.–4. (Answers will vary.)
5. (Answer should be twice as large as answer for question 4.)
6. 30

SHEET 19-2:

7. 25 glasses
8. Use a food that has a much higher U.S. RDA value for Vitamin C.
9. You would add the three percentage figures for protein. (Since the three percentage values are placed on the chart horizontally, some students may have difficulty summing them. This is a good opportunity for students to practice mental addition.)

SHEET 19-3:

10. Since no single food has an adequate amount of all nutrients, you need to eat more than one food. Since most foods provide a good supply of some nutrients, you can combine different foods to get your U.S. RDA. Eating the same food all the time becomes boring. It is more fun to use foods in different combinations. People have different preferences, so a variety of foods increases the chance that each person will find something he or she likes.

SHEET 19-5:

1. table mustard   2. thousand island dressing

SHEET 19-6:

3. breakfast orange drink   5. wheat bread
4. orange juice   6. yellow cake mix

QUIZ SHEET 19-1:

1. 90 calories   5. 12 percent   9. d
2. 80 calories   6. 18 percent   10. a
3. carbohydrate   7. wheat bran
4. 3 servings   8. Vitamin B_{12}

UNIT 20: A Close Look at Food Advertising

QUIZ SHEET 20-1:

1. (Answers could be any three from the following: problem/solution, demonstration, personification, testimony, slice of life, jingles or catchy phrases, use of pleasure words, free gift, endorsement by a famous person, more is better, nutrition buzz words. See the description of each in the Teacher's Unit Introduction for Unit 20.)
2. (Answers could be two from the following: the need to feel important, the need to be loved, the need to be protected.)
3. (Answers will vary. Evaluate the paragraph for inclusion of criteria discussed in class.)